GW00374255

Review Questions for
NCLEX-RN

SEVENTH EDITION

Sandra F. Smith, RN, MS

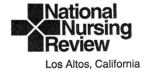

National Nursing Review

Los Altos, California

Copyright © 1995 by National Nursing Review

Manufactured in the United States of America. All rights reserved. No portion of this book
may be reproduced in any form or by any means without written permission of the pub-
lisher.

International Standard Book Number 0-917010-60-4

Composition: Forbes Mill Press
Printing and Binding: Quebecor Printing Kingsport

Copies of this book may be obtained from:

National Nursing Review
342 State Street, Suite 6
Los Altos, CA 94022
800.950.4095

1 2 3 4

Preface

During your nursing program, you have studied nursing theory and gained clinical experience. Now you face the important challenge of scoring sufficiently high on the National Council Licensure Examination to qualify for RN licensure. The objective of this book is to provide you with simulated NCLEX-RN questions so that you can be better prepared to pass your RN licensure examination.

Since 1976, National Nursing Review has published review books for the NCLEX-RN. Initially, we focused on providing comprehensive reviews of nursing content with a limited number of practice tests. However, faculty and students asked for more practice questions, so we published the first edition of this book in 1978. For this new seventh edition, the questions were completely updated, revised and reformatted to reflect the current NCLEX. A computer disk containing a simulated NCLEX exam is included to enable you to gain familiarity and comfort with the new CAT format and procedure.

The comprehensive tests and individual subject/clinical area questions serve two purposes: (1) to acquaint you with the type of questions to expect on the examination, and (2) to give you an opportunity to test and improve your knowledge of nurse-client clinical situations. The answers-and-rationale sections are intended to discourage rote memorization, but rather to reinforce learning by describing the underlying principles that tell you why the answers are right or wrong. The selection and presentation of content in this book are directed toward minimizing your review time and maximizing your test results.

Review Questions for NCLEX-RN is dedicated to the many nursing students who, after several years of classroom study and clinical experience, face the crucial examination for RN licensure. If this text and the accompanying computer disk help you prepare more fully and enter your test session with increased confidence, the project will be considered an unqualified success by the author.

Sandra F. Smith

Contents

I

PREPARING FOR NCLEX-RN

RN Licensure Procedures

The Purpose of NCLEX

The NCLEX-RN measures the licensure candidate's competence to perform safe and effective entry-level nursing practice. The boards of nursing in all 50 states, the District of Columbia, and the U.S. territories of Guam, the Virgin Islands, American Samoa, Puerto Rico, and the Northern Mariana Islands administer this screening test as developed by the National Council of State Boards of Nursing (NCSBN). This system of licensure provides protection for health care consumers and defines common entry-level standards throughout the U.S. In order to take the NCLEX, the candidate for licensure applies to the board of nursing in the state or jurisdiction in which the candidate plans to practice nursing. A complete list of the State Boards of Nursing is included as Appendix 1.

The NCLEX-RN Test Plan Framework

The NCSBN is responsible to provide its member boards of nursing with a psychometrically sound and legally defensible licensure examination. The purpose of the NCLEX-RN is to separate licensure candidates into two groups: those who can demonstrate minimal competence to perform safe and effective entry-level nursing care, and those who cannot. Although administration of the test via computerized adaptive testing (CAT) is a new procedure implemented in 1994, the basic test plan that provides the framework for presenting the questions has remained essentially unchanged since 1988. The NCSBN contracts with clinical nurses and nurse educators to write questions (referred to as test items) that test your ability to apply your knowledge of nursing. The test questions focus on job tasks normally performed by entry-level RNs during their first 6 to 12 months on the job. The NCSBN identifies these tasks by conducting extensive surveys, called job analyses, about every three years. It is entirely possible that your RN program may have included instruction on certain tasks that are not considered to be entry level by the NCSBN's job surveys. It is also possible that your RN program may **not** have provided you with instruction on some of the tasks about which questions have been included in the current test pool.

The job analysis studies are also used to help validate the test plan and to provide the basis for the proportional distribution of questions among the various subjects covered by the test. The test's two most significant conceptual areas are the Nursing Process and Client Needs. The following sections describe each phase of the Nursing Process, define the four broad categories of Client Needs, and list the 11 subcategories of Client Needs.

The Nursing Process

The phases of the Nursing Process that are measured by NCLEX-RN include Assessment, Analysis, Planning, Implementation, and Evaluation. The accompanying chart shows the percentage of questions that are allocated to each phase.

The Nursing Process—Question Allocation

- Assessment   17 to 23%
- Analysis   17 to 23%
- Planning   17 to 23%
- Implementation   17 to 23%
- Evaluation   17 to 23%

The nursing process is a frequently used, but often misunderstood, term. By definition, *process* is a series of actions that lead toward a particular result. When attached to *nursing*, the term *Nursing Process* becomes a general description of a nurse's job: assessing, analyzing, planning, implementing, and evaluating. Ideally, this process of decision-making results in optimal health care for the clients to which the nurse applies the process. While the five steps can be described separately and in logical order, it is obvious that in practice the steps will overlap and events may not always occur in the order listed above, especially when the unexpected happens. However, for purposes of understanding the NCLEX test plan, it is appropriate to work through each phase in a logical progression.

The five phases of the nursing process will be presented, defined and illustrated. A model of each phase will assist you to visualize how individual components can be translated into direct nursing actions or behaviors.

Assessment

The assessment phase refers to the establishment of a data base for a specific client. Assessment requires skilled observation, reasoning, and a theoretical knowledge base to gather and differentiate data, verify data and document findings. The nurse gathers information relevant to the client and then assigns meaning to this data. Assessment is a very critical phase, because all the other steps in the nursing process depend on the accuracy and reliability of the assessment process.

A model of the assessment phase is illustrated below.

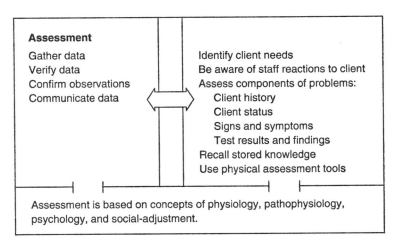

Assessment

Gather data   Identify client needs
Verify data   Be aware of staff reactions to client
Confirm observations   Assess components of problems:
Communicate data   Client history
                                   Client status
                                   Signs and symptoms
                                   Test results and findings
                               Recall stored knowledge
                               Use physical assessment tools

Assessment is based on concepts of physiology, pathophysiology, psychology, and social-adjustment.

An example of the assessment phase of the nursing process is in the sample question that follows.

A priority nursing assessment in the first 15 minutes of care for a client who has suffered a head injury and has just been brought into the emergency room would be to
1. Determine the scope and extent of the client's injury.
2. Contact family members.
3. Obtain baseline pulse and blood pressure.
4. Complete a respiratory assessment.

The answer is (4). Evaluating respiratory status is always a priority assessment. While contacting family members and determining the nature and scope of the client's injury are important, respiratory assessment will always have a higher priority.

Analysis/Nursing Diagnosis

The analysis phase focuses on the comprehension and interpretation of data collected during assessment for the purpose of goal formulation. This phase includes identification of client needs and the setting of goals, followed by the development of a plan of action for goal achievement.

A model of the analysis phase is depicted below.

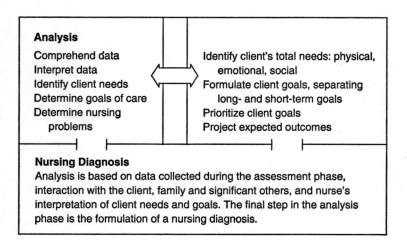

Analysis

Comprehend data
Interpret data
Identify client needs
Determine goals of care
Determine nursing
   problems

Identify client's total needs: physical,
   emotional, social
Formulate client goals, separating
   long- and short-term goals
Prioritize client goals
Project expected outcomes

Nursing Diagnosis

Analysis is based on data collected during the assessment phase, interaction with the client, family and significant others, and nurse's interpretation of client needs and goals. The final step in the analysis phase is the formulation of a nursing diagnosis.

Analysis questions focus on the understanding or interpretation of data necessary to formulate a nursing diagnosis.

The nurse has completed a postpartum assessment on a client two hours after delivery of a normal newborn. The client is restless, her pulse is 100 and weak, and her blood pressure is 100/68 with a soft fundus. From these assessment findings, the nursing diagnosis would be

1. Breathing Pattern, Ineffective.
2. Fluid volume Deficit, High Risk.
3. Cardiac Output, Decreased.
4. Infection, High Risk.

Answer is (2). Fluid Volume Deficit, High Risk is the most appropriate nursing diagnosis. The nurse would suspect hemorrhage based on the abnormal vital signs and soft fundus, perhaps caused by a laceration with subsequent bleeding.

Planning

The planning phase refers to the identification of nursing actions that are strategies to achieve the goals of care. This phase of the nursing process also includes nursing measures for the delivery of care. Clients may be involved in this planning phase.

A model of the planning phase appears below.

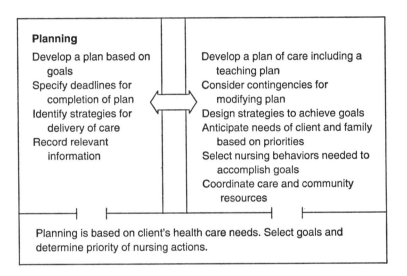

Planning

Develop a plan based on goals
Specify deadlines for completion of plan
Identify strategies for delivery of care
Record relevant information

Develop a plan of care including a teaching plan
Consider contingencies for modifying plan
Design strategies to achieve goals
Anticipate needs of client and family based on priorities
Select nursing behaviors needed to accomplish goals
Coordinate care and community resources

Planning is based on client's health care needs. Select goals and determine priority of nursing actions.

A planning question will focus on the development of a plan of care individualized for a specific client. For example

To facilitate the breathing of a 12 month old with bronchiolitis, the nursing care plan will include caring for the child in an environment of
1. Warm mist with oxygen.
2. Cool, moist oxygen.
3. Humidified oxygen.
4. Oxygen therapy with no mist.

The answer is (2). Cool, moist oxygen is the supportive therapy of choice for bronchiolitis. Warm mist from the shower may be administered for croup if the child is at home. Humidified oxygen is administered for pneumonia.

Implementation

The fourth phase of the nursing process is the implementation, or intervention, phase. It explicitly describes the action component of the nursing process. This phase involves initiating and completing those nursing actions necessary to accomplish the identified client goals.

A model of the implementation phase is illustrated.

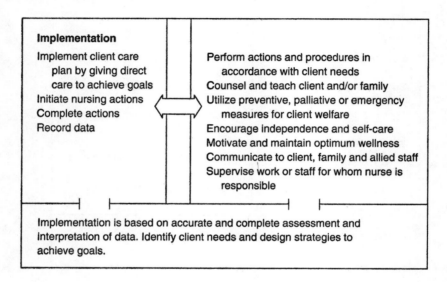

Implementation

Implement client care
    plan by giving direct
    care to achieve goals
Initiate nursing actions
Complete actions
Record data

Perform actions and procedures in
    accordance with client needs
Counsel and teach client and/or family
Utilize preventive, palliative or emergency
    measures for client welfare
Encourage independence and self-care
Motivate and maintain optimum wellness
Communicate to client, family and allied staff
Supervise work or staff for whom nurse is
    responsible

Implementation is based on accurate and complete assessment and interpretation of data. Identify client needs and design strategies to achieve goals.

Implementation of the plan involves giving direct care to the client to accomplish the specified goal. For example:

A 32-year-old female client was admitted in active labor to labor and delivery. Contractions are every two minutes, lasting 50 to 60 seconds. She is 6 cm dilated and 100 percent effaced. The fetal heart rate is 140 and regular, and the client's blood pressure is 80/40. Based on these findings, the first nursing action would be to

1. Place the client in Trendelenburg's position.
2. Take the blood pressure again to be sure it was accurate.
3. Call the physician immediately.
4. Turn the client on her side and check her blood pressure.

The answer is (4). The low blood pressure is likely due to supine hypotensive syndrome. Impaired venous return results when a gravid uterus presses on the ascending vena cava. Turning the client on her side will relieve the pressure from the interior vena cava and thus raise her blood pressure. Notify the physician if this intervention is not successful.

Evaluation

The final phase of the nursing process is evaluation, or determining the extent to which the plan or identified goals were achieved. Evaluation is the examination of the outcome of the nursing interventions. This process is extremely important because without this step, the nursing plan cannot be evaluated and adapted to the client's ongoing needs.

A model of the evaluation phase appears below.

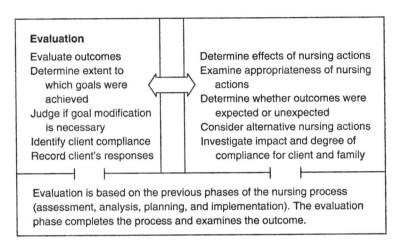

Evaluation

Evaluate outcomes
Determine extent to
    which goals were
    achieved
Judge if goal modification
    is necessary
Identify client compliance
Record client's responses

Determine effects of nursing actions
Examine appropriateness of nursing
    actions
Determine whether outcomes were
    expected or unexpected
Consider alternative nursing actions
Investigate impact and degree of
    compliance for client and family

Evaluation is based on the previous phases of the nursing process
(assessment, analysis, planning, and implementation). The evaluation
phase completes the process and examines the outcome.

During the evaluation phase, the outcome of a nursing action is examined and the extent to which the goal was achieved is determined. For example, in the previous situation, the initial nursing intervention was to position the client on her side and check her blood pressure.

In evaluating this action (or if the outcome of the intervention is successful), the nurse would expect which of the following client outcomes?
1. The client's blood pressure will remain the same and not drop any further.
2. The client's blood pressure will rise.
3. The blood pressure will not change, but the client will begin to feel better and breathe easier.
4. The fetal heart rate will return to normal.

The answer is (2). Relieving pressure from the inferior vena cava will cause the blood pressure to rise if a positive outcome of the intervention is achieved, so answers (1) and (3) are incorrect. If blood pressure does not rise, then the physician should be notified immediately. The fetal heart rate is already normal, so answer (4) is wrong.

Client Needs

The basic health needs of clients are grouped under four broad categories that are weighted according to the results of the *1992–93 RN Job Analysis Study* conducted by the National Council of State Boards of Nursing. The weight assigned to each category is reflected in the percentage of questions you will find on the NCLEX noted in the accompanying chart.

Client Needs—Question Allocation	
• Safe, Effective Care Environment	15 to 21%
• Physiological Integrity	46 to 54%
• Psychosocial Integrity	8 to 16%
• Health Promotion and Maintenance	17 to 23%

Safe, Effective Care Environment
To assist in meeting the client's needs in this area, the nurse must be able to provide the following:

- Coordinated Care
- Environmental Safety
- Safe and Effective Treatment and Procedures †

Physiological Integrity
To assist in meeting the client's needs for physiological integrity—this includes acute and/or chronically recurring physiological conditions, as well as potential complications—the nurse must be able to provide nursing care in the following areas:

- Physiological Adaptation
- Reduction of Risk Potential †
- Provision of Basic Care †

Psychosocial Integrity
To assist in meeting the client's needs for psychosocial integrity during periods of illness and common health problems that occur throughout the life cycle, the nurse must be able to provide nursing care in the following areas:

- Psychosocial Adaptation
- Coping/Adaptation †

Health Promotion and Maintenance

To assist in meeting the client's needs for health promotion and maintenance throughout the life cycle, the nurse must be able to provide nursing care in the following areas:

- Growth and Development through the Life Span
- Self-Care and Integrity of Support Systems †
- Prevention and Early Treatment of Disease

† Indicates areas of greater job importance; therefore, more emphasis is given to presenting questions in these subcategories.

Adapted from *NCLEX-RN™ Test Plan,* National Council of State Boards of Nursing, Chicago, to be implemented October 1995.

Computerized Adaptive Testing

With the introduction of Computerized Adaptive Testing (CAT) in 1994, the procedures for taking the NCLEX changed radically from prior protocol. The major new elements include:

1. Locating test sites throughout the U.S. where candidates make appointments to take the test on an individual basis.
2. Presenting the test on a computer screen rather than in a printed test booklet. The candidate makes answer selections by pressing keys on a computer keyboard instead of marking an answer sheet with a pencil.
3. Each candidate's test is unique because the computer selects each subsequent question based upon the candidate's prior answers.
4. Providing test results to each candidate soon after the test session and allowing candidates who fail NCLEX to retake the test within a short period of time.

The Advantages of CAT

CAT is described as providing a more comfortable and convenient way to take NCLEX. The testing environment at a Sylvan Technology Center will be similar to a small classroom or learning laboratory in contrast to a large hall or convention center with the distractions and tension associated with a large group of candidates taking the test simultaneously. From a procedural standpoint, the advantages of CAT are defined as:

1. A more efficient way to test and measure competency than the prior pencil and paper test format.

2. Reduction of testing time to a maximum of five hours in one session, including the tutorial procedure when you start and rest breaks you take during your test period.

3. Greater security and the avoidance of inconvenience to candidates if security measures break down.

4. Year-round testing schedules that provide applicants with greater flexibility and convenience than the prior twice-per-year system.

5. Substantial reduction in the elapsed time between applying to take NCLEX and receiving your results.

The Administrative Organizations for NCLEX CAT

Three organizations are involved with administering NCLEX: (1) boards of nursing from each state or jurisdiction, (2) the Educational Testing Service (ETS), and (3) Sylvan Learning Systems. As a candidate for licensure, it will help you to know the role of each organization.

As described earlier in this section, the NCSBN designs the test plan, conducts the job analysis, and sets the passing standard. The Educational Testing Service formulates the test questions to conform to the National Council's Test Plan. ETS maintains a test pool of several thousand questions written by specially selected item writers approved by the state boards of nursing. All NCLEX questions are drawn from this test pool. You will make an appointment with and physically take the NCLEX at a Sylvan Technology Center. Approximately 200 of these centers are available throughout the U.S. for NCLEX testing.

Application Procedures for the NCLEX CAT

After the state (jurisdiction) in which you plan to practice accepts your application and verifies your eligibility to take the NCLEX, you will receive an Authorization to Test and other information that includes the locations and telephone numbers of the Sylvan Technology Centers. You will then contact a test center of your choice to make an appointment to take the test. The test center does not need to be located in the state to which you have applied for licensure. As a first time test taker, you should be able to schedule your appointment within 30 days of your call. Read all instructions carefully, especially noting the items that you must take with you to the test center.

Taking the NCLEX CAT

Upon arriving at the Sylvan Technology Center, you will present your Authorization to Test and two forms of identification, both signed and one with a photo. A driver's license, school or employee I.D., and passport are the most accepted forms. A social security card is an example of an unacceptable proof of identity. At check-in, you will be photographed and thumb printed. Before commencing the test questions, you will complete a brief computer tutorial to make certain that you are comfortable with the keyboard procedures. The National Council advises that no prior computer experience is necessary for CAT.

The Number and Types of Questions on CAT

Two types of questions appear on NCLEX. The *real* questions test your competency and safety and provide the basis for your pass or fail score. The *tryout* questions are items being field tested for future NCLEX exams. You have no way of knowing the difference between *real* and *tryout* questions.

The minimum number of questions for each candidate will be 60 *real* and 15 *tryout* for a total of 75. The National Council maintains that the essential Test Plan categories can be covered by 60 carefully selected questions. The maximum number of *real* questions will be 250, so by adding the 15 *tryouts*, you could answer a total of 265 items.

CAT does not allow you to skip questions, change answers, or go back to look at questions already answered. Each question has an assigned degree of difficulty. Based on your prior answers—correct or incorrect—the computer selects the next question. Therefore, you must answer each question as it is presented. Because the computer draws from a large pool of questions, each candidate's test is unique. There is no absolute passing score in terms of the number or percent of questions that you must answer correctly in order to pass.

After you have answered the minimum number of questions, your test continues until the computer software calculates with a 95% degree of confidence that you fall into the safe/competent group or that you do not. Although there is no minimum amount of time for your test, the maximum allowable test duration is five hours, including your computer tutorial and rest breaks. A mandatory rest break of 10 minutes is required after two hours of testing and an optional break is available after the next one and one-half hours.

Because the number of questions is flexible, from a minimum of 75 to a maximum of 265, there is no optimal amount of time you should spend per question. However, because you won't know how long it will take you to reach the point where the computer stops presenting questions, it is not wise to spend several minutes on many questions. If you don't know the answer, guess and move on rather than spend five minutes and risk becoming immobilized.

Getting Your Test Results

The results of your test will be electronically transmitted from the Sylvan Technology Center where you take the test to Educational Testing Service in

Princeton, New Jersey, for processing. Within 48 hours, ETS will forward your results to the board of nursing to which you applied for licensure. Your results—pass or fail—will be sent to you by the board of nursing. A failure report will be accompanied by a diagnostic analysis to help you identify your specific areas of weakness. The time required for the board of nursing to notify the candidate will vary from state to state.

NCLEX-RN CAT Quick Reference

Test Location: Sylvan Technology Centers

Minimum Number of Questions: 75

Maximum Number of Questions: 265

Minimum Testing Time: None

Maximum Testing Time: 5 hours

Appendix 1. Directory of Boards of Nursing

Executive Officer
Board of Nursing
P.O. Box 303900
Montgomery, Alabama 36130-3900

Executive Secretary
Alaska Board of Nursing
3601 C Street, Suite 722
Anchorage, Alaska 99503

Secretary
Health Services Regulatory Board
LBJ Tropical Medical Center
Pago Pago, American Samoa 96799

Executive Director
Arizona State Board of Nursing
2001 W. Camelback, Suite 350
Phoenix, Arizona 85015

Executive Director
Arkansas State Board of Nursing
1123 South University, Suite 800
Little Rock, Arkansas 72204

Executive Officer
Board of Registered Nursing
P.O. Box 944210
Sacramento, California 95814

Program Administrator
Colorado State Board of Nursing
1560 Broadway, Suite 670
Denver, Colorado 80202

Executive Officer
Department of Health Services
150 Washington Street
Hartford, Connecticut 06106

Executive Director
Delaware Board of Nursing
O'Neill Building, P. O. Box 1401
Dover, Delaware 19901

Chairperson
District of Columbia
Board of Nursing
614 H Street NW
Washington, DC 20013

Executive Director
Florida State Board of Nursing
111 E. Coastline Drive East
Jacksonville, Florida 32202

Executive Director
Georgia Board of Nursing
166 Pryor Street SW
Atlanta, Georgia 30303

Administrator
Guam Board of Nurse Examiners
P. O. Box 2816
Agana, Guam 96910

Executive Secretary
Hawaii Board of Nursing
Box 3469
Honolulu, Hawaii 99503

Executive Director
Idaho State Board of Nursing
280 N. 8th Street, #210
Boise, Idaho 83720

Nursing Education Coordinator
Dept. of Professional Regulations
320 W. Washington Street
Springfield, Illinois 62786

Board Administration
Indiana State Board of Nursing
402 W. Washington Street
Indianapolis, Indiana 46204

Executive Director
Iowa Board of Nursing
1223 E. Court Avenue
Des Moines, Iowa 50319

Executive Administrator
Kansas State Board of Nursing
900 SW Jackson Street, Suite 551S
Topeka, Kansas 66612-1256

Executive Director
Kentucky Board of Nursing
312 Whittington Parkway, Suite 300
Louisville, Kentucky 40222-7000

Executive Director
Louisiana State Board of Nursing
912 Pere Marquette Building
New Orleans, Louisiana 70112

Executive Director
Maine State Board of Nursing
35 Anthony Avenue
State House Station 158
Augusta, Maine 04333-0158

Executive Director
Maryland Board of Nursing
4140 Patterson Avenue
Baltimore, Maryland 21215-2254

Executive Secretary
Board of Registration in Nursing
100 Cambridge Street, Room 150
Boston, Massachusetts 02202

Nursing Consultant
Michigan Board of Nursing
P. O. Box 30018, 611 West Ottawa
Lansing, Michigan 48909

Executive Director
Minnesota Board of Nursing
2700 University Avenue, West 108
St. Paul, Minnesota 55114

Commissioner
Mississippi Board of Nursing
P. O. Box 2336
Jackson, Mississippi 39211

Executive Director
Missouri State Board of Nursing
3605 Missouri Boulevard
Jefferson City, Missouri 65102

Executive Director
Montana State Board of Nursing
111 Jackson, Arcade Building
Helena, Montana 59620-0407

Associate Director
Bureau of Examining Board
P. O. Box 95007
Lincoln, Nebraska 68509

Executive Director
Nevada State Board of Nursing
2670 Chandler #9
Las Vegas, Nevada 89210

Executive Director
State Board of Nursing
Division of Public Health
6 Hazen Drive
Concord, New Hampshire 03301

Executive Director
New Jersey Board of Nursing
P. O. Box 45010
Newark, New Jersey 07101

Executive Director
New Mexico Board of Nursing
4253 Montgomery NE, Suite 130
Albuquerque, New Mexico 87109

Executive Secretary
New York State Board of Nursing
The Cultural Center, Room 3023
Albany, New York 12230

Executive Director
North Carolina Board of Nursing
P. O. Box 2129
Raleigh, North Carolina 27602

Executive Director
North Dakota Board of Nursing
919 S. 7th Street, Suite 504
Bismarck, North Dakota 58504-5881

Executive Director
Ohio Board of Nursing
77 S. High Street, 17th Floor
Columbus, Ohio 43266-0316

Executive Director
Oklahoma Board of Nursing
2915 N. Classen Boulevard, Suite 524
Oklahoma City, Oklahoma 73106

Executive Director
Oregon State Board of Nursing
800 NE Oregon Street, #25
Portland, Oregon 97232

Executive Secretary
Pennsylvania State Board of Nursing
P. O. Box 2649
Harrisburg, Pennsylvania 17105

Director
Council on Higher Education of PR
P.O. Box F University Station
Rio Piedras, Puerto Rico 00931

Director
Board of Nurse Registration
3 Capital Hill
Providence, Rhode Island 02908

Executive Director
South Carolina Board of Nursing
220 Executive Center Drive, Suite 220
Columbia, South Carolina 29210

Executive Specialist
South Dakota Board of Nursing
3307 South Lincoln
Sioux Falls, South Dakota 57105

Executive Director
Tennessee Board of Nursing
283 Plus Park Boulevard
Nashville, Tennessee 37217

Executive Director
Texas Board of Nurse Examiners
9101 Burnet Road, Suite 105
Austin, Texas 78752

Executive Administration
Utah State Board of Nursing
160 East 300 South, Box 45805
Salt Lake City, Utah 84145

Executive Director
Vermont Board of Nursing
Licensing and Registration Division
109 State Street
Montpelier, Vermont 05602

Executive Secretary
Virgin Islands Board of
Nurse Licensure
P. O. Box 4247
St. Thomas, Virgin Islands 00803

Executive Director
Virginia State Board of Nursing
6606 W. Broad Street, 4th Floor
Richmond, Virginia 23230-1717

Executive Director
Washington State Board of Nursing
1300 Quince Street, EY-27
Olympia, Washington 98504

Executive Secretary
Board of Examiners for Registered
Nurses
101 Dee Drive
Charleston, West Virginia 25311-1620

Administrative Officer
Wisconsin Department of
Regulation & Licensing
P. O. Box 8935
Madison, Wisconsin 57208-8935

Executive Director
State of Wyoming Board of Nursing
2301 Central Avenue, Barrett
Building
Cheyenne, Wyoming 82002

II

GUIDELINES FOR EFFECTIVE TEST TAKING

Test-Taking Strategies

Research has shown that NCLEX-RN candidates who fully understand test construction and who have become familiar with appropriate test-taking strategies score higher than candidates with a similar knowledge base who approach an examination without adequate skill in test-taking techniques. Fear of the unknown can contribute to pretest anxiety, and confusion at the test site can increase this anxiety. This section identifies and describes test-taking guidelines that have proven to be very helpful to candidates for RN licensure.

First, it is important to realize that a multiple choice test is very different from other types of tests such as essay, matching, and true/false. In multiple choice exams, the question is called the **stem**. The stem is followed by four alternative answers. One answer is correct, and the other three are referred to as **distractors** because they distract your attention from identifying and selecting the correct answer. It is important to understand that the distractors are not necessarily wrong, but rather they may not be **as** correct or **as** complete as the right answer. The multiple choice questions in this book are similar in format, subject matter, length, and degree of difficulty to those contained in the NCLEX-RN. The answers to the multiple-choice questions are accompanied by rationale or an identification of the underlying principle. The answer sections provide you with an added learning experience; if you understand the basic principles of nursing content, you can transfer these principles to the clinical situations contained in the NCLEX-RN. Furthermore, the comprehensive tests will provide a basis for understanding the process of selecting the "best" answer to a question.

The following guidelines will help you become better prepared to deal with various question types and to more efficiently compare and evaluate the answer selections.

Guideline #1 Do not read extra meaning into the question.

In effective test construction, the stem is direct and to the point. The question asks for one particular response, and you should not read other information into the question. Often you will find questions that require "common sense" answers. Reading into these questions, making interpretations, or searching for subtle hidden meanings is not advised. Your first action is to ask yourself, "What is the question asking?" Look for key words or phrases to help you understand. It is important to have the central point clearly in your mind before considering the distractors.

Guideline #2 Understand exactly what the stem is asking before considering the distractors.

Make very sure you read the stem correctly. Notice particularly the way the question is phrased. Is it asking for the most important or the *first* response? It is asking you for factual information, conceptual information, or nursing judgment? One of the most important principles in test taking is understanding precisely what the question is asking.

Guideline #3 Rephrase the question in your own words.

Another technique for assessing the stem and interpreting the question correctly is to rephrase the question so that it is very clear in your own mind. Rephrasing the stem of the question in your own language can assist you to read the question correctly and, in turn, choose the appropriate response. This is particularly important when you are faced with a difficult and/or confusing question.

> The nurse in the newborn nursery is unable to insert a tube into a newborn's stomach; she has met resistance with each attempt. Tracheoesophageal fistula with atresia is suspected. An important assessment is

To clearly understand the question, restate the condition in your own words: "With tracheoesophageal fistula, I know that there is a connection between the esophagus and the trachea." Then rephrase the question: "If there is an overflow of liquid into the larynx and trachea, what signs would I be likely to observe?" The answer is excessive drooling, choking, and coughing during the feeding.

Placing the question in a framework that you understand will enable you to cut through extraneous data to the heart of the stem. Also, stating the question as a process—what assessment is important for a baby who has tracheoesophageal fistula with atresia—will allow you to follow the process to a logical conclusion (usually the correct answer). If possible, think of the correct answer before considering the distractors. If you do not know the answer, the following cues to working with distractors may prove helpful.

Guideline #4 When analyzing the distractors, isolate what is important in the answer alternatives from what is not important relative to the question.

Distractors are various alternatives chosen to be as close as possible to the right answer. In good test construction, all of the distractors are similar, should be feasible and reasonable, and should apply directly to the stem. Also, all of the distractors may contain correct information, but not be the right choice for the specific question that is asked. One method of helping you choose the correct answer is to ask yourself whether each alternative is true or false in relation to the stem.

> Which one of the following characteristics is not found with parents who abuse their children?
> 1. They have very low impulse control.   TRUE
> 2. They are socially isolated and lonely people.   TRUE
> 3. They have realistic expectations of their children.   FALSE
> 4. Often they were abused as children.   TRUE

Asking yourself which of the distractors is true or false is a shortcut method of answering the question. It forces you to keep looking at the stem. Otherwise you are trying to judge all of the choices at once. After you have completed the true-false process, remember to go back to the stem and ask yourself if your choice does, in fact, answer the question.

Guideline #5 After choosing the correct answer alternative and separating it from the distractors, go back to the stem and make sure your choice does, in fact, answer the question.

An answer alternative may be correct as it stands by itself, but if the question asks for the first nursing action, you need to separate first from later nursing interventions. Too many candidates fail to recheck the answer with the stem, and they answer the question incorrectly.

Guideline #6 Use the "process of elimination" technique.

Examine each alternative and ask yourself, "Is this answer right?" or "Is this answer logical?" Try to eliminate at least one or more distractors. If you can eliminate one or two distractors, it will be easier to identify the correct answer. The "process of elimination" is one of the most effective test-taking strategies.

Guideline #7 When answering a difficult question, utilize your total body of knowledge.

When you come across a difficult question and you cannot immediately identify the answer, go back to your body of knowledge and draw on the information that you **do** know about the condition. Suppose you were asked a question about the most important equipment to have in the room when a patient returned from surgery. You would know that brain surgery would require different equipment from lung surgery, especially when you consider the potential complications. Even if you don't know the answer immediately, by taking your time to analyze the situation, recalling the information you have learned about that condition, and applying this information to the specific situation presented in the question, you should be able to arrive at the correct answer. Also, if you are unfamiliar with the disease or disorder and cannot choose the right nursing action, try to generalize to other situations. Even though you don't know exactly what **to do**, you might know what **not** to do. The elimination of one distractor substantially increases the odds of your selecting the correct answer.

To summarize the concept of generalizing, remember, if you don't know or recognize the specific condition, try to identify a general principle and apply it to that situation.

Guideline #8 The ability to guess correctly is both a skill and an art.

Because the NCLEX-RN exam requires you to answer each question before proceeding to the next one, you may, on occasion, have to guess. Guessing is an art in itself, and since you only have a 25% chance of guessing correctly, let's look at several strategies that may increase your odds.

1. Try to eliminate at least one (or more if possible) distractor, as this will increase your chances of guessing correctly.
2. Examine the distractors, and if one is the exact opposite of another (you know that unlimited fluid intake and restricted fluid intake cannot both be correct), choose the one that seems most logical.
3. Try to identify the underlying principle that supports the question. If you can answer the question, "What is this question trying to determine that I know?", you might then be able to guess the correct answer. This strategy is especially true with a psychosocial question.
4. Look at the way the alternatives are presented. Are two answers very close? Often when this occurs, the ability to discriminate will show evidence of judgment. Check to see if one, more than the other, is the best choice for the question.
5. Examine the alternatives for logic. Are some distractors just not logical? Are some distractors correct in themselves, but do not have anything to

do with the question? If so, eliminate these and concentrate on the remaining alternatives.

6. Finally, use your intuition. If you cannot choose an alternative by using logic, allow yourself to feel which one might be right. Often your sub-conscious mind will choose correctly (based on all the conscious knowl-edge you have, of course), so simply let yourself feel which alternative might be right.

Guideline #9 Choosing an answer from a "hunch."

During a test, frequently you may come to a question and not know the answer immediately, but have an inner feeling or a hunch that a particular alternative is the right answer. Do you depend on this "hunch"? Current research supports the conclusion that hunches are often correct, for they are based on rapid subcon-scious connections in the brain. In other words, going through logical, rational steps is not the only way to arrive at the answer. Your stored knowledge, recall and experience can combine to assist you in arriving at the correct answer. So, if you have an initial hunch, go with it. **Do not** change the answer if, upon reflec-tion, it just doesn't seem right. On the other hand, if you re-read the question and note information you previously missed, for example, the age of the client or diagnosis related to diet, then you may feel it is appropriate to change your answer selection. With additional information or a definite conclusion, rather than a "feeling," it is a good test-taking strategy to change an answer. Remember, however, when taking the NCLEX/CAT, you cannot go back and change the answer to a question once you have moved on to the next question. Therefore, you must be careful to make certain of your choice.

Guideline #10 Choosing the best answer from a strategy point-of-view.

Frequently, the most comprehensive answer is the best choice. For example, if two alternatives seem reasonable but one answer includes the other (i.e., it is more detailed, extends the first, or is more comprehensive), then this answer would be the best choice.

Guideline #11 Understanding the question helps in choosing the answer.

Carefully read each question. Determine what the question is really asking. Sometimes details are extraneous. Mentally underline important factors; pay attention to key terms and phrases. For example, do not misread *grams* as *mil-ligrams*. Read the question as it is stated, not as you would like it to be stated. The questions will test your ability to analyze a clinical situation and to apply your nursing knowledge. Do not look for a pattern in the answer key—there is none. For example, if you have already answered several consecutive questions with a #2, do not hesitate to answer the next question in sequence with a #2 if you think that is the right answer. Evaluate the possible answers in relation to the stem (the question), not to other answers. Choose the answer that best fits that question rather than an answer that sounds good by itself.

Guidelines for Answering Psychosocial Questions

The current test plan incorporates the psychosocial aspect of the illness, treatment, or client care plan. The psychosocial focus will be a central thread throughout the clinical areas: medical and surgical nursing, maternity and pediatric nursing. In other words, even though a question may be coded *medical* and deal with a client who has recently had a myocardial infarction, it is possible that the actual content of the question will relate to psychosocial nursing, rather than straight medical nursing. When you encounter psychosocial or communication-oriented questions, remember the following communication principles.

1. *Responses that focus on feelings.* All clients at some time find it difficult to express their feelings whether they have a terminal illness, a new baby, a somatic illness, or are scheduled for elective surgery. Any nursing response that elicits these feelings is therapeutic, so listen and pay attention to client cues. When the client needs to discuss fears, concerns, or angry feelings, then encourage their expression. If a client states he is afraid of dying, encourage talking about fears of dying (be specific), not just fears (general response).

2. *Responses that are honest and direct.* It is important that the nurse be honest in her responses to encourage trust and build a therapeutic relationship. Dishonesty will never support trust and a firm relationship. So, if a client asks you a question, give an honest response.

3. *Responses that indicate acceptance of the client.* Accept the client where and how he is regardless of his condition or verbalizations. In fact, you should not reject the client, even if you could not accept his behavior.

4. *Responses that pick up or relate to cues.* Responding to an important cue is an essential therapeutic technique if the nurse is to focus on the client and maintain a goal-focused interaction. Respond to "feeling level" cues rather than "cognitive" or superficial cues from the client.

Maximizing Your Review Time

A common source of test anxiety is the fear of not being sufficiently prepared to pass the test. This is very common among RN licensure candidates for a variety of reasons including:

1. Limited time available for review between the completion of final examinations and your appointment to take the NCLEX-RN.
2. Difficulty in motivation to begin concentrated study following the emotional and physical drain of finishing nursing school.
3. Inability to sort out and organize vast quantities of material to which you have been exposed during nursing school.
4. Absence of a defined study plan that includes a systematic review.
5. Lack of self-knowledge of your own strengths and weaknesses in terms of categories or subjects tested by the NCLEX-RN.
6. Uncertainty regarding the NCLEX-RN test plan, subject emphasis, or scoring procedures.
7. Lack of confidence that nursing school instruction effectively prepared you for the licensure examination.

There are many other reasons why candidates feel less than totally confident regarding NCLEX-RN, but the above list summarizes the major sources of test anxiety. Of course, when the candidate has high test anxiety, he or she may have difficulty even getting started on an effective review program.

You want your review program to be effective and efficient. By effective, we mean that the program works—you enter the test site with calmness and confidence, and you pass. By efficient, we refer to the relationship between the results and the cost in time and money to achieve them.

The following recommendations illustrate ways that you can achieve maximum results for the amount of time invested.

1. Plan your study and review periods at regular intervals for best efficiency.
    a. Arrange to study when mentally alert; if you study during periods of mental and physical fatigue, your efficiency is reduced.
    b. When studying, use short breaks at relatively frequent intervals. Breaks used as rewards for hard work serve as incentives for continued concentrated effort.

2. Identify your strengths and weaknesses to enable you to efficiently focus your review time.
    a. Consider your past performance on classroom tests and written clinical applications of factual material. Learn from past errors on tests by studying corrected material.

b. Systematically eliminate your weaknesses. Allow sufficient time for repeated review of those areas that continue to pose problems.

3. Familiarize yourself with the examination format and multiple choice tests.
   a. Study the format used for NCLEX-RN so that you will know the different ways in which questions are asked. For example, you must know how to deal with clinical situations and multiple-choice questions.
   b. Practice answering the questions in this book. Become familiar with how NCLEX questions are worded. Read the rationales that accompany the answers.

4. Apply time management to taking multiple-choice tests. The total time allotment for you to complete your NCLEX/CAT is five hours. However, it is still important that you practice time management with test questions, so that you are programmed not to spend too much time on any one question. You can prepare yourself to accomplish this by allotting 1 minute per question as you take practice tests. At the rate of 1 minute per question, you will be able to answer 265 questions in just under 4 1/2 hours. This allows you the additional time to complete your computer tutorial and to take your required break. However, the NCLEX/CAT appears to be designed to measure your competency in substantially fewer than the maximum of 265 questions.

5. Systematically study the material contained in a review book. You will find a complete review of nursing content in *Sandra Smith's Review for NCLEX-RN*.
   a. First gain a general impression of the chapter, or content unit, to be reviewed. Skim over the entire section. Observe how the material is organized and identify the main ideas.
   b. Systematically read through the material and, as appropriate, relate the content to the nursing process. Visualize the situations from a nurse-client decision making basis.
   c. Carefully read and study the tables and appendices where much factual background data is summarized. Using these quick reference sources will reduce time-consuming searches of textbooks or personal notes.
   d. Mark important material and note subjects that you do not know thoroughly for additional review.

6. Follow up on your priority areas.
   a. Set priorities on the material that is to be learned or reviewed. Identify the most crucial sections and underline the essential thoughts.
   b. Review what you have read. Ask yourself to think of examples that illustrate the main points you have studied. Recall examples from your own clinical experience or from clinical cases about which you have read.

c. Solidify newly learned material by writing down the main ideas or by explaining the major points to another person.

7. Test yourself on what you have learned.
    a. Answer the practice questions in this review book.
    b. Study the answers and their rationale. Concentrate on understanding the underlying principles and reasons for the answers.
    c. Acquire the flexibility to answer questions phrased in different ways over the same wide range of content. Important concepts may be tested repeatedly in exams, but the questions will be worded differently.
    d. Use the disk attached to the inside back cover of this book to answer questions so that you become familiar with the computer screen format and the keyboard procedures for answering questions.

At the Test Session

Students who are relaxed and confident while taking tests have a distinct advantage over those who become extremely anxious when taking an important exam. Achieving the maximum testing effectiveness involves your mental attitude as well as your knowledge of specific testing techniques. The following suggestions will help you maximize your testing effectiveness.

1. General readiness is a key to success.
    Prepare the night before the test. Assemble the materials that you must take to the test site as specified in your instructions. Get a good night's rest. Don't stay up all night learning new material. Avoid the use of stimulants or depressants, either of which may affect your ability to think clearly during the test. Approach the test with confidence and the determination to do your best. Think positively and concentrate on all you *do* know rather than on what you think you *do not* know.

2. On the day of the exam, get yourself together.
    Eat a solid breakfast. Protein will provide needed energy. Allow ample time to travel to the testing site, including time to park, and to check in. Choose a location in the testing room where you are least likely to be distracted.

3. Scoring well on the examination.
    As you start your test, check the time periodically, and maintain a good rate of progression. Do not spend too much time on any one question so that you become anxious and immobilized. If you do not know the answer, choose one of the alternatives. Do not waste time by struggling with questions that totally perplex you.

Computer Testing Tips

1. Answer each question. If you don't recognize a correct answer among the four choices, use your test-taking skills or, if necessary, make your best guess.
2. Be certain of your answer selection before pressing the "Enter" key a second time to confirm your choice. You cannot change your answers to prior questions.
3. Take your time and carefully read the questions and answer choices. You have 5 hours and the maximum number of questions you will be asked is 265.
4. Do not become immobilized by any one question. Spending 5 to 10 minutes on a question will probably make you more nervous and less attentive as you proceed.
5. The test center will provide you with scratch paper and a pencil. Use them when you encounter questions that require calculations.
6. Take a nutritious snack and perhaps bottled water with you. At the test center you will be assigned a locker where you must leave your personal items. After two hours of testing, you will have a mandatory rest break of 10 minutes.

Using Your Computer Disk

A 3.5" IBM compatible computer disk has been placed in an envelope inside the back cover of this book. The purposes of the practice disk include the following:

1. To provide you with simulated NCLEX/CAT questions so you can rehearse taking NCLEX on the computer. This includes your reading questions (stem and distractors) as they will be displayed on the computer screen, rather than seeing them printed in a test booklet.
2. To enable you to become familiar with the computer procedures that you will follow when you take NCLEX. The computer keys used to display questions and select and confirm answers on your practice disk are the same keys as you will use when you take NCLEX.
3. To give you useful feedback when you complete the simulated NCLEX test. You will be able to obtain a Performance Summary that will help you identify your strengths and weaknesses in terms of the Nursing Process, Client Needs and Clinical Areas.
4. To identify the specific questions you missed so you can review their rationales. This will help you understand the principles that underlie the correct answers.

5. To enable you to experience additional practice. You will be able to erase the answers on your disk and retake the simulated tests at a later date.

In summary, the information presented in this chapter provides you with guidelines and strategies, not absolutes. Always use your own judgment, knowledge, and nursing experience. These assets will serve you well in passing the NCLEX-RN. You have the background, education, and knowledge to pass these exams. Let your own creative abilities come through. Be confident that you will pass and, in fact, you will.

III

COMPREHENSIVE TESTS

Comprehensive Test 1

1. A 56-year-old male client is admitted to the coronary care unit with a diagnosis of myocardial infarction. He is placed on a cardiac monitor and has an IV of D_5W at a "keep open" rate. The nurse's priority concern is to assess for

   1. Apical pulse rate.
   2. Chest pain.
   3. Respiratory rate.
   4. Blood pressure increase.

2. The physician orders laboratory tests for a client with a suspected myocardial infarction. Which of the following lab findings would indicate that there has been myocardial damage?

   1. Elevated CPK-MB.
   2. Decreased CPK, SGOT.
   3. Elevated total CPK and elevated SGOT.
   4. Elevated SGOT and LDH.

3. A physician orders 2 mg per minute of Lidocaine for a client. Using 500 ml D_5W and 2 grams of Lidocaine, the nurse will administer how many ml's per minute?

   1. 1 ml.
   2. 0.75 ml.
   3. 0.50 ml.
   4. 0.25 ml.

4. A low-sodium diet is ordered for a client. The nurse will know he understands his low-sodium diet restrictions when he chooses a menu of

   1. Smoked turkey, mashed potatoes, spinach, and apple juice.
   2. Crab on rice, green beans, and Sanka.
   3. Lamb chop, mint jelly, rice, beets, and low fat milk.
   4. Roast beef, baked potato, squash, and Sanka.

5. A mother asks the nurse when her child's immunizations will start. The most appropriate response is to tell her

   1. Four months.
   2. Anytime after birth.
   3. Six months.
   4. Two months.

6. Before administering an immunization to a child, the nurse will assess for a primary contraindication, which is

   1. Impetigo.
   2. Failure to thrive.
   3. Congenital heart disease.
   4. Cystic fibrosis.

7. A six month old is brought to the clinic with a suspected diagnosis of cerebral palsy. In the initial assessment of his developmental

status, the nurse would be likely to find that he

1. Tracks an object with his eyes.
2. Needs to be propped to sit up.
3. Smiles when he sees his mother.
4. Indicates presence of a pincer grasp.

8. A 41-year-old client has had recurrent dull flank pain, nausea and vomiting for 24 hours. He is admitted to the hospital for a genitourinary work-up. Which of the following orders written by his physician would be considered a priority and thus carried out promptly?

1. Keep accurate intake and output records.
2. Strain all urine.
3. Record temperature every four hours.
4. Administer an antiemetic every four hours.

9. Which of the following clinical manifestations would indicate that a client has developed a complication following a cystoscopy?

1. Difficulty voiding.
2. Pink-tinged urine.
3. Burning on urination.
4. Development of a chill.

10. A newly pregnant client is unsure of the date of her last menstrual period (LMP). Means other than Nägele's rule will be used to determine the estimated date of delivery. The nurse would expect the physician to estimate the date by

1. Hearing the first audible fetal heart tone with a fetoscope.
2. Serial estriols.

3. Ultrasonography.
4. The nonstress test.

11. One of the vital signs that will be monitored throughout the pregnancy is blood pressure. An accurate graph of blood pressure is very important. The best position for taking blood pressure is

1. Left arm, supine position.
2. Right arm, sitting position.
3. Left arm, left lateral recumbent.
4. Same arm and position each time taken by the same person.

12. An 18 month old is admitted to the hospital with suspected Hirschsprung's disease. His weight is 8.5 kg, placing him at the 10th percentile on the growth grid. The diagnostic test the nurse would expect the physician to order is a/an

1. Barium swallow.
2. Abdominal sonogram.
3. Rectal biopsy.
4. Sigmoidoscopy.

13. During the preoperative period before surgery for Hirschsprung's disease, a priority nursing intervention will focus on

1. Maintaining the child's attachment to his parents.
2. Demonstrating correct administration of tap water enemas to his parents.
3. Providing a high-calorie diet.
4. Promoting adequate rest and sleep.

14. A female client, age 36, states she has been depressed and anxious. Her mood is one of sadness and gloom and she is requesting

medication. During the admission interview, the priority assessment is the client's

1. Living situation.
2. Coping mechanisms.
3. Suicide potential.
4. Support systems.

15. In a psychiatric setting, to develop a working relationship with a client, the nurse knows that goal setting is vital. To ensure that the goal is attainable, it must

    1. Be mutually set by the client and the nurse.
    2. Have observable outcomes.
    3. Be flexible and changeable as appropriate to the situation.
    4. Be set by the nurse and agreed to by the client.

16. A depressed client tells the nurse that most of the time she has no anger toward her husband and rarely says anything negative, but he is always angry with her. She may be using the defense mechanism of

    1. Denial.
    2. Sublimation.
    3. Projection.
    4. Fantasizing.

17. A female client is to be discharged on diazepam (Valium) 5 mg tid. The nurse will know she understands the side effects of Valium when the client says she is aware that

    1. Ingestion of alcohol potentiates the action of diazepam.
    2. Valium will help make her problems more manageable.

    3. She may not feel the action of the drug for two to three weeks.
    4. She should not eat cheese, chocolate, or wine while taking the drug.

18. During a pregnant client's visit, the nurse assesses her for signs of increasing eclampsia or pregnancy induced hypertension (PIH). If it is present, the nurse will observe

    1. Edema of the hands, feet, and face.
    2. Glycosuria.
    3. Tachycardia.
    4. Polyuria.

19. The nurse knows that the client understands the principles of managing Type I diabetes when he says that he maintains his health status with

    1. Oral hypoglycemics.
    2. A diabetic diet (ADA) regimen.
    3. Weight reduction.
    4. Insulin injections.

20. Assessing a client with the diagnosis of duodenal ulcer and diabetes, the nurse would expect to find the contributing factor that is directly related to both duodenal ulcers and uncontrolled diabetes. This contributing factor is

    1. A change in diet.
    2. High stress.
    3. Poor insulin control.
    4. A vitamin B_{12} deficiency.

21. The physician determines that a diabetic Type I client requires a subtotal gastric resection. In planning his postoperative

care, the nurse will be aware that the plan will take into account

1. A disruption in metabolic control.
2. An increased need for insulin.
3. An increased need for carbohydrates.
4. The onset of long term complications.

22. The mother of a 1-month-old infant comes to the well-baby clinic. During a counseling session, the nurse learns that the mother often props the baby's bottle because the baby wiggles a lot. An appropriate response would be

1. "It is probably a good idea to prop the bottle until you feel more comfortable holding the baby."
2. "It is not a good idea to do this because the baby could choke on the formula."
3. "Do you have a fear of dropping the baby?"
4. "You need to hold the baby when you are feeding her."

23. A 57-year-old male is admitted for an endocrine work-up. The provisional diagnosis is Cushing's syndrome. Among the tests scheduled are fasting blood sugar, electrolytes, plasma ACTH level, and urinary 17-ketosteroids. Considering the lab tests that were ordered, the nurse would expect to assess the client and find

1. Nervous exhaustion, hypertension, diaphoresis, heat intolerance.
2. Moon face, hirsutism, emotional lability, weight gain.
3. Increased cardiac output, heat intolerance, muscle fatigue, weight loss.
4. Hypothermia, inactivity, weight gain, constipation.

24. A client is scheduled for a unilateral adrenalectomy. In developing goals for postoperative care, the nurse would

1. Instruct him in daily steroid administration.
2. Teach him signs and symptoms of hypoglycemia.
3. Plan a diet low in protein and sodium.
4. Maintain skin integrity.

25. The nurse is assessing a normal infant. A Moro reflex, present at birth, is described as

1. Sudden, generalized, symmetrical movement with the legs drawn up together.
2. Rapid movement of the arm and leg on the side opposite the stimulation.
3. Slow, generalized, random activity of the whole body followed by a rigid positioning of the extremities.
4. Rapid movement of all the extremities with no fixed pattern.

26. A new mother asks the nurse about nutrition instructions for breast-feeding. The nurse explains that the diet should include

1. Four to five glasses of milk a day.
2. Restricted salt intake.
3. Low-calorie foods.
4. Restricted fat intake.

27. A new mother being discharged wishes to know what would be the best contraception for her, assuming she continues to breast-feed? The nurse will explain that the method of birth control that is contraindicated is

1. Oral contraceptive.
2. The sponge.
3. The diaphragm.
4. Foam and condoms.

28. A client tells the nurse she missed one menstrual cycle and her next cycle resulted in a slight amount of flow. She has not been pregnant before, but has had several sexual partners over the last year. Considering the history of her menstrual cycle, the nurse suspects she may have a tubal pregnancy. What is the appropriate intervention?

    1. Ask the physician to see the client immediately.
    2. Ask her if there is a familial history of tubal pregnancies.
    3. Examine her abdomen to determine if there is unilateral pelvic pain over a mass.
    4. Take her vital signs to determine if there are any abnormalities present.

29. The postoperative period is a very emotional time for a client following surgery for a tubal pregnancy. Which of the following comments would be the most therapeutic for the nurse to make to the client?

    1. "You're doing just fine so there is no need to worry like this."
    2. "Why are you crying?"
    3. "It really will be best for you if you can stop crying and think about something pleasant."
    4. "Crying is a good release, but perhaps you would like to talk about why you're crying."

30. A wife will be involved in providing nursing care for her husband who has had multiple sclerosis for 20 years. Which of the following nursing care measures would be most appropriate to include in the teaching sessions?

    1. Exercises that promote muscle strengthening and decrease tremors.
    2. Instruction in weight control.
    3. Side effects of routine medications.
    4. Importance of regular bowel and bladder evacuation.

31. When performing a neurological examination on a client who has seizures, which of the following assessments would be considered the most important or useful part of the examination?

    1. Reflexes.
    2. Pupil size.
    3. Pain response.
    4. Muscle strength.

32. While bathing a client, he tells the nurse the red spots he sees before his eyes just before a seizure occurs are starting right now. The initial nursing action is to

    1. Call the physician immediately.
    2. Start an IV for drug therapy.
    3. Turn him on his right side.
    4. Place a folded washcloth between his teeth.

33. A 20-year-old male is admitted to the hospital with the diagnosis of acute schizophrenia. Assessing his behavior, the nurse determines that he is hallucinating when there is

    1. A sensory experience without foundation in reality.
    2. A distortion of real auditory or visual perception.
    3. A voice that is heard by the client but not by others.
    4. An idea without foundation in reality.

34. A schizophrenic client becomes more withdrawn and suspicious of other clients. He constantly tries to argue with the nursing staff that several of the clients are "out to get him." The best nursing response to this behavior is to

   1. Ignore the behavior and it will diminish.
   2. Disagree with the client so that his fears won't be confirmed.
   3. Avoid disagreeing with the client and get him involved with an activity.
   4. Attempt to move rapidly into a nurse-client relationship to establish trust.

35. After one month in the hospital, a schizophrenic client states that voices are telling him he will die tonight, and asks the nurse if this is true. His statement and question indicate that he

   1. Is not improving and may be getting worse.
   2. Will begin to enter the manic phase of his illness.
   3. Is questioning the hallucination and wants reassurance from the nurse.
   4. Has a poor prognosis.

36. A 24 month old is admitted to the hospital with the diagnosis of bacterial meningitis. The nurse will assess for the presenting signs and symptoms that probably include

   1. Seizures, poor feeding, positive Kernig's sign.
   2. Poor feeding, vomiting, irritability, fever.
   3. Bulging fontanels, apnea, headache.
   4. Combativeness, seizures, apnea.

37. The priority nursing intervention for a child with meningitis is to

   1. Frequently take vital signs and perform neuro checks.
   2. Encourage fluids.
   3. Administer antibiotics as ordered according to schedule.
   4. Maintain respiratory isolation.

38. A client with a gunshot wound to the chest had a right-sided pneumothorax. The physician inserted two chest tubes into the pleural cavity, and connected the water-seal drainage system to a walled-in-suction. To assist in chest drainage, the nurse will place the client in the position of

   1. High-Fowler's.
   2. Supine.
   3. Right-side, low-Fowler's.
   4. Left-side, semi-Fowler's.

39. The purpose of the water-seal chamber is to

   1. Apply positive pressure on the water-seal drainage system to re-expand the lung.
   2. Apply a seal to keep air from being drawn back into the pleural space.
   3. Apply negative pressure to the lung to re-expand the lung.
   4. Drain secretions from the chest cavity to assist in re-expansion of the lung.

40. A client, age 11, is brought to the hospital by his parents and receives a diagnosis of acute rheumatic fever. While the nurse is assessing his heart sounds, she keeps in mind that the cardiac structure most susceptible to damage is the

   1. Ventricle.
   2. Atrium.
   3. Tricuspid valve.
   4. Mitral valve.

41. A client on the unit becomes agitated and assaultive when stressed. The nurse learns in report that his family did not visit him, and when making rounds, finds him with clenched fists, pacing the hall. The best strategy for dealing with his behavior would first be to

    1. Discuss with the client how he feels about his family not coming to visit him.
    2. Ask the client to come to the day room where you can better observe him in case he becomes more agitated.
    3. Invite the client to join you in an activity that you know he finds relaxing.
    4. Ignore the body language of anger and allow the client to pace off his anxiety.

42. A female client, age 65, is admitted to the outpatient setting for laser therapy as a result of progressive visual field loss and optic nerve damage. Her diagnosis is glaucoma. The following drug group used to lower intraocular pressure in glaucoma is

    1. Mydriatic.
    2. Miotic.
    3. Antibiotic.
    4. Antidiuretic.

43. While eating in the cafeteria, the nurse hears someone yell, "Help! My husband is choking!" The first intervention is to

    1. Give him an abdominal thrust.
    2. Give him a back blow.
    3. Establish an airway.
    4. Ask him, "Can you talk?"

44. Reviewing the chart before sending a surgical client to the operating room, nursing responsibilities would include notifying the physician if the

    1. Erythrocyte count is 6 mil/cu mm.
    2. Leukocyte count is 5,500/cu mm.
    3. Hemoglobin is 14 gm/dl.
    4. Platelet count is 100,000 ul.

45. A client was admitted to the hospital four hours ago with a head injury, incurred when he fell off a ladder. The nurse observes his restlessness and understands that it is probably caused by

    1. Decreased intracranial pressure.
    2. Cerebral anoxia.
    3. Dehydration.
    4. Pain.

46. Which of the following clinical manifestations is a late indication that a client is developing increased intracranial pressure (ICP) following a head injury?

    1. Restlessness.
    2. Increased blood pressure.
    3. Decreased pulse rate.
    4. Widened pulse pressure.

47. A female client, age 63, is admitted to the hospital. Her chart states that she has had a myocardial infarction that has progressed to cardiogenic shock. Which of the following parameters would indicate that cardiogenic shock is developing?

    1. A widening pulse pressure.
    2. Slow respiratory rate.
    3. Bradyarrhythmias.
    4. Decreasing arterial blood pressure.

48. Which one of the following conditions is a common cause of cardiogenic shock?

    1. Fluid overload.

2. Electrolyte imbalance.
3. Left ventricular failure.
4. Constrictive pericarditis.

49. Based on the nurse's knowledge of cardiogenic shock, the physician is most likely to order a medication that would

1. Dilate veins.
2. Decrease cardiac contractility.
3. Increase peripheral vascular resistance.
4. Increase heart rate.

50. An 18 year old is admitted to a psychiatric unit with a tentative diagnosis of antisocial personality. He recently physically assaulted his 16-year-old girlfriend when she wanted to break up with him. Assessing him, the nurse knows that a person with antisocial personality disorder can be described as

1. An individual of high intelligence who attempts to cope through manipulation.
2. A person with good superego development who manipulates others for the fun of it.
3. A person who appears very reasonable but who is highly manipulative.
4. A person who manipulates out of fear of punishment.

51. After a client with the diagnosis of personality disorder attended one group session on a psychiatric unit, he refused to attend any others even though he had contracted to go to group therapy. The appropriate nursing action is to

1. Renegotiate the contract to eliminate group therapy.
2. Take away a privilege until he keeps his agreement.

3. Discuss the treatment plan with his physician.
4. Try to talk him into coming to the next session.

52. A client with otosclerosis is admitted to the hospital. A stapedectomy is scheduled for the next day. The nurse understands that the primary purpose of this surgery is to

1. Decrease tinnitus.
2. Increase hearing.
3. Decrease vertigo.
4. Decrease pain.

53. Immediately following a stapedectomy, the priority nursing action is to

1. Turn and deep breathe the client.
2. Put the siderails up.
3. Check for drainage.
4. Test hearing capability.

54. A client, 12 weeks pregnant, comes to the clinic for Evaluating. She tells the nurse that although her boyfriend and her family have accepted the pregnancy, and they are planning to be married, she is not sure she is happy about having a baby. A therapeutic response from the nurse would be

1. "Are you thinking about an abortion?"
2. "Both your boyfriend and your family have accepted the pregnancy?"
3. "I can understand that. You did originally come in for contraception."
4. "That's a common response in early pregnancy. Would you like to talk more about it?"

55. A 47-year-old client is admitted to the hospital with a three-day history of severe, burn-

ing abdominal pain in the left epigastric area. His admitting diagnosis is suspected peptic ulcer disease. Based on nursing knowledge, which of the following questions will reveal the most information concerning the source of the pain?

1. How long does the pain last?
2. Does exercise bring on the pain?
3. Do certain foods cause the pain?
4. When does the pain occur?

56. A client is scheduled for a gastroduodenoscopy and the nurse will prepare him for this procedure. Preprocedure instructions would include information that during the procedure he will be

1. Heavily sedated.
2. Given a local anesthetic to ease the discomfort.
3. Asked to assist by coughing.
4. Asked to assist by performing a Valsalva maneuver.

57. A client with severe burns on his upper extremities is scheduled to go to surgery for debridement and application of homografts. The nurse is aware that the graft will come from

1. The client's own skin.
2. Cadaver skin.
3. Pig skin.
4. Artificial skin.

58. Nursing care in the first 24 hours following skin grafting will include

1. Maintaining a pressure dressing on the grafted area.
2. Monitoring continuous antibiotic irrigations to the grafted area.
3. Changing the dressings every four hours using sterile technique.
4. Irrigating the drains placed in the burn area every four hours with sterile saline solution.

59. A client has been brought to the immediate treatment center by the police for attacking his neighbor with a knife. His admitting diagnosis was schizophrenia. Beginning the admission process, the first nursing action would be to

1. Search the client for concealed weapons.
2. Ask the client how he is feeling.
3. Introduce herself to the client.
4. Get the client settled on the unit.

60. A 48-year-old female has been experiencing irregular menstrual periods, hot flashes, and mood swings for the last 15 months. She has come to the clinic for her yearly checkup and says she has a number of questions. Her first question is, "When can I stop using birth control methods?" The most appropriate reply for the nurse to give her is

1. "Anytime now because your periods have been irregular for more than 12 months."
2. "You should use a birth control method until your 50th birthday."
3. "It depends on whether or not you are still sexually active."
4. "You should use a birth control method until you have missed your period for 24 consecutive months."

61. During a counseling session at a GYN clinic, the client asks the nurse about using replacement hormones. The best nursing response would be

1. "What results would you expect from estrogen replacement therapy?"
2. "Are you aware of the increased risk of developing cancer with estrogen replacement therapy?"
3. "Estrogen replacement therapy may help you with your symptoms."
4. "Estrogen and progesterone replacement therapy will help control hot flashes and atrophic vaginitis."

62. Evaluating a 52-year-old female client's ongoing GYN status as she is in the menopause period, the nurse knows that there are certain danger signals. The most important sign the nurse would tell the client to report is

   1. Painful intercourse.
   2. Decreased libido.
   3. Spotting after periods cease.
   4. Increasing hot flashes.

63. A 56-year-old male client has been admitted to the hospital with the diagnosis of angina pectoris. He is scheduled to have a cardiac catheterization. Assessing the client, the nurse notices that there is a wandering baseline on the EKG monitor with an unclear EKG pattern. The initial nursing intervention will be to

   1. Begin CPR.
   2. Check the monitor leads.
   3. Give lidocaine per physician orders.
   4. Call a code.

64. A client returned one hour ago from the catheterization lab where he underwent a right- and left-sided heart catheterization. He is lying quietly in bed. The nurse has finished checking the groin catheter insertion site and his vital signs, when the client begins to raise the head of his bed. The initial nursing action will be to

   1. Explain that he must not move his leg for 12 hours, thus the head of the bed may not be elevated.
   2. Elevate his affected leg on a pillow and allow him to raise the head of the bed to a position of comfort.
   3. Allow him to raise the head of the bed no more than a semi-Fowler's position.
   4. Explain that the head of the bed should not be elevated because the groin site must be kept flat.

65. A client is admitted with a history of hemoptysis for the past several days. Several of the migrant workers with whom he lives have recently been diagnosed as having pulmonary tuberculosis. After questioning him about the hemoptysis, what additional question will the nurse ask during the admission nursing history?

   1. "Do you have frequent episodes of shortness of breath?"
   2. "Have you lost weight over the past few months?"
   3. "Do you awaken with a high temperature that subsides by early afternoon?"
   4. "Do you have a productive cough with sputum that is greenish-yellow in color?"

66. Planning a home visit to the neighbors and family of a client with the diagnosis of tuberculosis, which one of the people who is either infected or at high risk will *not* receive Isoniazid (INH) and vitamin B_6 prophylactically?

   1. A person on long-term steroid therapy.

2. A 5-year-old child who has a positive skin test.
3. Friends of a child with a positive skin test.
4. A person with a positive x-ray but negative sputum smear.

67. A newborn infant is admitted to the neonatal ICU immediately after birth. A large, bulging, purplish mass protrudes through a defect in the spinal column. Diagnosis of meningomyelocele is made. The most important nursing objective in treating this infant prior to surgical correction is prevention of

1. External rotation of the hips.
2. Urinary tract infection.
3. Hydrocephalus.
4. Infection of the lesion.

68. A three month old requires a shunting procedure for hydrocephalus. Postoperatively, the nurse will assess for all of the following signs/symptoms. Which one is most indicative of a potential complication?

1. Positive Babinski's sign.
2. Decreased blood pressure.
3. Increase in head circumference.
4. Narrow pulse pressure.

69. A 23-year-old female develops lupus erythematosus and is admitted to the hospital for a general work-up. With this collagen disease, one of the most distinguishing signs the nurse will assess for is

1. Leukoplakia.
2. Butterfly rash over nose and cheeks.
3. Generalized dermatitis.
4. Chloasma.

70. A female client, age 40, has just arrived at the "walk-in" psychiatric clinic. She tells the reception nurse that she feels overwhelmed and depressed. She fears she is going crazy. The first priority in making a plan for this client is to

1. Help her develop strength areas for coping mechanisms.
2. Clarify the problem and help her integrate the "triggering" event.
3. Make an accurate assessment of the problem and focus on the "here and now."
4. Help explore the available situational supports in the client's life.

71. A female client has come to the clinic for contraception because she and her boyfriend have been sexually active and she wants to be sure she doesn't become pregnant. The most appropriate first nursing assessment is to ask

1. "Have you and your boyfriend discussed the method of contraception you would prefer?"
2. "Have you and your boyfriend discussed when you will be 'ready' to get married?"
3. "When did you say your last period was?"
4. "Would you like to check to see if you are pregnant?."

72. An infant, five months old, is diagnosed with infantile eczema. The nurse understands that this condition is

1. A result of sensitivity to some substance.
2. Caused by staphylococcus aureus.
3. A parasitic skin disease.
4. Caused by poor hygiene.

73. A 54-year-old male client has been treated medically for the past seven years for increasingly severe diverticulosis. Two days ago he had emergency surgery for a ruptured diverticulum. The procedure performed was a double-barrel colostomy. The purpose for making two colostomy openings rather than one is to

1. Alternate use for irrigation so neither opening becomes excoriated.
2. Leave a nonfunctioning portion of the colon which will be anastomosed at a later date.
3. Prevent infection during the healing process by increasing stool movement through the colon.
4. Prevent recurrence of diverticulum.

74. When a colostomy is placed in the transverse colon, the nurse can explain to the client that normal stool from the colostomy will be

1. Liquid.
2. Soft formed.
3. Mushy.
4. Hard formed.

75. In teaching the client how to regulate his colostomy, the nurse will explain to him that regulation is increased by

1. Irrigating the colostomy after breakfast every day.
2. Increasing his daily exercise.
3. Limiting fluid intake to 1500 ml/day.
4. Eating regular balanced meals.

76. A female client, age 33, was brought to hospital by her husband. Her admitting diagnosis is major depressive episode. She is started on Tofranil. On the third day after admission she is observed to be staggering, and she complains of drowsiness and blurred vision. The nurse action is to

1. Administer the prn Cogentin.
2. Hold the next scheduled dose of medication and report the changes.
3. Note the client's behavior and continue to observe.
4. Place the client in bed for safety.

77. A 25-year-old female client is admitted to the labor room on September 10. Her contractions are about 4 to 5 minutes apart and 30 seconds long. Based on the information, the nurse assesses that she is in which stage of labor?

1. Early first stage.
2. Transition.
3. Second stage.
4. Third stage.

78. A couple has attended Lamaze childbirth classes. Based on this information, during transition, the breathing pattern the nurse would encourage is

1. Slow, deep, abdominal pattern.
2. Slow, deep, chest breathing.
3. Shallow chest breathing at 20–30 times a minute.
4. Shallow chest breathing at 40–60 times a minute.

79. A client is admitted to the emergency room with bronchospasms. They are not relieved by aminophylline. Prednisone is prescribed. The nurse will advise the client to take this medication

1. Before meals.
2. After meals.
3. With orange juice.
4. With milk.

80. A male client, age 60, is coming to the out-patient clinic for an iridectomy. Following this iridectomy the nurse will expect the client to have

   1. Peripheral vision alterations.
   2. Central visual loss.
   3. Blurred vision.
   4. No visual changes.

81. As the nurse is checking urine output of a female client for the previous day, she realizes that the output is 850 ml in 24 hours. The nursing action is to

   1. Notify the physician.
   2. Record the amount on the I&O chart.
   3. Begin to force fluids at 3000 ml/day.
   4. Catheterize the client.

82. The nurse is caring for a cardiac client on bedrest who complains of a leg cramp. The nursing intervention is to

   1. Extend the foot.
   2. Dorsiflex the foot.
   3. Massage the leg.
   4. Flex the knee.

83. A male client, having broken his leg in two places, has just returned from the cast room. The nurse positions the casted extremity above the level of the heart. The rationale for this action is to

   1. Allow the cast to dry evenly.

2. Decrease venous pooling and edema.
3. Prevent cracking from pressure.
4. Make it more comfortable for the client.

84. A mother is about to take her 1-year-old child home from the hospital. The child was admitted one week previously with a diagnosis of croup. One of the home care techniques the nurse might teach the mother to use if her child begins to cough is to

   1. Take the child into the bathroom and turn the shower on hot.
   2. Give the child frequent doses of prescribed cough medicine.
   3. Do not allow the child outside in the cold air.
   4. Have the child breathe into a paper bag.

85. During a routine physical examination, the following reflexes are noted in 7-month-old child. Which of the following is an abnormal finding?

   1. Reciprocal kicking.
   2. Neck righting reflex.
   3. Rooting and sucking reflex.
   4. Moro reflex.

86. A three month old is admitted to the hospital with a diagnosis of chalasia. He has had severe weight loss because of frequent vomiting. To minimize vomiting, the nurse will place the infant

   1. In a prone position after feeding.
   2. On his abdomen with his head to one side.
   3. On his left side with his head elevated.
   4. On his right side with his head elevated.

87. A client is being seen at an intake interview in a crisis intervention clinic. The goal at this initial point in crisis treatment is to

   1. Reintegrate to the same level of functioning prior to the crisis situation.
   2. Reintegrate but retain elements of the crisis period to have a basis to continue therapy.
   3. Reintegrate at a higher level of functioning to derive benefit from the crisis.
   4. Gain insight into the cause of the crisis in order to prevent it from occurring again.

88. A depressed client tells the nurse, "Don't waste your time with me. Talk to someone who deserves it." The nurse's best response would be

   1. "Why do you say that? You should feel better about yourself."
   2. "Don't be concerned about that. I have plenty of time."
   3. "It isn't healthy for you to be alone so much."
   4. "I don't feel it's a waste of time. If you'd rather not talk, we'll just sit here."

89. A female client is experiencing an acute schizophrenic disorder and has refused to bathe or shower for several days. She states, "I'm so full of electricity, I'd die if water hits me." After building trust in the relationship, which of the following nursing responses is most therapeutic?

   1. "I shall help you wash if you like and no one else will be there."
   2. "No one will want to be around you if you don't wash."
   3. "I simply want you to feel better. I'm only trying to help."
   4. "I don't understand about the electricity and dying. Tell me about it."

90. A male client approaches a female a nurse and states, "I'm going out on pass this weekend. Will you go out with me Saturday night?" The nurse's response should be

   1. "No. We have a professional relationship and it would not be appropriate for us to date."
   2. "I have a boyfriend who wouldn't like it."
   3. "That's against the rules around here."
   4. "What did your physician say about being discharged?"

Comprehensive Test 1
Answers with Rationale

1. (2) The nurse's priority is to assess the client for pain. The presence of chest pain can cause the pulse rate to increase and blood pressure to drop. It can also increase client anxiety. The client is on a cardiac monitor; therefore, an apical pulse is not the priority action. Once his comfort has been established, apical pulse, blood pressure and heart sound determinations are appropriate.

    Nursing Process: Assessment
    Client Needs: Safe, Effective Care Environment
    Clinical Area: Medical Nursing

2. (1) Elevated CPK-MB, which rises within six hours when an MI has occurred, is indicative of myocardial damage. SGOT is not specific to heart disease alone and LDH is not as specific as answer (1) in the diagnosis of myocardial infarction, even though the level rises in 6–8 hours and persists longer.

    Nursing Process: Analysis
    Client Needs: Physiological Integrity
    Clinical Area: Medical Nursing

3. (3) Each 500 ml of IV fluid contains 2000 mg of Lidocaine. One ml of IV fluid contains 4 mg; therefore, the client will receive 0.5 ml per minute.

    Nursing Process: Implementation
    Client Needs: Safe, Effective Care Environment
    Clinical Area: Medical Nursing

4. (4) This menu provides the lowest amount of sodium. Turkey, shellfish, spinach, and beets are high in sodium, thus would not be included in a low-sodium diet.

    Nursing Process: Evaluation
    Client Needs: Health Promotion and Maintenance
    Clinical Area: Medical Nursing

5. (4) Two months is recommended by the American Academy of Pediatrics for beginning immunizations of DPT, OPV and HbCV, based upon acquired protection in utero. The infant's immune mechanisms

    Nursing Process: Planning
    Client Needs: Health Promotion and Maintenance
    Clinical Area: Pediatric Nursing

are considered too immature to respond with sufficient antibody production under the age of two months.

6. (1)   Children with active infections such as impetigo should not be immunized.

Nursing Process: Planning
Client Needs: Safe, Effective Care Environment
Clinical Area: Pediatric Nursing

7. (2)   At six months of age, the child should be able to sit by himself. This delayed developmental milestone is frequently seen in children with cerebral palsy. A neat pincer grasp is not expected until 10–11 months of age. The other two abilities would be present before six months of age.

Nursing Process: Analysis
Client Needs: Psychosocial Integrity
Clinical Area: Pediatric Nursing

8. (2)   The client has symptoms indicative of a urinary calculus; therefore, it is important to strain all the urine in order to detect if the stone has passed and confirm the diagnosis.

Nursing Process: Implementation
Client Needs: Safe, Effective Care Environment
Clinical Area: Medical Nursing

9. (4)   Cold chills could indicate the spread of infection throughout the urinary tract. Answers (2) and (3) might be present after the procedure, as would difficulty in voiding.

Nursing Process: Evaluation
Client Needs: Physiological Integrity
Clinical Area: Medical Nursing

10. (3)   Ultrasonography is the most accurate test of those listed for determining pregnancy, and can now be used as early as 5 weeks. Hearing the fetal heart tone is the safest means to determine EDD (previously called EDC). However, the heart rate cannot be heard until 20 weeks gestation. Serial estriols and the nonstress test are done later in pregnancy as methods of determining fetal status or fetal well-being.

Nursing Process: Planning
Client Needs: Health Promotion and Maintenance
Clinical Area: Maternity Nursing

11. (4)   Consistency of approach is the best, because the position as well as the arm used causes variations in the reading. The

Nursing Process: Planning
Client Needs: Health Promotion and Maintenance
Clinical Area: Maternity Nursing

best graph is obtained by using the same
approach over time.

12.   (3)   A definitive diagnosis is only made
with a microscopic exam of actual bowel
tissue indicating absence or reduced number of parasympathetic ganglion nerve
cells. A barium x-ray is the next choice,
which would show evidence of a narrow
intestine proximal to the anus with a dilated section above.

Nursing Process: Assessment
Client Needs: Safe, Effective Care Environment
Clinical Area: Pediatric Nursing

13.   (3)   The child will be placed on a low-
residue, high-calorie diet. Children with
aganglionic disease tend to be thin and
undernourished, despite their large and
distended abdomens. Improving the
child's nutritional status before surgery is
very important. (1) is always true, but not
the best answer. Tap water enemas can
cause water intoxication.

Nursing Process: Implementation
Client Needs: Safe, Effective Care Environment
Clinical Area: Pediatric Nursing

14.   (3)   It is of primary importance to assess
the suicide potential of clients presenting
symptoms of depression. The client is asking for medication that could be used to
overdose, so suicide potential is crucial to
assess. The other factors are also important
to assess, but are not the priority.

Nursing Process: Assessment
Client Needs: Safe, Effective Care Environment
Clinical Area: Psychiatric Nursing

15.   (1)   To ensure that goals are attainable
they must be set by both nurse and client.
The other answers are important but cannot be achieved without the mutually
agreed upon goals. All outcomes must be
measurable in order to determine whether
or not they have been achieved.

Nursing Process: Planning
Client Needs: Health Promotion and Maintenance
Clinical Area: Psychiatric Nursing

16.   (3)   The client may be denying the feelings that belong to her and projecting them
onto her husband. Depressed clients often
cannot express anger directly and either

Nursing Process: Analysis
Client Needs: Psychosocial Integrity
Clinical Area: Psychiatric Nursing

repress it, project it to others, or deny these feelings.

17. (1) It is very important for any client taking Valium to understand that Valium and alcohol may be a lethal combination. (2) is incorrect because the nurse cannot promise that the drug will make her problems more manageable. (3) is incorrect because Valium is fast acting. (4) is incorrect and refers to precautions taken with MAO inhibitors.

Nursing Process: Evaluation
Client Needs: Safe, Effective Care Environment
Clinical Area: Psychiatric Nursing

18. (1) Edema, proteinuria and hypertension are the three cardinal signs of preeclampsia. Normal urine output or oliguria occurs rather than polyuria.

Nursing Process: Assessment
Client Needs: Physiological Integrity
Clinical Area: Maternity Nursing

19. (4) The insulin dosage is generally given once or twice daily. It is either intermediate-acting insulin alone or in conjunction with a short-acting insulin. With Type I diabetes, the pancreatic beta cells are not producing insulin, thus insulin must be given. Diet is also important for both Type I and II; frequently a Type II diabetic can be controlled with a diabetic diet or with a combination of oral hypoglycemics and diet.

Nursing Process: Evaluation
Client Needs: Physiological Integrity
Clinical Area: Medical Nursing

20. (2) Psychogenic influences affect the development of peptic ulcers. Tension and stress cause an increase in the tonus of the vagus nerve leading to an increase in secretions. Stress in the diabetic client causes a rise in the blood glucose level.

Nursing Process: Analysis
Client Needs: Psychosocial Integrity
Clinical Area: Medical Nursing

21. (1) This is the most comprehensive answer. In addition to gastric resections, clients with a radical mastectomy, thoracotomy, or abdominal perineal resection experience extensive metabolic disturbances. The metabolic disturbance is

Nursing Process: Planning
Client Needs: Physiological Integrity
Clinical Area: Surgical Nursing

related to the effects of total stress the
client is experiencing.

22. (3) Before explaining the importance of
holding the baby to develop the mother-
child relationship, it is necessary to find
out how the mother is feeling and to identify her fears. All of the other responses
close off communication.

Nursing Process: Implementation
Client Needs: Psychosocial Integrity
Clinical Area: Pediatric Nursing

23. (2) Cushing's syndrome is characterized
by exaggeration of normal physiological
conditions generally shown by weight gain
and protein wasting. Answer (1) is caused
by adrenal medulla disease. Answer (3) is
caused by hyperthyroidism.

Nursing Process: Assessment
Client Needs: Physiological Integrity
Clinical Area: Medical Nursing

24. (1) Adrenalectomy necessitates replacement therapy with both glucocorticoids
and mineralocorticoids for up to six
months. Teaching the client about steroid
administration before the surgery will help
achieve goals after the surgery.

Nursing Process: Planning
Client Needs: Safe, Effective Care Environment
Clinical Area: Surgical Nursing

25. (1) This reflex is termed the Moro reflex,
also termed the startle reflex. This reflex is
present at birth, is symmetrical, and disap-
pears around four months of age.

Nursing Process: Assessment
Client Needs: Health Promotion and Maintenance
Clinical Area: Pediatric Nursing

26 (1) Lactating mothers need four to five
glasses of milk a day. They should never
be advised to restrict any nutrient or
attempt to diet during lactation.

Nursing Process: Implementation
Client Needs: Health Promotion and Maintenance
Clinical Area: Maternity Nursing

27. (1) The oral contraceptive suppresses
milk production, so while the mother continues breast-feeding, she should use
another method of contraception.

Nursing Process: Implementation
Client Needs: Health Promotion and Maintenance
Clinical Area: Maternity Nursing

28. (3) The triad associated with early ruptured extrauterine pregnancy includes the
menstrual cycle history, unilateral pelvic

Nursing Process: Assessment
Client Needs: Safe, Effective Care Environment
Clinical Area: Maternity Nursing

pain, and, additionally, presence of a
cul-de-sac mass.

29. (4) The nurse is acknowledging that it is
all right for the client to cry but also giving
her permission to express her feelings verbally if she chooses to do so. Answers (1)
and (3) close off communication and
answer (2) is so direct that it is nontherapeutic.

Nursing Process: Implementation
Client Needs: Psychosocial Integrity
Clinical Area: Maternity Nursing

30. (4) Bowel and bladder retention or incontinence is a major problem with clients
who have multiple sclerosis; therefore,
establishing a good routine for evacuation
is essential. Weight control is usually not a
problem. While exercising is important,
specific exercises for muscle strengthening
or decreasing tremors are not effective.
Multiple sclerosis clients do not take medication routinely.

Nursing Process: Planning
Client Needs: Safe, Effective Care Environment
Clinical Area: Medical Nursing

31. (2) Pupil size is a most important assessment. Usually reflexes are not as useful
due to the fact that the client may not be
responsive during a neurological examination. Pain response and muscle strength
are not specific enough to be considered
more useful than pupil size.

Nursing Process: Assessment
Client Needs: Safe, Effective Care Environment
Clinical Area: Medical Nursing

32. (4) The red spots represent the client's
aura and, therefore, the washcloth may be
placed between the teeth immediately,
before the seizure activity begins and the
jaws are clenched shut. This action, however, would be dependent on the facility's
policies. The nurse would also remove a
partial denture plate. If the seizure had
already started, the nurse would not
attempt to put anything between the teeth.
Turning the client should be carried out
after placement of the washcloth; this position will prevent airway occlusion.

Nursing Process: Implementation
Client Needs: Safe, Effective Care Environment
Clinical Area: Medical Nursing

33.   (1)   A hallucination is a sensory experience that has no basis in reality. Answer (2)
is an illusion; (3) may be taken as an example of a hallucination but is not as encom-
passing as (1); (4) is a delusion.

Nursing Process: Analysis
Client Needs: Psychosocial Integrity
Clinical Area: Psychiatric Nursing

34.   (3)   The best choice is to encourage the
client to become involved in an activity to
get his mind off the paranoid thoughts.
The nurse would also avoid power strug-
gles (as this increases anxiety). Answer (4)
is wrong because proceeding with nursing
therapy too rapidly will cause a suspicious
client to be more distrustful.

Nursing Process: Implementation
Client Needs: Safe, Effective Care Environment
Clinical Area: Psychiatric Nursing

35.   (3)   The client is actually improving
because he has the ability to question his
symptom; the nurse may reinforce this
strength; then she might stay with him and
help him discuss his fears. (4) is incorrect
as his prognosis cannot be calculated. (1)
and (2) are not substantiated by the data.

Nursing Process: Evaluation
Client Needs: Psychosocial Integrity
Clinical Area: Psychiatric Nursing

36.   (2)   The most common symptoms are listed in answer (2); in addition, there are
nucal-spinal rigidity and positive Kernig's
and Brudzinski's signs. Even though it is
present, Kernig's sign is difficult to elicit or
evaluate in young children and headache
is impossible to evaluate. These children
usually will not have a seizure and meningitis is not characterized by apnea.

Nursing Process: Assessment
Client Needs: Health Promotion and Maintenance
Clinical Area: Pediatric Nursing

37.   (3)   Even though all interventions will be
carried out, administering antibiotics is the
priority. Antibiotics are started after the
lumbar puncture is done and the organism
is identified.

Nursing Process: Planning
Client Needs: Safe, Effective Care Environment
Clinical Area: Pediatric Nursing

38.   (4)   Positioning a client on the left side
will assist in drainage and semi-Fowler's
will assist in breathing. The client can usually be turned to both sides and back.

Nursing Process: Implementation
Client Needs: Safe, Effective Care Environment
Clinical Area: Surgical Nursing

39. (2) The water-seal chamber acts as a seal to keep air from being drawn into the pleural space. When the chest has been opened, a vacuum must be applied to the chest to reestablish negative pressure.

Nursing Process: Analysis
Client Needs: Physiological Integrity
Clinical Area: Surgical Nursing

40. (4) The mitral and aortic valves are most susceptible to damage as a result of this inflammatory disease. The disease has declined in the last 30 years.

Nursing Process: Analysis
Client Needs: Physiological Integrity
Clinical Area: Pediatric Nursing

41. (1) Helping the client verbalize will reduce his tension. Later, or in addition, engaging him in an activity which he finds relaxing will help avoid possible assaultive behavior, because stress reduction and assaultive behavior are incompatible. The body language is an important cue, and it is important to pick it up.

Nursing Process: Planning
Client Needs: Safe, Effective Care Environment
Clinical Area: Psychiatric Nursing

42. (2) Miotics constrict the pupil and increase aqueous outflow which leads to a reduction of intraocular pressure. Mydriatics dilate the pupils and would increase intraocular pressure. A carbonic anhydrase inhibitor is used in some types of glaucoma.

Nursing Process: Planning
Client Needs: Health Promotion and Maintenance
Clinical Area: Medical Nursing

43. (4) By asking, "Can you talk?" the nurse establishes that the person has something in his airway. If he is able to answer, he is not choking. A person is unable to talk when choking.

Nursing Process: Implementation
Client Needs: Safe, Effective Care Environment
Clinical Area: Medical Nursing

44. (4) All of the other reports are within normal range. The low platelet count signifies thrombocytopenia. Bleeding can result from this low platelet count and the cause should be researched before surgery.

Nursing Process: Analysis
Client Needs: Physiological Integrity
Clinical Area: Surgical Nursing

45. (2) Cerebral anoxia occurs frequently in severe trauma to the brain. A blood clot or edema can cause an interruption of the

Nursing Process: Analysis
Client Needs: Physiological Integrity
Clinical Area: Medical Nursing

blood circulation, which alters oxygen supply to the tissue. Reduced oxygen causes anoxia.

46.   (4)   Widened pulse pressure is a late sign. Restlessness is the earliest sign of increased intracranial pressure and is due to compression of the brain from edema or hemorrhage (or both) causing hypoxia. Blood pressure and pulse changes are not the earliest clinical manifestation of increased intracranial pressure.

Nursing Process: Analysis
Client Needs: Physiological Integrity
Clinical Area: Medical Nursing

47.   (4)   As the left ventricle fails in its pumping action, the blood pressure will fall. A widened pulse pressure (the difference between systolic and diastolic pressures) is indicative of decreased peripheral vascular resistance. As the heart fails, the pulse increases in an attempt to circulate more blood, and the respiratory rate increases in order to take in more oxygen.

Nursing Process: Analysis
Client Needs: Physiological Integrity
Clinical Area: Medical Nursing

48.   (3)   When the pump of the heart (left ventricle) is damaged, it cannot eject a normal cardiac output and the circulatory system begins to fail. Fluid overload would cause a weak left ventricle to fail, but a normal myocardium would stretch and contract with increased force to handle the increased fluid. Electrolyte imbalances can cause cardiac decompensation by way of arrhythmias (potassium) and decreased force of contraction (calcium).

Nursing Process: Analysis
Client Needs: Physiological Integrity
Clinical Area: Medical Nursing

49.   (3)   The goal of therapy in cardiogenic shock is to increase circulating oxygenated blood to the vital organs. This is accomplished by increasing peripheral vascular resistance with medication. By so doing, less blood is pooled in the periphery; thus, more blood is available for the major organs.

Nursing Process: Planning
Client Needs: Physiological Integrity
Clinical Area: Medical Nursing

50. (3) The client's ability to behave within normal standards and yet be highly manipulative is characteristic of the antisocial personality. This makes it difficult not only to work with the client, but at times to diagnose him. His superego is poorly developed. He may or may not have a high IQ.

Nursing Process: Analysis
Client Needs: Psychosocial Integrity
Clinical Area: Psychiatric Nursing

51. (2) Using a behavior modification plan, this type of client will benefit from negative reinforcement. When he keeps to the agreement, his privileges will be restored. Trying to talk him into attending group is nontherapeutic.

Nursing Process: Implementation
Client Needs: Psychosocial Integrity
Clinical Area: Psychiatric Nursing

52. (2) When the stapes are removed and the procedure is completed, the client can usually hear.

Nursing Process: Analysis
Client Needs: Physiological Integrity
Clinical Area: Surgical Nursing

53. (2) The issue is safety, thus the siderails should be up. Clients can sometimes experience vertigo and could fall from bed. Finally, clients should not be turned postoperatively unless there is a specific order to do so.

Nursing Process: Implementation
Client Needs: Safe, Effective Care Environment
Clinical Area: Surgical Nursing

54. (4) This statement reassures and acknowledges her feelings and allows for further exploration of her feelings. Both (1) and (3) answers are not on target and answer (2), while opening up the communication, does not deal with the client's conflict.

Nursing Process: Implementation
Client Needs: Psychosocial Integrity
Clinical Area: Maternity Nursing

55. (4) The symptoms of peptic ulcers are due to mucosal inflammation. There is usually pain when the stomach is empty: one to three hours after meals in gastric ulcers and three to four hours after meals in duodenal ulcers. The other questions already make the assumption that the client has ulcer disease. The pattern of the

Nursing Process: Assessment
Client Needs: Physiological Integrity
Clinical Area: Medical Nursing

pain will help to determine whether or not he does have ulcer disease.

56. (2) A gastroduodenoscopy is the visualization of the esophagus, stomach, and duodenum through a flexible tube inserted orally. The exam is not a comfortable one because the muscles of the gastrointestinal tract have spasms as the tube is passed. This causes difficulty swallowing. The client is usually given a local anesthetic to the posterior pharynx to reduce the discomfort during the passage of the tube. He will not be heavily sedated because he must be able to assist by swallowing. Coughing or performing a Valsalva maneuver would impede the passage of the tube.

Nursing Process: Planning
Client Needs: Safe, Effective Care Environment
Clinical Area: Medical Nursing

57. (2) A homograft is skin from another human, not from the client. An autograft is skin from the client himself. A heterograft is skin from a nonhuman source.

Nursing Process: Planning
Client Needs: Physiological Integrity
Clinical Area: Medical Nursing

58. (1) The pressure dressing is used to prevent fluid accumulation under the graft site as well as to promote immobilization of the affected area. Drains are frequently placed under the skin flap to promote drainage. The drains are attached to suction; they are not irrigated.

Nursing Process: Planning
Client Needs: Safe, Effective Care Environment
Clinical Area: Surgical Nursing

59. (3) It is important for the nurse to introduce herself and make contact, rather than search the client for weapons, ask how he is feeling, or get the client settled. Introduction is acknowledgment and the first step in establishing a relationship.

Nursing Process: Implementation
Client Needs: Safe, Effective Care Environment
Clinical Area: Psychiatric Nursing

60. (4) Usually 24 months after menstruation ceases is advised as the length of time a woman should continue using birth control to avoid pregnancy. It is important to

Nursing Process: Implementation
Client Needs: Health Promotion and Maintenance
Clinical Area: Maternity Nursing

reinforce the possibility of pregnancy in the presence of irregular menses.

61. (1) While all responses are correct, the best approach is to assess the client's reason for the question. When the nurse understands the client's baseline knowledge, she can plan how to develop the counseling in a logical manner to assist the client in decision making.

Nursing Process: Assessment
Client Needs: Psychosocial Integrity
Clinical Area: Maternity Nursing

62. (3) Although spotting is hard to determine when periods are irregular, it should be reported, as spotting or bleeding may be the first sign of uterine/cervical cancer. Decreased libido and increasing hot flashes often accompany menopause, as does painful intercourse caused by dryness of the vaginal wall resulting from decreased estrogen levels.

Nursing Process: Evaluation
Client Needs: Health Promotion and Maintenance
Clinical Area: Maternity Nursing

63. (2) The nurse's first action should be to inspect equipment for malfunctioning. There is no evidence of cardiac arrest or PVCs, so beginning CPR or calling a code or administering lidocaine is not appropriate at this time.

Nursing Process: Implementation
Client Needs: Safe, Effective Care Environment
Clinical Area: Surgical Nursing

64. (4) In order to ensure femoral arterial clot formation, the groin area should be kept flat for 12 hours following a cardiac catheterization. The client may move his leg, but the leg should be kept flat (no pillows) and straight.

Nursing Process: Implementation
Client Needs: Safe, Effective Care Environment
Clinical Area: Surgical Nursing

65. (2) Weight loss is an indicator of tuberculosis. Additional signs and symptoms of tuberculosis are usually minimal but do include anorexia, fatigue, afternoon fever, cough, and hemoptysis.

Nursing Process: Assessment
Client Needs: Safe, Effective Care Environment
Clinical Area: Medical Nursing

66. (4) If the chest x-ray is positive, the client will be placed on therapeutic drug therapy, not prophylactic therapy. All of the other

Nursing Process: Planning
Client Needs: Safe, Effective Care Environment
Clinical Area: Medical Nursing

people will be placed on preventive therapy, so that those people who are infected with tuberculosis will not develop the active clinical disease.

67.   (4)   Though (1) and (2) are important, an infection of the lesion will often lead to meningitis. (3) is incorrect because the nurse cannot prevent hydrocephalus, but only observe for its potential development.

Nursing Process: Planning
Client Needs: Physiological Integrity
Clinical Area: Pediatric Nursing

68.   (3)   An increase in head circumference is a potential complication of the shunting procedure. A 3-month-old child will have a positive Babinski. Other signs of a complication developing are increased blood pressure and widening pulse pressure.

Nursing Process: Assessment
Client Needs: Physiological Integrity
Clinical Area: Pediatric Nursing

69.   (2)   The butterfly rash is a discoid, localized scaling, erythematous skin eruption that is a very common sign of lupus. Chloasma occurs with use of birth control pills. Leukoplakia are lesions on the mucous membrane of the mouth, often a precursor of cancer of the oral cavity.

Nursing Process: Assessment
Client Needs: Physiological Integrity
Clinical Area: Medical Nursing

70.   (3)   While all the alternatives would be included in the course of crisis therapy, making an assessment of the exact problem and staying in the "here and now" would be the first priority. Clarifying the problem would also be appropriate, but integration would come later.

Nursing Process: Planning
Client Needs: Psychosocial Integrity
Clinical Area: Psychiatric Nursing

71.   (3)   Before raising her anxiety by checking to see if she might be pregnant, it is appropriate to check the data base and validate the dates. The next focus will be question (1). Answer (2) is inappropriate considering the data presented.

Nursing Process: Assessment
Client Needs: Safe, Effective Care Environment
Clinical Area: Maternity Nursing

72.   (1)   Infantile eczema is usually seen in children with allergic tendencies. Symptoms often occur in children four

Nursing Process: Analysis
Client Needs: Physiological Integrity
Clinical Area: Pediatric Nursing

months to four years old. Poor hygiene or a parasite may make eczema worse but does not cause it. It is also not caused by staphylococcus aureus.

73. (2) A double-barrel colostomy, often done for diverticulitis, leaves a nonfunctioning portion of the colon so it will heal. The colon cannot heal when feces are moving through it. The colostomy is left three weeks to six months before it is reanastomosed.

Nursing Process: Analysis
Client Needs: Physiological Integrity
Clinical Area: Surgical Nursing

74. (3) Stool gets increasingly firm as it progresses through the colon. At the ileocecal valve, it is liquid; in the transverse colon, it is mushy; and in the sigmoid colon, it is solid.

Nursing Process: Implementation
Client Needs: Physiological Integrity
Clinical Area: Surgical Nursing

75. (4) A routine of regular balanced meals will produce stools of consistent volume, consistency and frequency. Stools with these characteristics are most easily regulated. Irrigation, if needed at all, can be done whenever it is most convenient for the client.

Nursing Process: Implementation
Client Needs: Physiological Integrity
Clinical Area: Surgical Nursing

76. (2) The nursing action for any untoward side effects of a medication is to hold the next dose until the client's response can be evaluated. In this case, tricyclics may cause significant changes in cardiac function. Cogentin is often given with an antipsychotic drug, not an antidepressive drug, for extra-pyramidal side effects.

Nursing Process: Implementation
Client Needs: Safe, Effective Care Environment
Clinical Area: Psychiatric Nursing

77. (1) Contractions in early first stage are usually more than 3 minutes apart and less than 45 seconds long.

Nursing Process: Assessment
Client Needs: Safe, Effective Care Environment
Clinical Area: Maternity Nursing

78. (3) Shallow chest breathing, slightly faster than a normal rate, is the pattern used most in transition. Slow breathing,

Nursing Process: Implementation
Client Needs: Health Promotion and Maintenance
Clinical Area: Maternity Nursing

while effective for some women during transition, is usually most effective in earlier labor. Supporting a more rapid rate of 40–60 times a minute is not physiologically sound, and could lead to hyperventilation.

79. (4) Prednisone may cause a stress ulcer so it should be taken with milk to protect the lining of the stomach. Certain foods taken at mealtime may interfere with the absorption of iron, so it is more effective to take the supplement with milk. Iron is given with orange juice.

Nursing Process: Implementation
Client Needs: Health Promotion and Maintenance
Clinical Area: Medical Nursing

80. (4) An iridectomy is done for the purpose of increasing the outflow of aqueous humor. There is no change in vision with this procedure.

Nursing Process: Evaluation
Client Needs: Physiological Integrity
Clinical Area: Surgical Nursing

81. (1) It is important to notify the physician because less than 60 ml/hour is indicative of a potential problem, either dehydration or kidney failure. The physician will probably order a fluid challenge test to determine the source of the problem before ordering more fluids.

Nursing Process: Implementation
Client Needs: Safe, Effective Care Environment
Clinical Area: Medical Nursing

82. (2) The most appropriate action is to use dorsiflexion to release the foot cramp. Massage and flexing the knee would not be done because both actions would be contraindicated in any potential case of thrombophlebitis.

Nursing Process: Implementation
Client Needs: Safe, Effective Care Environment
Clinical Area: Medical Nursing

83. (2) Positioning the cast above the level of the heart would increase venous flow to the heart, decrease pooling and reduce edema. This position does not influence cast drying or cracking.

Nursing Process: Evaluation
Client Needs: Safe, Effective Care Environment
Clinical Area: Surgical Nursing

84. (1) Warm, moist air reduces epiglottic edema and helps relieve coughing. Cough medicine may or may not be prescribed.

Nursing Process: Implementation
Client Needs: Health Promotion and Maintenance
Clinical Area: Pediatric Nursing

Breathing into a paper bag is suggested for hyperventilation. Cold air might trigger coughing so it is not a good idea, but answer (1) is more correct.

85.   (4)   The Moro reflex begins to fade at the third or fourth month and, therefore, should not be present. All of the other reflexes are normal for this age child.

Nursing Process: Assessment
Client Needs: Physiological Integrity
Clinical Area: Pediatric Nursing

86.   (4)   The greater curvature of the stomach is toward the left side, so being positioned on the right side creates less pressure on the stomach. Elevation of the head decreases tendency to vomit.

Nursing Process: Implementation
Client Needs: Safe, Effective Care Environment
Clinical Area: Pediatric Nursing

87.   (1)   The level of functioning the client returns to is dependent upon variables such as age at onset, past psychiatric history, and how quickly treatment is instituted. The goal, however, is always to return the client to the precrisis level of functioning. The nurse might suggest that therapy continue after the crisis, but the rest of answer (2) makes it wrong. Answer (4) is incorrect because gaining insight is not a goal of crisis intervention.

Nursing Process: Planning
Client Needs: Safe, Effective Care Environment
Clinical Area: Psychiatric Nursing

88.   (4)   The nurse should not accept the client's assessment of unworthiness, but should respond in a way that does not make the client "wrong" for expressing this assessment. It will not be helpful if the client is "wrong" or has to defend the correctness of a poor self-appraisal.

Nursing Process: Implementation
Client Needs: Psychosocial Integrity
Clinical Area: Psychiatric Nursing

89.   (1)   Depending on the circumstances, any of the other approaches might encourage interaction and problem-solving regarding the client's personal hygiene. Answer (2) is inappropriate because in the acute stage of a schizophrenic reaction, interaction with others is very difficult. Because the client

Nursing Process: Implementation
Client Needs: Safe, Effective Care Environment
Clinical Area: Psychiatric Nursing

probably wants to withdraw from interpersonal relationships, the threat of isolation may actually be very appealing. Any statement like "I'm only trying to help" may instill guilt in the client and is not therapeutic. Answer (4) is a clarifying statement, but may be threatening at this time.

90. (1) The best response is a clear, direct message that dating is not proper in the nurse-client working relationship. The nurse should follow this by encouraging the client to talk about his feelings and to explore alternative ways that he could seek female companionship.

Nursing Process: Implementation
Client Needs: Psychosocial Integrity
Clinical Area: Psychiatric Nursing

Comprehensive Test 2

1. A client with an obstruction just proximal to her old ileostomy stoma is admitted to the hospital. She has had the ileostomy for six months. Which one of the following conditions is considered a major complication and should be anticipated in the client's care plan?

   1. Infection.
   2. Diarrhea.
   3. Fluid and electrolyte imbalance.
   4. Constipation.

2. A dietary goal for a client postsurgery is to support tissue repair. The nurse will know the client understands dietary principles to achieve this goal when she increases her intake of

   1. Fats.
   2. Carbohydrates.
   3. Incomplete proteins.
   4. Amino acids.

3. A young male, age 11 months, has been a robust, thriving boy. Recently, his appetite has been poor, and he has vomited frequently. He is admitted to the unit after his parents brought him to the hospital following an episode when he suddenly shrieked loudly, pulled his knees to his chest, and seemed to be in acute pain. Assessing the client, the nurse recognizes that this behavior

   1. Is indicative of poisoning.

   2. Indicates presence of parasites.
   3. Indicates acute appendicitis.
   4. Is typical of intussusception.

4. A client is admitted with the diagnosis of glomerulonephritis. He was initially treated with dietary, fluid, and electrolyte restrictions but now has recurrent hypertension and edema. Evaluating the client's lab results in relationship to his disease process, the nurse would expect to find increased

   1. Serum sodium.
   2. Red blood cells.
   3. BUN.
   4. White blood cells.

5. For a client with severe cirrhosis, the physician orders lactulose 30 ml via nasogastric tube. After administering the lactulose, the nurse expects to note an increase in

   1. Constipation.
   2. Diarrhea.
   3. Nausea.
   4. Urine output.

6. A client with cirrhosis has blood test results returned that indicate a prothrombin time of 30 seconds. The nurse would expect the physician to order

   1. Vitamin K.
   2. Heparin.

3. Coumadin.
4. Ferrous sulfate.

7. A client with cirrhosis has ascites that has diminished but complains that he cannot rest during the day and asks the nurse for a sedative to help him sleep. The best nursing response is to say

   1. "Sedatives are processed in the liver and, because your liver is affected by your condition, they would be dangerous to take."
   2. "I'll notify your physician."
   3. "Sedatives are contraindicated because they could depress your respirations."
   4. "I'll see what I can do to get you a medication to help you sleep."

8. When a client with severely decreased liver function due to cirrhosis selects a snack, the choice that indicates he understands his dietary requirements is a

   1. Peanut butter sandwich.
   2. Banana.
   3. Hard boiled egg.
   4. Portion of cheese and crackers.

9. An 81-year-old client is in a long-term care facility. His family couldn't cope with him at home after his senile dementia progressed to the stage where he would wander away and his behavior was unpredictable. Late one night, the nurse finds the client wandering around the halls. He says he is looking for his wife. The nursing approach should be to

   1. Use a matter-of-fact attitude as you help him back to his room.
   2. Remind him about staying in his room.

3. Remind him of where he is and assess why he is having difficulty sleeping.
4. Allow him to sleep in the dayroom so he will not disturb the other clients.

10. Planning activities of daily living for a client with the diagnosis of Alzheimer's, it is essential that the nursing staff

    1. Encourage the client to do as much of his own care as possible.
    2. Assume that the client needs to have the staff take responsibility for his daily care.
    3. Make the client responsible for his own care.
    4. Assign another client to assist the client and socialize with him.

11. An elderly client with the diagnosis of Alzheimer's disease is assigned to a reminiscence group. The nurse knows that the purpose of this type of group is to

    1. Orient him to reality.
    2. Obtain feedback and encouragement from other clients.
    3. Decrease his isolation and loneliness.
    4. Provide the nurse with more information about his memory gaps.

12. A 56-year-old male client is in the ICU and is being prepared to have a CVP inserted. As the physician attaches IV tubing to the hub of the needle, the nurse instructs the client to perform the Valsalva's maneuver. The purpose of this procedure is to

    1. Avoid infiltration of the vein.
    2. Alleviate pain during the procedure.
    3. Prevent an air embolism from occurring.
    4. Assist with catheter advancement.

13. The nurse is monitoring the client when there is a sudden change in the CVP reading. The first nursing action is to

   1. Check whether the client's position has changed.
   2. Take the client's vital signs.
   3. Have the client do the Valsalva's maneuver.
   4. Call the physician immediately.

14. A four month old is diagnosed with hemophilia B. The nurse's understanding of this illness is that it is usually transmitted

   1. By sex-linked genes from the father to his son.
   2. By the Y chromosome from mother to son.
   3. Through a dominant gene of the mother to her son.
   4. By an asymptomatic mother to her son.

15. As a preventative measure, the nurse should teach a child's parents that hemophiliacs

   1. Need to continually be careful not to bruise their skin.
   2. May participate in sports but must use protective gear.
   3. Should not take aspirin in any form, phenothiazines, Indocin, or Butazolidin.
   4. Need to rigorously brush their teeth to ensure good dental hygiene and strong gums.

16. A female client was admitted to the hospital with a diagnosis of pernicious anemia. In counseling the client, the nurse would discuss the major therapeutic treatment that she will receive which is

   1. Packed cells.
   2. B_{12} injections.
   3. Folic acid.
   4. Diet therapy with iron.

17. A 32-year-old client in active labor was admitted through the emergency room. She is having contractions every 2 minutes, lasting 50 to 60 seconds. A vaginal exam shows she is 6 cm dilated and 100 percent effaced. After the exam, the FHR is 140 and regular and her blood pressure 80/40. The first nursing action would be to

   1. Place the client in knee-chest position.
   2. Take the blood pressure again to check accuracy.
   3. Call the physician immediately.
   4. Turn the client on her side and check her blood pressure.

18. The nurse knows that it is important to facilitate bonding between mother and infant soon after birth; thus, delaying giving the infant erythromycin will facilitate bonding. The latest the nurse can wait before instilling this medication is

   1. Fifteen minutes after birth.
   2. Thirty minutes after birth.
   3. One to two hours after birth.
   4. Four hours after birth.

19. A client is admitted to the hospital, diagnosed with liver failure after chemical exposure during an industrial accident. An early indication of liver failure that the nurse would assess for is

   1. Coma.
   2. Liver flap.

3. Sluggish verbal responses.
4. Stupor.

20. Assessing a client, the nurse determines that he is in the early stages of prehepatic coma. The nurse notifies the physician of these findings, expecting which of the following medications to be discontinued?

    1. Neomycin.
    2. Vitamin K.
    3. Lactulose.
    4. Morphine.

21. An elderly client has developed acute left-sided heart failure. The nurse understands that the best description of this condition is

    1. Fluid accumulation in pulmonary interstitial tissues as a result of fluid being forced into the pulmonary circulation.
    2. Blood backing up in the systemic circulation leading to fluid accumulation in the periphery and heart as a result of increased peripheral resistance.
    3. Fluid sequestered in the liver causing increased portal pressure and increased venous return to the heart.
    4. Blood and fluid increasing in amount throughout the heart and pulmonary vasculature as a result of vasoconstriction of the arteries.

22. The nursing action most important to include in a care plan for a client with congestive heart failure is

    1. Allow exercise and out-of-bed ad lib.
    2. Maintain alternate rest and exercise periods.

3. Provide frequent exercise periods to prevent loss of muscle tone.
4. Maintain bedrest at all times.

23. Assessing a client with heart disease, the sign that indicates left-sided heart failure rather than right-sided heart failure is

    1. Sacral edema.
    2. Hepatomegaly.
    3. Increased pulmonary artery wedge pressure.
    4. Jugular venous distention.

24. Client education is an important modality in the care of clients with bulbar type myasthenia gravis chronic conditions. When teaching the client about her medications, the nurse should include information from the drug classification of

    1. Anticholinergics.
    2. Stimulants.
    3. Anticholinesterase.
    4. Cholinesterase.

25. A client with myasthenia gravis should be cautioned against taking certain drugs because they could cause complications of the disease. One of these potentially dangerous drugs is

    1. Penicillin.
    2. Neomycin.
    3. Neostigmine.
    4. Tensilon.

26. The nurse understands that a primary cause of bronchiolitis in a 12 month old is

    1. An acute episode of laryngeal spasm.

2. Laryngeal edema and congestion.
3. Consolidation of a lobe of the lung.
4. Blockage of air from air sacs.

27. A 12-month-old child is admitted to the pediatric unit with suspected bronchiolitis. An important symptom the nurse would assess for is

    1. Retractions and inspiratory stridor.
    2. Flaring of nostrils and expiratory stridor with wheezing and grunting.
    3. Rapid, shallow respirations accompanied by severe, subcostal retractions.
    4. Elevated temperature and expiratory stridor.

28. A client was admitted to the psychiatric unit with the diagnosis of compulsive disorder. She paces up and down the hall 20 times before she carries out any activity and continually states she must get these ideas out of her mind. The nurse understands that the client's anxiety is associated with the

    1. Performance of certain repetitive acts.
    2. Persistence of undesired thoughts or ideas.
    3. Interference from other clients which she experiences while pacing.
    4. Personality characteristics of insecurity, guilt, and sensitivity.

29. A client with compulsive disorder has a schedule of pacing before any activity and often arrives late to meals and does not have time to finish eating. The appropriate nursing action would be to

    1. Plan to provide her meals later and after the other clients have eaten.

2. Notify the client that it is one-half hour before the meal so she can begin her pacing.
3. Interrupt the pacing and insist the client come to meals with everyone else.
4. Allow her to continue as is, but provide her access to the kitchen.

30. While the nurse is talking with a client who has an obsessive-compulsive diagnosis, she tearfully asks the nurse, "Do you think I'm crazy?" The nurse's best response would be

    1. "That depends on your definition of crazy."
    2. "I think you're upset, but not crazy."
    3. "You're obviously concerned about such a thought."
    4. "You're upset. Let's talk about something else."

31. Counseling a client who suspects she is pregnant, the nurse knows that a common early sign of pregnancy is

    1. Amenorrhea.
    2. Morning sickness.
    3. Breast tenderness.
    4. Menorrhagia.

32. On her second visit to the maternity clinic, it is determined that a client is experiencing hyperemesis gravidarum. The nurse knows that this condition is manifested by pernicious vomiting. A dangerous side effect nurse will assess for is

    1. Metabolic acidosis.
    2. Metabolic alkalosis.
    3. Respiratory acidosis.
    4. Respiratory alkalosis.

33. The nurse walks into a new mother's room to check on how she is doing with the new baby, and finds her squeezing the baby's nose. She looks up and laughs and says, "It's funny. I thought only teenagers got pimples." The best response is

    1. "No, anyone can have pimples at any age. We just seem to associate it with teenagers."
    2. "It's best not to squeeze the baby's nose. You should apply warm compresses instead."
    3. "You had better not do that until we run a culture to see what they are."
    4. "It's not necessary to squeeze. The blemishes are clogged oil (sebaceous) glands and will go away on their own."

34. A tumor of the thyroid gland was diagnosed during a client's work-up. Before surgery could be performed, the client developed thyroid storm. This condition is best described as

    1. A type of shock where the blood pressure increases and the client goes into a cardiovascular collapse.
    2. Infection leading to a systemic infection.
    3. Thyroid overactivity which causes severe tachycardia, delirium, and extreme irritability.
    4. Severe dehydration due to overzealous administration of SSKI drops and cortisone preparations.

35. A client is admitted to the hospital for a thyroidectomy. His preoperative care will most likely include

    1. Low sodium diet.
    2. SSKI drops.

    3. Force fluids to 3500 ml/day for one week.
    4. Synthroid on a daily basis.

36. A client has a subtotal thyroidectomy and is returned from the recovery room. Immediate postoperative care would include correct positioning. The appropriate position is

    1. Semi-Fowler's with neck erect.
    2. High-Fowler's with neck extended.
    3. Semi-Fowler's with neck flexed.
    4. Sims' with neck extended.

37. Gathering data for the differential diagnosis of organic dementia, the nurse will focus on

    1. A set delusional system with hallucinatory overtones.
    2. Withdrawal alternating with manic behavior.
    3. Loss of intellectual abilities which interfere with social or occupational functioning.
    4. Clouded state of consciousness with decreased ability to communicate.

38. A client, age 70, was brought to the psychiatric unit and admitted with the tentative diagnosis of organic brain syndrome, dementia type. He had poor judgment, emotional lability, and, at times, seemed to forget events that had just occurred. Assessing his condition, the nurse would expect that his prognosis would be

    1. Good, because the organic condition usually tends to be reversible.
    2. Favorable, because the symptoms are not closely related to the client's basic personality.

3. Poor, because the condition is progressive and irreversible.

4. Poor, because the disease onset is abrupt and slowly reversible.

39. Establishing a plan of care for a client with organic brain syndrome, the nurse would include

    1. An active, stimulating environment.
    2. Total physical care.
    3. Frequent reality orientation.
    4. Freedom to choose his own diet.

40. A 25-year-old client is pregnant for the first time. Which of the following complaints from a client would be considered an abnormal presumptive sign of pregnancy?

    1. Breast tenderness.
    2. Increased vaginal discharge.
    3. Painful urination.
    4. Nausea.

41. A client in late pregnancy asks the nurse to check her breasts because she has noted a discharge. The nurse explains that colostrum can appear from the nipple as early as

    1. The beginning of labor.
    2. Two hours postpartum.
    3. Twelve weeks gestation.
    4. Thirty-two weeks gestation.

42. A 30-year-old client is admitted to the hospital with the diagnosis of hemorrhoids. While taking the health history, the nurse would identify associated conditions that could be the causative factor in the development of the client's hemorrhoids. Which one of the

following is the most likely condition experienced by the client?

    1. Paralytic ileus.
    2. Irritable colon.
    3. Chronic constipation.
    4. Portal hypertension.

43. A mother enters the room to find her 18 month old experiencing generalized body twitching. The mother becomes very frightened, picks the child up, and runs to the neighbors. A safer action that the nurse can teach the mother for the future would be to

    1. Place a spoon or comb in the child's mouth to prevent the tongue from occluding the airway.
    2. Elevate the child's head with a pillow to prevent airway occlusion.
    3. Place the child on her abdomen to prevent aspiration.
    4. Place the child on her side to prevent airway obstruction.

44. A 20-year-old female client is admitted in a comatose state to the emergency room. Her vital signs are BP 140/80, P 110, R 30 and labored. She has a flushed face. No relatives are present to give a history. Whenever a client is admitted comatose to the emergency room without apparent trauma, an early assessment should be made for

    1. Diabetes mellitus.
    2. Renal failure.
    3. Hypoglycemia.
    4. Metabolic alkalosis.

45. A clinical manifestation that would be observed early in ketoacidosis is

1. Polyuria.
2. Acetone odor to breath.
3. Kussmaul breathing.
4. Sensorium change.

46. A client takes 22 units of NPH insulin at 7:30 A.M. each day. At which time should the nurse assess her for signs of restlessness, memory lapses and headache?

    1. 8:30 A.M.
    2. 10:30 A.M.
    3. 3:30 P.M.
    4. 5:00 A.M.

47. Drug abuse is a major problem in the United States today. Which of the following factors is a predictor of rehabilitation from drug addiction?

    1. Women seem to be more successful.
    2. Persons who were younger at the onset of their addiction have more success.
    3. Persons who began for "kicks" have a greater success rate.
    4. A strong identification with a peer group aids in drug abstinence.

48. A female client, age 75 and diagnosed with COPD, has been admitted to the hospital. Her physician prescribed Aminophylline IV infusion 2 mg/minute. The nurse will evaluate the effectiveness of Aminophylline by observing for decreased

    1. Mucus production.
    2. Respiratory distress.
    3. Pulse rate.
    4. Rales.

49. A pregnant client, age 20, arrives at the emergency room. As the nurse assesses the client's condition, she observes that her membranes have spontaneously ruptured and the umbilical cord is protruding from her vagina. The first intervention is to

    1. Administer ordered oxygen at 4 L/minute.
    2. Check the fetal heart rate.
    3. Notify the physician.
    4. Place the client in knee-chest position.

50. A client has been admitted to the nursing unit with a tentative diagnosis of urinary tract infection. The nurse knows that the most important factor influencing ascending infection is

    1. Inadequate fluid intake.
    2. The obstruction of free urine flow.
    3. A change in pH.
    4. The presence of microorganisms.

51. A male client was admitted for an upper bowel obstruction. Following surgery, he came back with a #15 Levin nasogastric (NG) tube. One of the first nursing actions is to check his NG tube, which the nurse knows must be attached to

    1. Continuous low suction.
    2. Continuous high suction.
    3. Intermittent low suction.
    4. Intermittent high suction.

52. The most accurate method of checking placement of the nasogastric (NG) tube is to

    1. Place the end of the tube in a glass of water and observe for bubbles.
    2. Inject air into the tube, and with a stethoscope positioned over the stomach, listen for a popping sound.

3. Aspirate the gastric contents and check it with litmus paper.
4. Aspirate the gastric contents and determine whether the amount exceeds 20 ml of fluid.

53. A client with a Foley catheter has orders for irrigation of the bladder. The nursing measure the nurse would utilize to ensure catheter patency is to

1. Irrigate the bladder using a solution of sterile water.
2. Instill air into the catheter to push any mucus out of the catheter tip.
3. Insert 10–20 ml of aqueous Zephiran into the bladder and then siphon it out.
4. Irrigate the bladder with sterile normal saline.

54. A client has orders for an IV of D_5W to infuse at 50 ml/hour. Analyzing the IV fluid orders, the nurse would consider that an IV of D_5W has enough calories to provide

1. Insufficient caloric intake for a 24 hour period.
2. Sufficient carbohydrates to maintain homeostasis.
3. Insufficient protein for tissue repair.
4. Sufficient caloric intake over a 24 hour period.

55. A nurse at an outdoor music festival is asked to help a woman in the early stage of delivery. Evaluating the situation, the nurse determines that the baby is beginning to crown and that the best decision is to send someone for help while assisting the mother. The first nursing action would be to

1. Tell the mother to gently cross her legs to hold the baby back until help comes.
2. Allow the head to deliver and watch for tearing of the perineum.
3. Tell the mother not to push and let the baby deliver with the contractions.
4. Support the perineum to prevent tearing as the delivering head presents.

56. In an emergency delivery, which of the following principles best explains why the nurse would not cut the cord?

1. It is the physician's responsibility to cut the cord.
2. Cutting the cord under emergency conditions might lead to hemorrhage.
3. Cutting the cord under emergency conditions might lead to infection.
4. The nurse has not been trained in the proper procedure.

57. The nurse is assigned a 4-year-old child with a cyanotic heart defect who has a lack of energy, frequent infections, and manifests clubbing of her fingers and toes. Which one of the following statements accurately describes cyanotic congenital cardiac lesions?

1. Cyanotic lesions present with right-to-left intracardiac shunting.
2. There is no correlation between the amount of blood shunted away from the lungs and the amount of reduced hemoglobin in systemic circulation.
3. Supplemental oxygen will significantly improve oxygen saturation levels in children with cyanotic lesions.
4. The hematocrit drops with progressing severity of the disease.

58. A 3-year-old child is diagnosed as having tetralogy of Fallot. In making an assessment, the nurse would expect her to

1. Favor squatting.
2. Have normal growth patterns.
3. Be acyanotic except with exertion.
4. Have an audible murmur.

59. A nine year old has just returned from the cardiac catheterization lab. This procedure was performed via the left femoral vein. Which one of the following clinical manifestations would indicate a complication of this procedure?

1. Apical pulse is 130; femoral pulse is 120.
2. Child is asking for a lot of fluids to drink.
3. Diastolic pressures are decreasing rapidly.
4. Hypothermia is present.

60. A 31-year-old gravida 3 para 2 is 34 weeks pregnant. She has been admitted in premature labor with her membranes intact. Her cervix is 40 percent effaced and 1 cm dilated. The client is anxious and obviously upset. The nurse assigned to care for this client would do which of the following nursing actions first?

1. Assist her into bed and maintain bedrest.
2. Put her in Fowler's position for comfort.
3. Help her express her fears.
4. Apply an external fetal monitor.

61. The physician orders an intravenous infusion of Ritodrine for a client in premature labor in an attempt to stop the contractions. Because Ritodrine is a Beta-sympathomimetic agent that causes muscle relaxation, the nurse will monitor closely for

1. Hypertension and tachycardia.
2. Hypotension and tachycardia.
3. Tachycardia with irregular pulse.
4. Bradycardia with regular pulse.

62. A 45-year-old client is admitted to the psychiatric unit smelling of alcohol and saying that he is being pursued by animals, which he can both see and feel touching him. In assessing this client, the nurse knows that his signs and symptoms indicate that the cause of his condition is

1. Acute hallucinations.
2. Schizophrenia.
3. Delirium tremens.
4. Withdrawal from alcohol.

63. After five days of delirium tremens, the client has no further hallucinations, tremors, diaphoresis, or illusions. He seeks permission from the nurse before undertaking his own personal care, such as bathing and eating, and he sometimes asks the nurse where the bathroom and dining room are located. These requests indicate that this client

1. Is ready for discharge, because he is out of bed and ready to do these things for himself.
2. May be starting to have a recurrence of delirium tremens.
3. Is somewhat disoriented but functioning very independently because he is feeding and bathing himself.
4. Is exhibiting dependency and is somewhat disoriented.

64. A 55-year-old client with a long history of alcohol abuse and cirrhosis of the liver is being admitted to the hospital. He has ascites and jaundice, with a blood pressure

of 140/80, pulse 82, respirations 26, and temperature 99° F rectally. Providing adequate fluid intake for this client, the nurse would expect his orders to include an IV of

1. $D_{10}W$.
2. D_5W.
3. $D_5/.2$ NS with KCl.
4. $D_5/.45$ NS.

65 Evaluating a client's condition who has just received Lasix, the nurse would observe for which major side effect of the drug?

1. Dyspnea.
2. Tachycardia.
3. Muscular weakness.
4. Headache.

66. A 43-year-old male is brought to the mental health unit by the police for vandalizing his neighbor's car, but says that it was his neighbor's fault. He seems bright, articulate and oriented upon admission. The diagnosis is paranoid disorder. A person with a paranoid disorder can be described as exhibiting

1. Delusions that are less established.
2. None of the other classical symptoms of schizophrenia, such as "the 4 As."
3. Delusions that are usually more bizarre than schizophrenic delusions.
4. Emotions and behavior not appropriate to the content of the delusional system.

67. In planning for discharge of a client with paranoid disorder, it is most important that the team evaluate which of the following areas?

1. The client's potential for violence.
2. The insights the client has gained.

3. The effectiveness of the client's discharge medication.
4. A referral to a community mental health agency.

68. While bathing a one year old, the nurse feels a large mass in the abdominal area and notices that his diaper is soiled with pinkish tinged urine. The initial nursing action is to

1. Assess if the tumor has spread to the lymph nodes.
2. Immediately notify the physician.
3. Continue the assessment by observing his behavior indicating pain on palpation.
4. Gently palpate the abdominal mass to determine if it is a Wilms' tumor.

69. Considering the physical developmental period of a one year old, hospitalization may affect or delay his progression with

1. Crawling.
2. Running.
3. Walking.
4. Sitting.

70. A 21-year-old client was injured in a motor-cycle accident yesterday. As a treatment for his fractured right femur, Kirschner wires were inserted and he was placed in balanced suspension traction. The position that will best promote healing is

1. Supine and flat to keep the traction in place.
2. With his right leg flat on the bed to promote the effectiveness of the traction.
3. In semi-Fowler's to prevent the traction from slipping.
4. With his right leg positioned at a 20 degree angle to maintain traction pull.

71. It is the nursing responsibility to monitor the oxygen level in an incubator of a premature infant. The highest safe level of oxygen the nurse will administer to premature infants is

1. 25 percent.
2. 40 percent.
3. 55 percent.
4. 70 percent.

72. Respiratory acidosis, a serious complication of respiratory distress syndrome (RDS) occurring in infants, occurs as a result of

1. Retention of carbon dioxide due to inadequate ventilation.
2. Retention of oxygen due to inadequate ventilation.
3. Poor exchange of oxygen and carbon dioxide in the lungs.
4. Pulmonary hyperperfusion.

73. The nurse explains to a new mother that the condition of small for gestational age (SGA) is caused by

1. Placental insufficiency.
2. Maternal obesity.
3. Primipara.
4. Genetic predisposition.

74. Which of the following child care practices makes a one year old more likely to get middle ear infections than other children?

1. Drinking a bottle of milk while supine in her crib.
2. Using Q-tips for cleaning ears.
3. Getting her ears wet during her bath.
4. Using oil drops in her ears once a week.

75. If otitis media becomes a chronic problem, which one of the following complications should the nurse observe for?

1. Tonsillitis.
2. Sepsis.
3. Sore throat.
4. Hearing loss.

76. For a client with a detached retina, the preoperative nursing care plan will include

1. Bathroom privileges with assistance.
2. Turn, cough and deep breathe.
3. Keep both eyes bandaged.
4. Turn to the left side only.

77. The first postoperative day following surgery for a detached retina, the nursing care plan will include the intervention to

1. Turn, cough and deep breathe every two hours.
2. Allow the client up out of bed ad lib.
3. Allow the eye patch removed during the day.
4. Give a bed bath.

78. A 48-year-old client admitted with a diagnosis of depression quietly sits by herself, gazing out the window and occasionally crying. Her husband says that her personal neglect is recent and really started after their last child left home for college. This client's personality prior to the illness probably resembled a woman who

1. Had a very organized household and often put her husband's and children's wishes ahead of her own.
2. Kept a neat house and was indecisive most of the time.

3. Was not inclined toward much recreation and who often thought of suicide.

4. Focused her activity exclusively around her children and who lived with an unresolved relationship with her parents.

79. A client took a medication overdose soon after admission to the hospital. She has now been returned from ICU to a room on the psychiatric unit. Upon seeing the nurse who admitted her, the client looks down at the floor and mumbles, "Hello." The nurse's best initial statement is

1. "You have been transferred back to this unit. This is your new room."
2. "Hello. I see that in ICU you've been getting a light diet. How does your stomach feel now?"
3. "I was upset when I found you had tried to kill yourself."
4. "Would you like to talk about what happened?"

80. A female client who is 37 weeks pregnant presents to the labor room with vaginal bleeding and a tentative diagnosis of partial placenta previa. Following a nursing assessment, the priority intervention is to

1. Immediately call the physician.
2. Prepare for an emergency C-section.
3. Place the client in a side-lying position.
4. Complete a pelvic exam to determine progress of labor.

81. Following a cesarean section, the priority nursing care includes

1. Observing for presence of hematuria.
2. Monitoring vital signs for hypertension.

3. Checking the client's fundus and lochia.
4. Monitoring for signs of infection.

82. Because of the large fluid and electrolyte loss from massive burns, the client will receive 18,000 ml of fluid in the first 24 hours. According to the Parkland formula (4 ml/kg body weight/percent of body burn), how much fluid should the nurse be prepared to give in the first eight hours?

1. 600 ml/hour.
2. 750 ml/hour.
3. 1125 ml/hour.
4. 1238 ml/hour.

83. Monitoring a burned client's fluid replacement, the fluid that is commonly used for the first 24 hours is

1. 5% Dextrose in water.
2. 5% Dextrose in normal saline.
3. Normal saline.
4. Ringer's lactate.

84. There are two basic types of respiratory tract injuries associated with burns: smoke inhalation and upper airway injuries. In a client with an upper airway burn, the nurse would expect to assess

1. Hoarseness and stridor.
2. Pulmonary parenchymal dysfunction.
3. Sootlike secretions.
4. Cherry-red lips.

85. A 57-year-old client has benign prostatic hypertrophy and is being admitted for a transurethral resection (TUR). Preoperative nursing care will include which of the following interventions?

1. Discussion of the surgical intervention and the fact that it causes impotence.
2. Decreased fluid intake for at least two days to prevent bladder irritability.
3. Keep client NPO for at least 18 hours to prevent bowel evacuation during the surgical procedure.
4. Discussion of hygienic care of the penis before surgery.

86. The complication that the nurse will evaluate for following a transurethral resection (TUR) is

1. Hemorrhage.
2. Infection.
3. Urinary retention.
4. Adhesions of the neck of the bladder.

87. While awaiting surgery for repair of a cleft lip in a 2-month-old child, the parents need instruction in what to expect. The primary problem they should be counseled to expect is

1. The infant's irritability.
2. Frequent upper respiratory tract infections.
3. Food returning through the nose.
4. Lack of normal dental development.

88. Of the following, the nursing intervention most important in the postoperative nursing care for a 2-month-old child with a repair of cleft lip is

1. Feeding her with a rubber-tipped syringe.
2. Suctioning the nasopharynx frequently.
3. Keeping the suture area clean.
4. Removing elbow restraints frequently.

89. Following abdominal surgery for removal of a benign tumor, the nurse observes that the dressing is wet with serosanguineous drainage. After changing the dressing, the nurse checks the chart and learns that the client's dressing was changed four hours previously and the same drainage was charted. The appropriate conclusion is that

1. This kind and amount of drainage is to be expected after abdominal surgery.
2. This amount of drainage is frequently a sign of impending dehiscence.
3. The serosanguineous drainage means that he is losing too much blood.
4. The dressing should be changed more frequently than every four hours.

90. Postabdominal surgery, the client is able to choose a daily menu. The nurse will know he understands his diet when he chooses

1. According to his own individual needs and similar to his preoperative diet.
2. Low fiber with 2000 ml fluids daily.
3. High fiber with 2000–3000 ml fluids and supplemental vitamin K.
4. Regular diet with no milk products.

Comprehensive Test 2
Answers with Rationale

1. (3) Due to the extreme loss of fluids from the high colon interruption, fluid and electrolyte imbalance is the most common complication. The lower colon reabsorbs a major portion of the fluid, whereas the upper colon does not have this function. A great potassium loss also occurs, as it is found in large amounts in the upper colon.

   Nursing Process: Planning
   Client Needs: Physiological Integrity
   Clinical Area: Surgical Nursing

2. (2) Carbohydrates are protein-sparing food sources. When present, they provide for energy and allow the proteins to be used for tissue repair.

   Nursing Process: Evaluation
   Client Needs: Physiological Integrity
   Clinical Area: Surgical Nursing

3. (4) The client's behavior, especially indicating pain, is typical of a child with intussusception. Other signs may be vomiting and bloody mucus in the stool. Appendicitis would evidence pain in the right lower quadrant of the abdomen. Neither poisoning nor parasites would present with this symptom pattern.

   Nursing Process: Analysis
   Client Needs: Physiological Integrity
   Clinical Area: Pediatric Nursing

4. (3) The potassium and BUN are increased due to the kidney's decreased ability to secrete these materials. Red blood cells are decreased due to the decreased production of erythropoietin, the factor that stimulates production of erythrocytes. Sodium is restricted but if diuresis is great, sodium replacement may be required.

   Nursing Process: Evaluation
   Client Needs: Physiological Integrity
   Clinical Area: Medical Nursing

5. (2) Lactulose is a synthetic disaccharide that the small intestine cannot utilize. It causes diarrhea by lowering the pH so that

   Nursing Process: Evaluation
   Client Needs: Physiological Integrity
   Clinical Area: Medical Nursing

the bacterial flora are changed in the bowel. The bacteria responsible for producing ammonia by acting on proteins are absent, so the ammonia level decreases.

6. (1)   A prothrombin time of 30 seconds indicates the clotting time is prolonged and bleeding could occur. The normal prothrombin time is 12–15 seconds. A vitamin K injection will increase the synthesis of prothrombin by the liver.

Nursing Process: Planning
Client Needs: Physiological Integrity
Clinical Area: Medical Nursing

7. (1)   While answer (3) is true, the best response is (1), giving him the facts. Sedatives are metabolized by the liver. The client cannot tolerate these drugs because of his defective hepatic function. He would have very high levels of the drug in his blood for a prolonged period of time. Other options, such as relaxation techniques, are important to try before resorting to drugs.

Nursing Process: Implementation
Client Needs: Health Promotion and Maintenance
Clinical Area: Medical Nursing

8. 17.   (2) Carbohydrates are one of the mainstays of the cirrhotic client's diet. The liver can metabolize only very small amounts of protein, so usually only 50 grams of protein is allowed per day (normal diet is 80 grams per day). All of the other choices contain protein.

Nursing Process: Evaluation
Client Needs: Health Promotion and Maintenance
Clinical Area: Medical Nursing

9. (3)   This answer orients the client to time and place in addition to assessing the underlying cause of his sleep disturbance. Answer (2) is only a short-term solution, and (4) does not focus on his problem but on other client needs.

Nursing Process: Implementation
Client Needs: Psychosocial Integrity
Clinical Area: Psychiatric Nursing

10. (1)   The nursing care plan needs to be based on the client level of functioning and to reinforce independence and self-care as appropriate. Answer (2) creates an atmosphere of dependence while (3) totally ignores the client's realistic dependence

Nursing Process: Planning
Client Needs: Safe, Effective Care Environment
Clinical Area: Psychiatric Nursing

needs. Answer (4) places the responsibility for the client's care onto another client.

11.   (3)   The purpose of reminiscence is to allow the client to interact with others in a way that is easy and comfortable for him. Answers (2) and (4) may be true but are not the major focus of this type of group. Answer (1) may also be true, especially if the focus is "here and now," but it is not the main purpose of the group.

Nursing Process: Analysis
Client Needs: Psychosocial Integrity
Clinical Area: Psychiatric Nursing

12.   (3)   The rationale for a Valsalva's procedure is to prevent air from entering the catheter, thus reducing the risk of an air embolism. None of the other answers is accurate.

Nursing Process: Analysis
Client Needs: Physiological Integrity
Clinical Area: Surgical Nursing

13.   (1)   If the client's position has recently changed, it could alter the CVP reading. The first nursing action is to check for this and repeat the reading. Depending on the source of the reading change, the nurse would then notify the physician.

Nursing Process: Implementation
Client Needs: Safe, Effective Care Environment
Clinical Area: Medical Nursing

14.   (4)   Classic hemophilia is transmitted by an asymptomatic female carrier and affects sons; therefore, it is carried on the X chromosome and is recessive.

Nursing Process: Analysis
Client Needs: Physiological Integrity
Clinical Area: Pediatric Nursing

15.   (3)   Aspirin may cause bleeding. Hemophiliacs should not be given IM injections nor engage in contact sports. They also need excellent dental hygiene and should use very soft brushes on their teeth rather than stiff bristle brushes.

Nursing Process: Implementation
Client Needs: Health Promotion and Maintenance
Clinical Area: Pediatric Nursing

16.   (2)   Without the intrinsic factor, B_{12} cannot be absorbed if taken orally. When the body's store of B_{12} is used up, the client shows signs of anemia and B_{12} injections must be administered to correct the deficiency.

Nursing Process: Implementation
Client Needs: Health Promotion and Maintenance
Clinical Area: Medical Nursing

17. (4) The low blood pressure is likely due to supine hypotensive syndrome. Turning the client on her side will relieve the pressure from the inferior vena cava. After this action, the nurse will repeat the blood pressure reading.

Nursing Process: Implementation
Client Needs: Safe, Effective Care Environment
Clinical Area: Maternity Nursing

18. (3) Erythromycin, a broad spectrum antibiotic, (or silver nitrate) can be instilled up to two hours after delivery without the infant's eyes being harmed.

Nursing Process: Analysis
Client Needs: Safe, Effective Care Environment
Clinical Area: Maternity Nursing

19. (3) Memory impairment, decreased attention, decreased concentration, and slow response rate all indicate the onset of brain impairment. The other signs, (1), (2), (4), occur later in this condition.

Nursing Process: Assessment
Client Needs: Physiological Integrity
Clinical Area: Medical Nursing

20. (4) The first three drugs may improve the client's condition, but morphine is detoxified by the liver and may further increase CNS depression.

Nursing Process: Planning
Client Needs: Physiological Integrity
Clinical Area: Medical Nursing

21. (1) Left-sided heart failure results in pulmonary interstitial fluid accumulation. Other terms for left-sided heart failure include forward heart failure and low-output failure. Right-sided heart failure is a result of increased pulmonary artery pressure leading to blood damming back in the systemic circulation.

Nursing Process: Analysis
Client Needs: Physiological Integrity
Clinical Area: Medical Nursing

22. (4) When a client is experiencing heart failure, the heart cannot provide for the basic needs of the body; therefore, the client is maintained on bedrest until the heart is strengthened.

Nursing Process: Planning
Client Needs: Health Promotion and Maintenance
Clinical Area: Medical Nursing

23. (3) Increased pulmonary artery pressure is the best indicator of left-sided failure indicating failure of the left ventricle to pump adequately. Increased CVP indicates only

Nursing Process: Analysis
Client Needs: Physiological Integrity
Clinical Area: Medical Nursing

the amount of circulating blood flow enter-ing the right side of the heart. Answers (1), (2) and (3) are signs of right-sided failure.

24. (3)   Anticholinesterase drugs are used to inactivate cholinesterase, which then allows acetylcholine to carry the nerve impulse across the myoneural junction. The only other drug group that might be ordered are steroids, usually given as a last resort.

Nursing Process: Implementation
Client Needs: Health Promotion and Maintenance
Clinical Area: Medical Nursing

25. (2)   Neomycin is an aminoglycoside and may cause muscle weakness; for example, in the respiratory system or in swallowing, etc. Also, the client should avoid strepto-mycin and gentamicin because they block neuromuscular transmission. Neostigmine is an anticholinesterase drug, one of the drugs used for myasthenia.

Nursing Process: Implementation
Client Needs: Health Promotion and Maintenance
Clinical Area: Medical Nursing

26. (4)   There is widespread inflammation of the bronchial mucous membrane. The mucosa swells, and a thick exudate is pro-duced. Air can enter the alveoli on inspira-tion, but is not expelled on expiration; it is trapped in the lungs and the chest becomes over-distended.

Nursing Process: Analysis
Client Needs: Physiological Integrity
Clinical Area: Pediatric Nursing

27. (2)   Low obstructive respiratory syndrome has expiratory stridor with a characteristic wheeze and grunt. The respirations are rapid and shallow because of severe lung distention, but retractions are mild. Increased temperature is more likely to be found in high obstructive respiratory con-ditions.

Nursing Process: Assessment
Client Needs: Physiological Integrity
Clinical Area: Pediatric Nursing

28. (2)   Anxiety is associated with the persis-tence of thoughts or ideas and is increased when the client cannot release it through a repetitive act such as pacing. The compul-sive, ritualistic actions reduce the anxiety.

Nursing Process: Analysis
Client Needs: Psychosocial Integrity
Clinical Area: Psychiatric Nursing

29.   (2)   It is important that the client be allowed to complete the ritual so the anxiety will be controlled. Giving her time to do this will meet the need to reduce anxiety through performing the ritual and good nutrition.

Nursing Process: Implementation
Client Needs: Safe, Effective Care Environment
Clinical Area: Psychiatric Nursing

30.   (3)   Rather than be evasive or attempt to answer a question for which there really is no answer, the nurse should encourage the client to express what she is thinking and feeling. This is most likely to be helpful in assisting her to deal with her fears.

Nursing Process: Implementation
Client Needs: Safe, Effective Care Environment
Clinical Area: Psychiatric Nursing

31.   (1)   Amenorrhea happens in almost all cases of early pregnancy, whereas morning sickness or breast tenderness may or may not occur. Answer (4), menorrhagia, refers to excessive menstrual bleeding.

Nursing Process: Analysis
Client Needs: Health Promotion and Maintenance
Clinical Area: Maternity Nursing

32.   (1)   With minimal vomiting, metabolic alkalosis develops. With protracted vomiting, the client becomes dehydrated, suffers electrolyte imbalance, and, if untreated, will develop metabolic acidosis from excessive loss of fluids from the GI tract.

Nursing Process: Evaluation
Client Needs: Physiological Integrity
Clinical Area: Maternity Nursing

33.   (4)   The pimples are milia, which are clogged sebaceous glands. These are a normal newborn feature and will soon disappear. The mother should be counseled not to squeeze these areas to avoid infection.

Nursing Process: Implementation
Client Needs: Health Promotion and Maintenance
Clinical Area: Maternity Nursing

34.   (3)   When clients are under severe stress or develop an infection, thyroid hormone is excreted in large amounts. This condition can lead to dehydration, high fever and the symptoms listed in answer (3).

Nursing Process: Analysis
Client Needs: Physiological Integrity
Clinical Area: Surgical Nursing

35.   (2)   Antithyroid drugs inhibit synthesis and release of thyroid hormone. SSKI is used prior to surgery to prevent thyroid

Nursing Process: Planning
Client Needs: Health Promotion and Maintenance
Clinical Area: Surgical Nursing

storm. SSKI also decreases vascularity of the gland which decreases risk of hemorrhage. Bedrest and a nutritious diet high in vitamins are included in the postoperative nursing care plan.

36. (1) Semi-Fowler's with the neck erect is the position of choice to maintain respiratory status. The objective is to decrease pressure on the suture line and prevent edema formation, which could cause respiratory distress.

Nursing Process: Implementation
Client Needs: Safe, Effective Care Environment
Clinical Area: Surgical Nursing

37. (3) Loss of intellectual abilities is a classic symptom of organic brain syndrome. The other answers may be characteristics of other psychiatric disorders but are not necessarily consistently seen in organic dementia.

Nursing Process: Assessment
Client Needs: Physiological Integrity
Clinical Area: Psychiatric Nursing

38. (3) Organic brain syndrome, dementia type has a poor prognosis, is usually progressive and irreversible, and the symptoms are closely related to the client's basic personality.

Nursing Process: Analysis
Client Needs: Physiological Integrity
Clinical Area: Psychiatric Nursing

39. (3) Frequent reality orientation is important for the client. The environment should be calm and controlled and the client encouraged to complete as many physical care activities as possible. (4) is incorrect because this client cannot use discrimination or make choices.

Nursing Process: Planning
Client Needs: Safe, Effective Care Environment
Clinical Area: Psychiatric Nursing

40. (3) Frequent urination is a normal sign of early pregnancy. Painful urination is abnormal and may indicate a urinary tract infection.

Nursing Process: Assessment
Client Needs: Physiological Integrity
Clinical Area: Maternity Nursing

41. (3) Colostrum, the forerunner of milk, can appear as early as the end of the first trimester.

Nursing Process: Analysis
Client Needs: Health Promotion and Maintenance
Clinical Area: Maternity Nursing

42.   (3)   Chronic constipation is a problem
with peristalsis and movement of gastrointestinal contents. This generally causes
pressure within the vein resulting in hemorrhoids.

Nursing Process: Analysis
Client Needs: Physiological Integrity
Clinical Area: Medical Nursing

43.   (4)   The child should be placed on her side
to prevent airway occlusion. Current practice is not to put any object into the mouth,
even a tongue blade, to prevent injury.

Nursing Process: Implementation
Client Needs: Safe, Effective Care Environment
Clinical Area: Pediatric Nursing

44.   (1)   Diabetes complications, such as
ketoacidosis, can occur rapidly, especially
if the client has an infection or has failed to
take insulin. When there is no evidence of
trauma, it is important to check for diabetes in a comatose client.

Nursing Process: Assessment
Client Needs: Physiological Integrity
Clinical Area: Medical Nursing

45.   (1)   Polyuria, polydipsia, and polyphagia
are early symptoms. The other conditions
occur later in ketoacidosis. As acetone is
liberated through the breakdown of fat, it
is volatile and is blown off by the lungs,
creating the characteristic fruity odor of
the breath.

Nursing Process: Assessment
Client Needs: Physiological Integrity
Clinical Area: Medical Nursing

46.   (3)   Intermediate insulin peaks from 8–12
hours after injection. 3:30 P.M. is the most
appropriate time to assess for signs of
insulin reaction.

Nursing Process: Assessment
Client Needs: Physiological Integrity
Clinical Area: Medical Nursing

47.   (1)   Besides women, people who began
taking drugs later in life are more successful at breaking the addictive pattern. Drug
addicts are experts at manipulating the
group while on the street. Unless the group
is adept at recognizing and confronting
manipulative behavior, group identification does not help the individual abstain.

Nursing Process: Analysis
Client Needs: Psychosocial Integrity
Clinical Area: Psychiatric Nursing

48.   (2)   Aminophylline causes bronchodilata-
tion and, therefore, increased oxygenation.
The client is more able to cough up secre-

Nursing Process: Evaluation
Client Needs: Physiological Integrity
Clinical Area: Medical Nursing

tions and the breath sounds will become more clear. The CNS is stimulated by this drug and the pulse rate may increase.

49. (4) Placing the client in knee-chest position will prevent more damage by getting the pressure off the cord. Answer (2) and (3), continuing to assess or notifying the physician, wastes time when a nursing action is indicated. A follow-up intervention may be to administer the oxygen.

Nursing Process: Implementation
Client Needs: Physiological Integrity
Clinical Area: Maternity Nursing

50. (2) Free flow of urine, together with large urine output and acidic pH, are antibacterial defenses. Health professionals should teach clients to test urine periodically and increase oral intake of foods that make the urine pH acidic.

Nursing Process: Analysis
Client Needs: Physiological Integrity
Clinical Area: Medical Nursing

51. (3) Intermittent low suction is most appropriate. Intermittent suction allows the mucosal wall of the stomach to drop away from the NG tube during periods when the suction is off. This action will prevent damage to the mucosal wall.

Nursing Process: Implementation
Client Needs: Safe, Effective Care Environment
Clinical Area: Surgical Nursing

52. (3) Aspirating stomach contents is the most accurate method, as litmus paper will indicate acid reaction. (2) is incorrect because it will be a "whooshing" sound if the tube has entered the stomach rather than the bronchus, and it is not as accurate a method.

Nursing Process: Implementation
Client Needs: Safe, Effective Care Environment
Clinical Area: Surgical Nursing

53. (4) Irrigating the bladder with sterile normal saline is the accepted action. It is never advisable to force fluids into any tubing to check for patency. Sterile water and aqueous Zephiran will affect the pH of the bladder as well as cause irritation. To check for patency, the nurse would not leave solution in the bladder; this is used only for instillation of medications.

Nursing Process: Implementation
Client Needs: Safe, Effective Care Environment
Clinical Area: Medical Nursing

54. (1) The D_5W solution of 50 ml/hr provides 1200 ml of IV fluid. Each bottle of 1000 ml provides approximately 200 calories; therefore, the 1200 ml will provide 240 calories. Each gram of carbohydrate provides approximately 4 calories per gram.

Nursing Process: Planning
Client Needs: Physiological Integrity
Clinical Area: Medical Nursing

55. (4) Applying gentle counter pressure will help prevent tears as the head delivers. Never hold the head back, but allow it to deliver naturally. Never instruct the mother to cross her legs to hold the baby back.

Nursing Process: Implementation
Client Needs: Safe, Effective Care Environment
Clinical Area: Maternity Nursing

56. (3) Because Wharton's jelly expands as it comes in contact with the air, there will be no bleeding from the placentae surface. Cutting the cord under emergency conditions could lead to infection.

Nursing Process: Analysis
Client Needs: Physiological Integrity
Clinical Area: Maternity Nursing

57. (1) Cyanosis occurs with right-to-left shunting because the blood that is shunted in this manner never comes in contact with the alveolar-capillary interface in the lung; hence, there is an increased amount of reduced hemoglobin or unoxygenated blood in the systemic circulation. The greater the amount of reduced hemoglobin the more visible/pervasive the cyanosis. Supplemental oxygen will improve oxygen saturation and the hematocrit rises.

Nursing Process: Analysis
Client Needs: Physiological Integrity
Clinical Area: Pediatric Nursing

58. (1) When a sudden onset of dyspnea, cyanosis and restlessness occurs, children with tetralogy develop a "hypoxic spell." Squatting is a spontaneous compensatory mechanism used by children to alleviate these spells. Squatting increases systemic resistance while decreasing backflow to the heart from the inferior vena cava. The decrease of systemic return makes relatively more oxygenated blood available to the body.

Nursing Process: Assessment
Client Needs: Physiological Integrity
Clinical Area: Pediatric Nursing

59.   (1)   A pulse deficit is indicative of an arrhythmia and may indicate occlusion of the left femoral artery (emboli formation). If systolic and diastolic pressures were hypotensive, it would indicate hemorrhage. Hypothermia is not relevant. Thirst is a result of being NPO, not a reaction to the procedure.

Nursing Process: Evaluation
Client Needs: Physiological Integrity
Clinical Area: Pediatric Nursing

60.   (1)   The nurse would first assist the client to bed and maintain bedrest. She is already 1 cm dilated—this process could go very fast. The other interventions would follow.

Nursing Process: Implementation
Client Needs: Safe, Effective Care Environment
Clinical Area: Maternity Nursing

61.   (3)   Ritodrine acts on type II Beta-adrenergic receptors resulting in uterine muscle relaxation. Cardiovascular complications can occur; therefore, the client should be closely assessed for signs of tachycardia and an irregular pulse. The fetus may also have a period of tachycardia so frequent FHTs are important.

Nursing Process: Evaluation
Client Needs: Safe, Effective Care Environment
Clinical Area: Maternity Nursing

62.   (3)   In DTs, the picture described by the client is common. This condition is the source of hallucinations, not schizophrenia. DTs or acute intoxication is not necessarily caused by withdrawal from alcohol, but from heavy alcohol intake without proper nutrients.

Nursing Process: Assessment
Client Needs: Physiological Integrity
Clinical Area: Psychiatric Nursing

63.   (4)   Seeking permission for simple tasks indicates dependent functioning. Forgetting where things are indicates persisting confusion, disorientation and need for structure. He is obviously not ready for discharge (1); nor is he functioning independently (3).

Nursing Process: Evaluation
Client Needs: Health Promotion and Maintenance
Clinical Area: Psychiatric Nursing

64.   (2)   The solution of choice is D_5W. There is no reason at this time to administer a 10% dextrose solution. Until the ascites is treat-

Nursing Process: Planning
Client Needs: Physiological Integrity
Clinical Area: Medical Nursing

ed, solutions containing sodium are contraindicated because they foster fluid retention.

65. (3) Lasix promotes diuresis by preventing sodium and chloride reabsorption in the kidney tubules. Potassium and water loss occurs as well. The potassium loss could cause muscle weakness. Only if there were an excessive water loss would the client become tachycardic and have a headache. Dyspnea is not associated with the use of Lasix.

Nursing Process: Evaluation
Client Needs: Physiological Integrity
Clinical Area: Medical Nursing

66. (2) Paranoid disorders are characterized by delusions of persecution but not by the other classic symptoms of schizophrenia, such as associative looseness, affective disturbance, autism, and ambivalence. Clients with this disorder have emotional behaviors that are appropriate to the content of the delusional system.

Nursing Process: Analysis
Client Needs: Psychosocial Integrity
Clinical Area: Psychiatric Nursing

67. (1) Although the other answers are important, it is critical that the client be evaluated for further violence potential. Ideas of persecution can lead to violence so this behavior must be evaluated.

Nursing Process: Evaluation
Client Needs: Health Promotion and Maintenance
Clinical Area: Psychiatric Nursing

68. (2) The physician should be notified immediately. A suspected Wilms' tumor should never be palpated more than necessary because of the potential for metastasis and should be treated immediately following discovery. It is really not a nursing responsibility to assess for lymph node enlargement.

Nursing Process: Implementation
Client Needs: Safe, Effective Care Environment
Clinical Area: Pediatric Nursing

69. (3) At 12 months, the child should be starting to walk. A hospitalization at this stage could delay this developmental stage. The child should sit by six months and already be crawling.

Nursing Process: Analysis
Client Needs: Psychosocial Integrity
Clinical Area: Pediatric Nursing

70. (4)   The affected leg should always be kept at an angle of at least 20 degrees from the bed. Weights are never lifted up; this action could undo all of the reduction that has already occurred.

Nursing Process: Planning
Client Needs: Safe, Effective Care Environment
Clinical Area: Surgical Nursing

71. (2)   Concentrations above 40 percent may cause damage to the retinas, which later may lead to severe sight limitation or blindness. Oxygen levels must be monitored carefully and the infant should not receive more than it needs.

Nursing Process: Implementation
Client Needs: Safe, Effective Care Environment
Clinical Area: Pediatric Nursing

72. (1)   Respiratory acidosis is specifically due to retention of carbon dioxide. This is a result of inadequate pulmonary ventilation caused by atelectasis which results when hyaline membrane develops in the bronchial tree.

Nursing Process: Analysis
Client Needs: Physiological Integrity
Clinical Area: Pediatric Nursing

73. (1)   Placental insufficiency is a primary cause of SGA. It may result from an embryonic placental deficiency, hypertension, maternal smoking, maternal malnutrition, aging, and other associated causes.

Nursing Process: Implementation
Client Needs: Physiological Integrity
Clinical Area: Maternity Nursing

74. (1)   Reflux of nasopharyngeal secretions into the middle ear can occur when a child swallows while lying in the supine position.

Nursing Process: Planning
Client Needs: Health Promotion and Maintenance
Clinical Area: Pediatric Nursing

75. (4)   Hearing loss can follow otitis media particularly if there were repeated episodes of otitis. Affected children should have audiometric follow-up.

Nursing Process: Evaluation
Client Needs: Safe, Effective Care Environment
Clinical Area: Pediatric Nursing

76. (3)   Both eyes are bandaged to prevent movement in either eye. When one eye moves, the other eye follows. By preventing movement, the extension of complications can be prevented. Positioning of clients is usually done with the area of detachment in a dependent position.

Nursing Process: Planning
Client Needs: Safe, Effective Care Environment
Clinical Area: Surgical Nursing

Deep breathing is done, but coughing
increases intraocular pressure and it
should be discouraged or prevented by use
of antitussives.

77.   (4)   A bath in bed is the most likely choice,   *Nursing Process:* Implementation
as the client will still have patches on both   *Client Needs:* Safe, Effective Care Environment
eyes and be on bedrest. Coughing could   *Clinical Area:* Surgical Nursing
increase intraocular pressure which could
lead to hemorrhage.

78.   (1)   Persons predisposed to middle-aged   *Nursing Process:* Analysis
depression tend to have been rigid and   *Client Needs:* Psychosocial Integrity
self-sacrificing and spent their personal   *Clinical Area:* Psychiatric Nursing
time meeting other people's needs. When
there is no longer a focus for their self-sac-
rifice, depression may ensue. They probably did not have a long history of depression or suicidal thoughts.

79.   (4)   Caring is conveyed through acknowl-   *Nursing Process:* Implementation
edgment. Asking the client if she would   *Client Needs:* Safe, Effective Care Environment
like to talk allows her the choice whether   *Clinical Area:* Psychiatric Nursing
or not to discuss the suicide attempt at this
time. Revealing personal feelings is inappropriate and ignoring the attempt will
close off communication.

80.   (3)   The priority intervention is to place   *Nursing Process:* Implementation
the client in a side-lying position to facili-   *Client Needs:* Safe, Effective Care Environment
tate uterine-placental perfusion. The physi-   *Clinical Area:* Maternity Nursing
cian should be notified after the client is
positioned. Depending on the severity of
the placenta previa, a C-section may be
imminent. Pelvic exams are to be avoided
to prevent additional bleeding.

81.   (3)   Bleeding is a common postoperative   *Nursing Process:* Planning
complication; therefore, monitoring the   *Client Needs:* Safe, Effective Care Environment
lochia will provide data to support a deci-   *Clinical Area:* Maternity Nursing
sion on whether hemorrhage is occurring.
Infection may occur later.

82. (3) The Parkland formula is calculated at 4 ml/kg body weight/percent of body burn; therefore, 4 ml x 90 kg x 50% = 18,000 ml. (Remember that it is only calculated to a total of 50% body burn.) He is to receive half of this fluid, or 1125 ml/hour, in the first eight hours to maintain the intravascular compartment.

Nursing Process: Planning
Client Needs: Physiological Integrity
Clinical Area: Medical Nursing

83. (4) Ringer's lactate is the fluid replacement of choice. Five percent dextrose solutions are not given in the first 24 hours because a stress-induced pseudodiabetes often occurs after major burns. Administration of more dextrose would increase the possibility of hyperosmolar disease. Many physicians do not order colloids to be given in the first 24 hours because the burn causes generalized increased capillary permeability. The colloids leak out of the burn area into areas such as the pulmonary interstitial spaces and may cause pulmonary edema.

Nursing Process: Planning
Client Needs: Physiological Integrity
Clinical Area: Medical Nursing

84. (1) Upper airway burns (to the head, neck, chest) cause local edema which may produce mechanical occlusion of the airway manifested by hoarseness and stridor. Smoke inhalation can cause parenchymal changes from superheated gases and/or toxic chemicals. The parenchyma is generally unaffected in upper airway burns.

Nursing Process: Assessment
Client Needs: Physiological Integrity
Clinical Area: Medical Nursing

85. (4) Usually, a shower with detergent soap is taken the night before and morning of surgery. Particular attention should be paid to cleansing around the glans to rid it of microorganisms. An increased fluid intake and a good diet are essential to prevent urinary tract infections postop. Clients are not impotent following surgery.

Nursing Process: Implementation
Client Needs: Safe, Effective Care Environment
Clinical Area: Surgical Nursing

86. (1) Hemorrhage is the major early complication due to the manipulation by the instrument in resecting away the prostatic tissue. The use of continuous drainage assists in preventing hemorrhage. Observation of the type of drainage facilitates early detection of excessive bleeding.

Nursing Process: Evaluation
Client Needs: Physiological Integrity
Clinical Area: Surgical Nursing

87. (3) In children with cleft lip, suction cannot be created for effective sucking and frequently formula accumulates in the mouth and returns through the nose. Otitis media is a major problem, but upper respiratory tract infections are not associated with this condition any more frequently than with other conditions. Lack of normal dental function does occur, but it is not a major problem at this stage of the infant's development.

Nursing Process: Analysis
Client Needs: Health Promotion and Maintenance
Clinical Area: Pediatric Nursing

88. (3) The suture area must be kept clean to prevent infection. Strain on the sutures must always be prevented by using a Logan Bar.

Nursing Process: Implementation
Client Needs: Safe, Effective Care Environment
Clinical Area: Pediatric Nursing

89. (2) After seven days the sutures have probably been removed, and the presence of serosanguineous wound drainage lasting a few hours to several days is nearly always a sign of impending dehiscence.

Nursing Process: Evaluation
Client Needs: Safe, Effective Care Environment
Clinical Area: Surgical Nursing

90. (1) Diets are individualized, and generally clients are able to eat the same foods they enjoyed preoperatively. Fresh fruits may cause diarrhea in some, but not all, individuals.

Nursing Process: Evaluation
Client Needs: Health Promotion and Maintenance
Clinical Area: Surgical Nursing

Comprehensive Test 3

1. Assessing a client who has possible carcinoma of the stomach, the nurse would understand that the symptoms of stomach cancer occur

   1. Early in the disease state before a tumor is palpable or visible on x-rays.
   2. When the tumor is large enough to be seen on x-rays but is not palpable.
   3. Usually after the disease has spread to other organs and is incurable.
   4. Only in the terminal stages of the disease.

2. A child, age two years, is brought to the emergency room by his father. He has bruises on his head, face and mouth, and reddened areas at his wrists. He appears fearful. The nurse suspects child abuse. The nurse should be aware that 75 percent of abused children are

   1. Under six months of age.
   2. Under three years of age.
   3. From three to five years old.
   4. Under two years of age.

3. The nurse should understand that parents who abuse their children usually

   1. Have adequate impulse control.
   2. Do not have unreasonable expectations of their child.
   3. Care what happens to their child.
   4. Blame themselves for the injury.

4. The nurse, counseling a client who may be pregnant, explains that urine pregnancy tests are based on the presence of

   1. Estrogen.
   2. Progesterone.
   3. Testosterone.
   4. Chorionic gonadotropin.

5. Reviewing a client's chart who has been diagnosed with CA of the stomach, laboratory test results consistent with this diagnosis would be

   1. SGOT 40.
   2. Serum ammonia 40 u/100 ml.
   3. Hgb 8 gm/100 ml; Hct 30%.
   4. WBC 10,000; Eosinophils 2%.

6. A 36-year-old client has a history of rheumatic heart disease with cardiac arrhythmias. She was diagnosed as having mitral valve stenosis. When she is admitted to the emergency room with a rapid, irregular heart rhythm, the nurse determines that the arrhythmia is most likely

   1. Ventricular flutter.
   2. Ventricular tachycardia.
   3. First degree A-V block.
   4. Atrial fibrillation.

7. A 22-year-old schizophrenic is scheduled for discharge after having been in the hospital

for three weeks. The last day there is a change in his behavior and he appears very anxious. The most likely cause of the sudden appearance of anxiety is

1. Exacerbation of the acute stage.
2. Reluctance to terminate the relationship with the nurse.
3. Concern about independence and living on his own.
4. Return of paranoid ideas caused by the anxiety.

8. A newly pregnant client asks the nurse why her physician told her to discontinue taking all unnecessary drugs during pregnancy. The nurse's reply, based on the understanding of the relationship between drugs and the fetus, is

1. "Your physician is just being safe. There is some research to support the belief that common drugs affect the fetus."
2. "Some drugs can cause deformity, but most do not pass on to the fetus."
3. "All drugs can cross the placental barrier and may be dangerous."
4. "Drugs should be avoided in pregnancy only during the last trimester."

9. Adequate nutrition is essential during early pregnancy for optimum fetal development. The nurse, in counseling a client, would recommend a daily diet that would include

1. Low roughage foods.
2. One fruit or vegetable high in vitamin C.
3. A low sodium diet.
4. 1500 calories.

10. The nurse will evaluate the client for a major complication that can occur from an arrhythmia, which is

1. Development of microemboli in the kidneys.
2. Cerebral vascular accident.
3. Respiratory distress.
4. Complete heart block.

11. When a client with the diagnosis of schizophrenia is having an anxiety attack before an impending discharge, which of the following nursing actions would be the most therapeutic?

1. Recommending to the psychiatrist that the client be kept in the hospital until he can control his anxiety.
2. Letting the client know that the nurse is aware he is having difficulty.
3. Assessing the degree to which the client wants to go home.
4. Telling the client that his behavior is inappropriate.

12. Following a fall from a tricycle, a two year old is assessed for increased intracranial pressure. The nurse would expect to identify

1. Narrowing pulse pressure, tachycardia.
2. Widening pulse pressure, headache.
3. Hypotension, tachypnea.
4. Tachycardia, hypertension.

13. When a child with increased intracranial pressure is treated with steroids and mannitol, his condition improves. Which of the following positions would be the most therapeutic for this child?

1. Semi-Fowler's position.
2. Sims' position.
3. Prone position.
4. Supine position.

14. A female client, pregnant for the first time, has been admitted in labor and is about 6 cm dilated. From a nursing assessment, the nurse knows that her water has broken and that the baby is in an oblique lie position. Understanding this, the nurse knows that she should assess for a

1. Prolapsed umbilical cord.
2. Quicker than normal labor.
3. Baby born feet first.
4. Baby born head first.

15. A 36-year-old client is brought to the hospital complaining of rapid heartbeat, diarrhea, dry mouth, and shortness of breath. She says that she feels like she is having a heart attack. The immediate nursing action will be to

1. Assess the client's physical and emotional state.
2. Implement an anxiety-reducing activity.
3. Analyze what triggered the symptoms.
4. Explore her behavior and feelings.

16. A 12 year old has just been returned to the unit following a tonsillectomy. A priority nursing intervention during the postoperative period is to

1. Administer oral analgesics every four hours.
2. Place the client in a semi-Fowler's position.
3. Apply warm compresses to the surgical site.
4. Provide cool water or apple juice to drink.

17. A 28-year-old male client is admitted to the hospital for a suspected brain tumor. While assessing this client, the nurse would keep in mind that the most reliable index of cerebral status is

1. Pupil response.
2. Deep tendon reflexes.
3. Muscle strength.
4. Level of consciousness.

18. A change in blood pressure that indicates increasing intracranial pressure occurs when the

1. Diastolic pressure rises rapidly.
2. Pulse pressure widens.
3. Diastolic pressure decreases.
4. Pulse pressure narrows.

19. The nurse would determine that a client is experiencing Cheyne-Stokes respiration when he has

1. Periods of hyperpnea alternating with periods of apnea.
2. Periods of tachypnea alternating with periods of apnea.
3. An increase in both rate and depth of respirations.
4. Deep, regular, sighing respirations.

20. Following a cerebral arteriogram, the nurse observes that the client may be having a reaction to the dye. The sign or symptom leading to this conclusion is

1. A severe headache.
2. Numbness of the extremities.
3. Hypertension.
4. Polyuria.

21. A four year old is diagnosed as being moderately retarded (evidencing cognitive

impairment). The nurse is aware that the child probably has an IQ that is

1. 20–35.
2. 35–55.
3. 50–65.
4. 65–80.

22. The type of training found to be very successful with mentally retarded children is

1. Structured.
2. Self-pacing.
3. Behavior modification.
4. Unstructured.

23. Following surgery for repair of an inguinal hernia, the nurse establishes a postoperative fluid intake goal for the client. The most appropriate amount would be

1. 500–700 ml/day.
2. 1000–1500 ml/day.
3. 2000–3000 ml/day.
4. 3000–3500 ml/day.

24. Basilar crackles are present in a client's lungs on auscultation. The nurse knows that these are discrete, noncontinuous sounds that are

1. Caused by the sudden opening of alveoli.
2. Usually more prominent during expiration.
3. Produced by air flow across passages narrowed by secretions.
4. Found primarily in the pleura.

25. A client has an IV running, orders for oxygen, prn orders for Lasix, and bedrest. After determining that the client has fluid overload, the first nursing action will be to

1. Administer the standing order for Lasix.
2. Place in Fowler's position to decrease venous return.
3. Turn the IV off to reduce fluid intake.
4. Administer O_2 for shortness of breath.

26. A client has an order for Lasix 40 mgm IV. Following the Lasix administration, the nurse will evaluate for one of the major complications that occurs with the loss of

1. Sodium chloride.
2. Potassium chloride.
3. Chloride.
4. Bicarbonate.

27. A pregnant client with diabetes is controlled by insulin. When she asks the nurse what will happen to her insulin requirements during pregnancy, the correct response is

1. "Because your case is so mild, you are likely not to need much insulin during your pregnancy."
2. "It's likely that as the pregnancy progresses to term you will need increased insulin."
3. "Every case is individual so there is really no way to know."
4. "If you follow the diet closely and don't gain too much weight, your insulin needs should stay about the same."

28. A diabetic client who has just learned that she is pregnant seems to be concerned about something. On further inquiry she asks the nurse what her pregnancy will be like. The best response is

1. "Because your diabetes is well-controlled, your pregnancy should be normal."

2. "It should go well, and toward the end we will do tests to see if you need to have an early delivery."

3. "It's hard to say for sure; everything should go well and your regular attendance at clinic will help ensure that everything is fine."

4. "It should be fairly normal. Tell me what you expect and what you know about diabetics and pregnancy."

29. The nurse in the newborn nursery understands that assessing a newborn with a diabetic mother, the insulin level would be

   1. Higher than in normal infants.
   2. Lower than in normal infants.
   3. The same as in normal infants.
   4. Varied from baby to baby.

30. In the nurse's first assessment of a client just admitted to the psychiatric unit with a tentative diagnosis of depressive episode, she seems very despondent and refuses to get out of bed. She says, "I've screwed everything up. It's hopeless. It's no use." The nurse should anticipate and plan that the client may

   1. Be able to utilize the next group therapy session.
   2. Need to be observed carefully as she might attempt to hurt herself.
   3. Became angry and hostile as time goes on.
   4. Begin to verbalize her feelings and this is the first step in rehabilitation.

31. The immediate medical/nursing management of a child admitted to the hospital for an acute asthma attack will include

1. Rigorous percussion and postural drainage, high concentrations of oxygen.
2. Metered-dose steroid inhaler, instruction in breathing exercises.
3. High-Fowler's position, low concentrations of oxygen.
4. Side-lying position, parenteral methotrexate.

32. Formulating a nursing care plan for a 9-year-old asthmatic child, the first priority would be to

   1. Accept that the physical symptoms are real.
   2. Provide a nonthreatening environment.
   3. Reduce demands on the child.
   4. Assess the total range of symptoms.

33. Assessing a client with arterial insufficiency, the nurse knows that the first test required to establish the diagnosis is

   1. Trendelenburg's exercise studies.
   2. Dye injection studies.
   3. Leg circumference measurements.
   4. Doppler ultrasound studies.

34. Assessing a client with arterial insufficiency, the nurse expects to find

   1. Edema of the affected extremity.
   2. Extreme pain on walking.
   3. Very cold extremity.
   4. Pallor of the affected extremity.

35. In developing a nursing care plan for a client with Raynaud's disease, it is essential to include

   1. Buerger-Allen exercises.
   2. Exercises to increase collateral circulation.

3. Thigh high TEDs at all times.
4. Side effects of drug therapy.

36. A new mother asks about the drops that are put in the baby's eyes at birth and whether or not all babies must have them. The nurse explains that

1. Silver nitrate or penicillin is used to prevent the infant from catching herpes.
2. Silver nitrate or erythromycin is required by state law to be administered to all newborns.
3. Sterile water and silver nitrate are used to cleanse the baby's eyes.
4. Liquid steroids are used to reduce inflammation of the eyes.

37. As the nurse is teaching a class on labor and delivery, she explains that engagement is a term used to describe the position of the infant's head during labor. Engagement occurs when the

1. Head is in the left occipital position for birth.
2. Head is at the level of the ischial spines.
3. Biparietal diameter of the head passes the inlet.
4. Head is visible on the perineal floor.

38. A client with a history of cholecystitis is now being admitted to the hospital for possible surgical intervention. The orders include NPO, IV therapy, and bedrest. In addition to assessing for nausea, vomiting and anorexia, the nurse should observe for pain

1. In the right lower quadrant.
2. After ingesting food.
3. Radiating to the left shoulder.
4. In the right upper quadrant.

39. The urinalysis report of a client with cholecystitis indicates that she has increased bilirubin, .03 mg urobilinogen, sp. gr. 1.018, and catecholamines 12 ug/dl. The conclusion of the nurse is that the urinalysis indicates

1. A normal report.
2. Dehydration.
3. Biliary obstruction.
4. Acute liver disease.

40. While monitoring a client's blood transfusion, the nurse determines that a hemolysis reaction is occurring. The first nursing intervention is to

1. Slow down the transfusion.
2. Administer IV Benadryl.
3. Stop the transfusion.
4. Notify the physician.

41. The nurse knows that in assessing a client who has started a blood transfusion, an early indication of a transfusion reaction is

1. Urticaria and laryngeal edema.
2. Dyspnea and hives.
3. Hematuria and bronchospasm.
4. Fever and chills.

42. A major goal of treatment for a five year old with Legg-Perthes disease is aimed at

1. Preventing deformity in the shaft of the femur.
2. Preventing degenerative changes in the knee joint.
3. Reducing muscle spasm.
4. Preventing pressure on the head of the femur.

43. For a 5-year-old child on two weeks of bedrest, the best activity would be

1. Listening to the radio or watching TV.
2. Telling stories with puppets.
3. Reading books and comics.
4. Putting together airplane models.

44. Peritoneal dialysis is begun as a temporary treatment measure for a client who has failing kidneys. Monitoring the initial dialysate return, the nurse will immediately notify the physician if the return is

1. Bloody.
2. Brown.
3. Absent.
4. Yellow.

45. The most common complication resulting from peritoneal dialysis is

1. Muscle cramps.
2. Peritonitis.
3. Respiratory distress.
4. Paralytic ileus.

46. A client is scheduled for a kidney transplant. A medication she will probably take on a long-term basis that will require specific client teaching to ensure compliance is

1. Corticosteroids.
2. Antibiotics.
3. Anticoagulants.
4. Gamma globulin.

47. A newly admitted client to the psychiatric unit dresses in a skimpy nightie and approaches the male nurse. She states she is "coming down" and just needs a little comforting and conversation. The best initial response by the nurse would be

1. "Please go put on your bathrobe and then we can talk."

2. "I'm very busy now. Maybe the other nurse can spend some time with you."
3. "What seems to be the problem?"
4. "What you are experiencing is very common. It should get better soon."

48. A schedule of Valium withdrawal is ordered by the physician. As the dose is decreased, the nurse will expect to observe the client experiencing

1. Decreased blood pressure.
2. Tremors and hyperactivity.
3. Increased appetite.
4. Grandiose ideation.

49. Three days after admission for alcoholism, a client is seen in the hospital parking lot talking to a male visitor. When approached by the nurse about her leaving the unit without permission, she laughs and says, "I needed to see my old man. He's squeamish about hospitals, and ten minutes is no big deal." The best initial nursing response is

1. "Next time ask a staff member to accompany you."
2. "You do not have pass privileges and your willingness to follow the rules is essential to your treatment program."
3. "I'm going to have to report your activities to the physician."
4. "I can understand needing to see your friend, but next time invite him to the unit."

50. A client is brought into the recovery room following spinal anesthesia for removal of a cyst. The assessment that indicates a complication of anesthesia is

1. Hiccoughs.

2. Numbness.
3. Headache.
4. No urge to void.

51. A client is ten weeks pregnant and comes into the clinic for prenatal counseling. One of the concerns is her nutrition. The nurse would counsel the client that during her pregnancy she needs more of which one of the following nutrients?

   1. Potassium.
   2. Protein.
   3. Iron.
   4. Vitamin D.

52. A client with emphysema has the following arterial blood gases (ABG) drawn.

	FIO$_2$	pH	pCO$_2$	HCO$_3$	pO$_2$
ABG 1:	21%	7.35	50	27	48
ABG 2:	6 L O$_2$ NP	7.29	70	29	140

Changes the nurse might observe in a client at the time the second ABG sample was obtained are a/an

   1. Improvement of hypoxemia, decreased cyanosis, increased alertness.
   2. Increase in acid-base imbalance, improvement of hypoxemia, somnolence, and coma.
   3. Decreased cyanosis, agitation, improvement of acid-base imbalance.
   4. Increase in acid-base imbalance, somnolence, increased cyanosis.

53. During a normal pregnancy, the nurse would expect the client's blood pressure to show

1. A steady, sustained rise throughout pregnancy.
2. No change from baseline throughout pregnancy.
3. A slight decrease in the second trimester.
4. A small increase in the third trimester.

54. A client's pregnancy has progressed to the third trimester and she is demonstrating pregnancy induced hypertension (PIH). Which of the following treatment approaches is commonly used in the management of PIH?

   1. Sodium restricted diet.
   2. High-protein diet.
   3. Diuretic therapy.
   4. Weight gain restriction.

55. A client on the psychiatric unit is always trying to manipulate the staff as a way of getting his needs met. Which response would indicate that the nurse understands the psychodynamic principle behind manipulation?

   1. "I will not allow you to manipulate me."
   2. "If this behavior does not stop, I will tell the doctor."
   3. "Let's talk about your manipulative behavior."
   4. "I will not take you to the dining room to buy cigarettes, but I will stay and talk with you."

56. A 58-year-old client with a diagnosis of schizophrenia, chronic undifferentiated type is taking 400 mg of Thorazine tid. The nurse notices on morning rounds that he is drooling and flapping when he walks. The best nursing action would be to

1. Provide activities away from other clients so he will not be embarrassed.
2. Call the physician immediately about the toxic effects of the drug.
3. Chart the observations and request that the physician call the unit.
4. Hold the client's noon dose of Thorazine.

57. If a client develops extrapyramidal side effects, the nurse would expect the physician to order

   1. Cogentin.
   2. Niamid.
   3. Ritalin.
   4. Atarax.

58. A concerned client asks the nurse what her Class I pap smear means. The appropriate response is that these results

   1. Show atypical cells present.
   2. Are strongly suggestive of malignancy.
   3. Show abnormal cells that may be malignant.
   4. Indicate that no abnormal or atypical cells were found.

59. When providing diversional activities for a child in isolation, it must be remembered that

   1. Articles brought to the unit should be washable or disposable.
   2. Articles are sent to Central Supply for gas sterilization before using.
   3. Toys should not have movable parts.
   4. Favorite toys will keep the child occupied for a longer period of time.

60. While on the unit one day, a nurse observes another nurse unlock the narcotic cabinet, look around, then put a vial of morphine sulfate in her pocket. The appropriate action under these circumstances is to

   1. Ignore the behavior this time, but keep your eye on the nurse.
   2. Confront the nurse and ask her why she is doing it.
   3. Tell the head nurse what you observed.
   4. Call the police, as you know taking narcotics is illegal.

61. A two year old has eaten half a bottle of his grandmother's ferrous sulfate tablets. They live 30 miles from the hospital. The first action is to tell the mother to

   1. Take the child to the hospital immediately.
   2. Give the child syrup of ipecac.
   3. Contact the poison control center by phone.
   4. Do nothing because vitamins are nonpoisonous.

62. The diet regimen usually prescribed for a child with noncomplicated acute glomerulonephritis is a

   1. Low sodium, high protein diet.
   2. Regular diet, no added salt.
   3. Low sodium, low protein diet.
   4. Low protein, low potassium diet.

63. The nurse realizes that the mother does not fully understand the significance of the effect the Rh factor will have on her future pregnancies. The nurse explains that the purpose of administering RhoGAM is to

prevent erythroblastosis fetalis in the next pregnancy, which could result in

1. Hydrops fetalis.
2. Hypobilirubinemia.
3. Congenital hypothermia.
4. Transient clotting difficulties.

64. A male client is admitted to the hospital and is diagnosed with kidney failure. The physician orders hemodialysis treatments. Immediately following hemodialysis, which of the following signs and symptoms would indicate the need to administer Dilantin, a prn medication?

1. Decreased blood pressure, rapid pulse.
2. Nausea, vomiting, twitching.
3. Pain and tingling at the access site.
4. Muscle cramps, headache.

65. The nurse would expect to find an improvement in which of the blood values as a result of the dialysis treatment?

1. High serum creatinine levels.
2. Low hemoglobin.
3. Hypocalcemia.
4. Hypokalemia.

66. A six-week-old baby is admitted to the hospital with a possible diagnosis of pyloric stenosis. While obtaining a nursing history, the nurse will chart other symptoms that the mother would have observed, such as

1. Bile-stained emesis, abrupt onset of projectile vomiting.
2. Gradual onset of projectile vomiting, weight loss.
3. Abdominal pain, vomiting.
4. Weight loss, abdominal pain.

67. In the preoperative period for correction of pyloric stenosis, nursing care for the baby will include placing him

1. In a prone position.
2. In semi-Fowler's position on his left side.
3. In Fowler's position or on his right side.
4. In Sims' position.

68. A female client is admitted to the therapeutic community with a diagnosis of conversion disorder with symptoms of aphonia. The nurse understands which of the following statements is true about conversion disorder?

1. Conversion disorders are consciously triggered.
2. A high level of anxiety underlies the symptom of aphasia.
3. The client's aphasia is always symbolic of a basic problem.
4. The client will exhibit increased affect proportionate to the severity of her symptoms.

69. A young man who accidentally came in contact with a high-tension electrical wire has a small injury on his right hand and on his left calf. When his family arrives at the hospital, they are understandably distraught and want to know exactly how he is and what will happen to him. The most therapeutic response is to say,

1. "He is doing well, although he may be in the hospital for some time."
2. "He has received an electrical burn. His condition is stable, and we will keep you informed of any change."
3. "He has received an electrical burn which caused coagulation of some tissues."
4. "He does not appear to have much damage and should be fine soon."

70. Burn clients require continuous emotional support. Evaluating the nursing care of this type of client, the nurse will know that the client will receive therapeutic support by which of the following nursing actions?

    1. The staff keeping his room neat and clean.
    2. Rotating the staff so he could have varied interactions.
    3. Reacting to him as an individual by spending time with him.
    4. Keeping family members aware of his condition.

71. A 58-year-old female client is in the hospital for the second time, diagnosed with myxedema. Considering the diagnosis, the initial assessment should reveal symptoms that include

    1. Bradycardia, heart failure, weight loss, diarrhea.
    2. Lethargy, weight gain, slow speech, decreased respiratory rate.
    3. Tachycardia, constipation, exophthalmos.
    4. Hypothermia, weight loss, increased respiratory rate.

72. Certain physiological changes will result from the therapy for myxedema. The symptoms that may indicate adverse changes in the body that the nurse should observe for are

    1. Increased respiratory excursion.
    2. Increased pulse and cardiac output.
    3. Hyperglycemia.
    4. Weight loss, nervousness and insomnia.

73. The nurse is assigned to work on a unit that has a group of autistic children as inpa-

tients. They have all been on the unit for at least six months and exhibit self-destructive and withdrawn behavior as well as bizarre responses. As a new member of the health team, the nurse knows that the first goal is to

    1. Set limits on their behavior so the children will perceive the nurse as an authority figure.
    2. Assess each child's individual developmental level so the nurse will have the data for realistic care plans.
    3. Understand that the children must be protected from self-destructive behavior.
    4. Establish some method of relating to the children, either verbal or nonverbal.

74. One day an autistic child of seven tells the male nurse that he is afraid because the nurse is a big person. The nurse would best respond to this communication by saying

    1. "I won't hurt you."
    2. "What are you afraid of?"
    3. "I wouldn't hurt you."
    4. "My bigness frightens you?"

75. Following surgery for hernia repair, nursing measures to prevent the complications of deep vein thrombophlebitis include

    1. Placing a pillow under the affected limb.
    2. Wearing thigh-high elastic hose at all times.
    3. Having the client out of bed several times per day.
    4. Lowering the foot of the bed.

76. Following delivery of a healthy baby, the nurse completes a postpartum assessment of the new mother. Which of the following

symptoms would be indicative of a full bladder?

1. Increased uterine contractions.
2. Decreased lochia.
3. Fundus 2F above umbilicus.
4. Pulse 52 beats/minute.

77. A 22-month-old child has just been admitted to the pediatric unit for a fractured right femur. Observing Bryant's traction to determine if it is properly assembled, the nurse will expect to see the

1. Moleskin taut and placed on either side of the lower leg to provide traction.
2. Weights attached to a pin which is inserted in the femur.
3. Pin site and weights aligned in a horizontal position.
4. Weights attached to skin traction and hung freely from the crib.

78. A client involved in a knifing was admitted through the emergency room and is now in the ICU. His admission assessment reveals shallow and rapid respirations, paradoxical pulse, CVP 15 cm H_2O, BP 90 mmHg systolic, skin cold and pale, urinary output 70 ml over the last two hours. From these findings, the nurse concludes that he may be developing

1. Hypovolemic shock.
2. Cardiac tamponade.
3. Sepsis.
4. Atelectasis.

79. A client the nurse is assessing appears to be having respiratory difficulty. The condition that leads the nurse to determine he is hypoxic is

1. Bradycardia.
2. Agitation.
3. Mucosal cyanosis.
4. Decreased blood pressure.

80. A 35-year-old client is 36 weeks pregnant and has been admitted to the obstetrical unit for continuous close observation. She confides to the nurse that she doesn't think she will ever be a mother and begins to cry. The best nursing response is to

1. Reassure her that advanced medical knowledge will detect any problems that may be present with this pregnancy.
2. Sit quietly with her and follow her cues.
3. Suggest that she discuss her fears with her physician.
4. Gently change the subject to something more positive.

81. A client, 36 weeks pregnant, is induced with oxytocin (Pitocin). One of the most important observations is the duration of the resting phase between the end of one contraction and the beginning of the next. The nurse knows that a resting phase should not be less than

1. 15 seconds.
2. 30 seconds.
3. 45 seconds.
4. 60 seconds.

82. A client has been admitted to the hospital with symptoms of weakness, weight loss and anorexia. The provisional diagnosis is cancer of the colon. The nurse observes that the client has remained very quiet. The nurse understands that her actions are probably due to

1. Trying to be a good client.
2. Denying the situation.
3. Shyness and fear of asking questions.
4. Feeling anger toward the hospital staff.

83. Evaluating the effectiveness of preoperative teaching before colostomy surgery, the nurse expects that the client will be able to

    1. Describe how the procedure will be done.
    2. Exhibit her acceptance of the surgery.
    3. Explain the function of the colostomy.
    4. Apply the colostomy bag correctly.

84. A 16 year old is hospitalized for adolescent adjustment problems. After assessing her, the nurse's first objective is to establish a nurse-client relationship. The next day the nurse is late for the appointment. Knowing that the client has difficulty assuming responsibility for her own behavior, the nurse would like to use this situation as an opportunity for role modeling. The most appropriate statement the nurse could make is

    1. "I'm late. I apologize."
    2. "Thank goodness you are still here; I just had a flat tire."
    3. "Oh, you are here. I thought we'd be arriving at the same time."
    4. "What do you mean you are angry with me? I bet you keep people waiting."

85. The nurse is assigned to do a home visit for a new mother one week postpartum. In the assessment, leg edema and a slight temperature are noted. Aside from advising her to see the physician immediately, the nurse would tell her that she should *not*

    1. Elevate the leg.

2. Apply warmth to the leg.
3. Decrease leg movement.
4. Gently massage the painful area of the leg.

86. A new mother is breast-feeding her infant and intends to do so until the baby is about a year old. She asks the nurse if childhood immunizations have to be given because she is breast-feeding. The best response is

    1. "Immunizations should start as soon as you begin to wean the baby."
    2. "Immunizations should begin as soon as possible because they will be needed for the childhood diseases you have not had."
    3. "If the baby was put to breast for the colostrum, they are not necessary until breast-feeding stops."
    4. "Immunizations should be given on the same schedule as nonbreast-fed babies."

87. Following laminectomy surgery, the client returns from the recovery room to the surgical unit. The nurse would anticipate that the most common complication following anesthesia would be

    1. Atelectasis.
    2. Pneumonia.
    3. Paralytic ileus.
    4. Edema.

88. Following surgery, a client has shallow respirations and he is restless. The best nursing procedure to prevent atelectasis is to have him deep breathe every two hours. The first nursing action before attempting to deep breathe the client is to

    1. Ask him if he feels like participating in the exercise.

2. Ask him to cooperate with the procedure.
3. Medicate him with his prn pain medication.
4. Turn him on his side to reduce pressure.

89. A client asks the nurse to again explain the purpose of the amniocentesis test. The nurse responds that one purpose of this test is to indicate the

    1. Accurate age of the fetus.
    2. Presence of certain congenital anomalies.
    3. Biparietal diameter of the fetal skull.
    4. Hormone content of the amniotic fluid.

90. A client is admitted to the surgical unit for a scheduled above-the-knee amputation with a delayed prosthesis fitting. Preoperatively, the nurse can best assist the client by instructing him to do

    1. Sit-up exercises.
    2. Upper body strengthening exercises.
    3. Strengthening exercises with his other leg.
    4. No exercises until the postoperative period.

Comprehensive Test 3
Answers with Rationale

1. (3) Usually the client experiences no symptoms until the growth spreads to nearby organs. At that time, he may experience nonspecific symptoms such as weight loss, flatulence, loss of appetite, and weakness. If the cancer metastasizes to the liver, jaundice with bleeding tendencies may occur.

    Nursing Process: Analysis
    Client Needs: Physiological Integrity
    Clinical Area: Medical Nursing

2. (2) Studies indicate that 75 percent of abused children are under the age of three years and 25 percent are under one year.

    Nursing Process: Analysis
    Client Needs: Health Promotion and Maintenance
    Clinical Area: Pediatric Nursing

3. (3) Parents who abuse their children often care very much about them, but they have very little understanding of how to deal with crises and the child's frustrating behavior. They have low impulse control (1) and unreasonable expectations (2) of their child. They do not usually blame themselves for injuries.

    Nursing Process: Analysis
    Client Needs: Health Promotion and Maintenance
    Clinical Area: Pediatric Nursing

4. (4) The presence of chorionic gonadotropin in the maternal plasma and its excretion in the urine are the basis for urinary immunologic pregnancy tests.

    Nursing Process: Implementation
    Client Needs: Health Promotion and Maintenance
    Clinical Area: Maternity Nursing

5. (3) The Hgb and Hct are decreased; normal serum levels for males are Hgb >12 and Hct 40–54%. These levels would be expected to be decreased if the client were bleeding from the area of the lesion. SGOT is an enzyme found mainly in the liver; the normal levels are 8–46 u/L in males, or 7–34 u/L in females. If there was liver

    Nursing Process: Analysis
    Client Needs: Physiological Integrity
    Clinical Area: Medical Nursing

involvement, the SGOT would be released into the blood and the levels would be increased. The WBC would increase if infection were present (normal range is 4500–11,000). The eosinophil count would increase in parasitic infestation, normal values for adults are 1%–4% (50–400 u/L).

6.   (4)   In atrial fibrillation, the atrial and ventricular rate are not equal. There are frequently two, three, or even four atrial beats for each ventricular response. Normal sinus rhythm has a regular rate with a normal P-R interval of 0.12–0.20 seconds. Atrial flutter would be irregular. Each QRS would be preceded by several flutter waves which are sawtooth in appearance. First-degree heart block would have the same appearance as normal sinus rhythm except that the conduction time from the SA node to the AV node is prolonged, revealing a prolonged P-R interval.

Nursing Process: Analysis
Client Needs: Physiological Integrity
Clinical Area: Medical Nursing

7.   (3)   While reluctance to terminate may be a source of anxiety, the fears around being independent and responsible for himself after discharge would most probably be the greatest source of anxiety in this client situation. Feeling anxious would not necessarily increase paranoid thinking.

Nursing Process: Analysis
Client Needs: Psychosocial Integrity
Clinical Area: Psychiatric Nursing

8.   (3)   All drugs may be expected to cross the placental barrier and are especially damaging during the first eight weeks, when fetal organogenesis is taking place. Drugs taken in later pregnancy may also affect the fetus, their effects not being known for years. Even drugs taken during labor may have a depressive effect upon the CNS of the fetus and may take several days to wear off. Nicotine from smoking may cause low birth weight infants as well as congenital defects.

Nursing Process: Implementation
Client Needs: Safe, Effective Care Environment
Clinical Area: Maternity Nursing

9. (2)   The diet must include at least one fruit or vegetable high in vitamin C, and should include a total of four fruits and vegetables. Pregnancy requires the addition of 300 calories a day over regular caloric intake, and 1500 calories a day would be inadequate. The recommended calories for someone aged 28 are 2300 a day. Research indicates that sodium is essential during pregnancy.

Nursing Process: Planning
Client Needs: Health Promotion and Maintenance
Clinical Area: Maternity Nursing

10. (2)   Because the atria do not fully empty, emboli can form there. These emboli then travel to the left ventricle and to the cerebral vessels. Microemboli occur in very small peripheral vessels. PVCs result from decreased myocardial oxygen and increased ventricular irritability. Complete heart block occurs from damage to the conduction system of the heart, which results from myocardial infarction.

Nursing Process: Evaluation
Client Needs: Physiological Integrity
Clinical Area: Medical Nursing

11. (2)   Providing the client the opportunity to discuss his feelings by letting him know the nurse is aware of his problem is the best approach. (1) is not helpful because learning to cope with life's difficulties requires that the client confront his problems and explore ways to cope successfully. Postponing the inevitable discharge not only postpones the problem but also gives the client the message that the nurse does not believe he can cope. Neither (3) nor (4) is appropriate.

Nursing Process: Implementation
Client Needs: Safe, Effective Care Environment
Clinical Area: Psychiatric Nursing

12. (2)   Increased intracranial pressure can manifest itself in a variety of ways. Widening pulse pressure and headache are classical manifestations. As the pressure increases, the child will become lethargic and lapse into a coma. The child will also be restless, irritable, crying and vital signs will change.

Nursing Process: Assessment
Client Needs: Physiological Integrity
Clinical Area: Pediatric Nursing

13.   (1)   Semi-Fowler's is the most therapeutic position. It is important to elevate the head of the bed to reduce intracranial pressure and assist with drainage of any excess fluid that may have accumulated.

Nursing Process: Planning
Client Needs: Health Promotion and Maintenance
Clinical Area: Pediatric Nursing

14.   (1)   Without head or breech to occlude the cervix when the water breaks, the cord is more likely to prolapse.

Nursing Process: Assessment
Client Needs: Physiological Integrity
Clinical Area: Maternity Nursing

15.   (1)   An assessment is vital before interventions can be planned. After the assessment is made, it would be important to decrease the client's anxiety level and find out what triggered the symptoms. (4) would be part of the long-term planning.

Nursing Process: Assessment
Client Needs: Safe, Effective Care Environment
Clinical Area: Medical Nursing

16.   (4)   Apple juice or water is given as soon as the client is awake and not hemorrhaging. Avoidance of citrus juices will prevent irritation of the operative site. The client should be placed on his abdomen or side to facilitate drainage and prevent aspiration. Ice bags are applied to the neck to prevent edema and bleeding.

Nursing Process: Implementation
Client Needs: Safe, Effective Care Environment
Clinical Area: Surgical Nursing

17.   (4)   The state or level of consciousness is the most reliable index of cerebral status.

Nursing Process: Assessment
Client Needs: Physiological Integrity
Clinical Area: Medical Nursing

18.   (2)   The systolic pressure increases to maintain adequate cerebral blood flow. The diastolic pressure does not increase. This results in a widened pulse pressure and indicates increasing intracranial pressure.

Nursing Process: Evaluation
Client Needs: Physiological Integrity
Clinical Area: Medical Nursing

19.   (1)   Periods of hyperpnea alternating with apnea is a breathing pattern that is easily missed if the client's respirations are not observed for a few minutes. It may indicate disorders of cerebral circulation, increased cerebral pressure, and/or injury to the brain tissue.

Nursing Process: Analysis
Client Needs: Physiological Integrity
Clinical Area: Medical Nursing

20. (2) Numbness of the extremities is a
symptom of delayed reaction. Respiratory
distress is a frequent early sign of anaphy-
lactic shock. The release of histamine causes major vascular and bronchial symptoms
in anaphylaxia.

Nursing Process: Analysis
Client Needs: Physiological Integrity
Clinical Area: Surgical Nursing

21. (2) The moderately retarded child has an
IQ between 35 and 55 and is considered
trainable. Mildly retarded children have
IQs between 50–70; profoundly retarded
children have IQs below 25.

Nursing Process: Analysis
Client Needs: Health Promotion and Maintenance
Clinical Area: Pediatric Nursing

22. (3) Behavior modification, with its immediate reward system, is best understood by
slow children and they have shown more
improvement and mastery with this type
of training than with any other.

Nursing Process: Planning
Client Needs: Psychosocial Integrity
Clinical Area: Pediatric Nursing

23. (3) 2000–3000 ml/day would be a good
maintenance postsurgery. The client's
body will require additional fluids over the
minimum due to fluid loss and the recovery process after surgery. Minimum fluid
intake is considered 1500 ml per day.

Nursing Process: Planning
Client Needs: Safe, Effective Care Environment
Clinical Area: Surgical Nursing

24. (1) Basilar crackles are usually heard during inspiration and are caused by sudden
opening of alveoli.

Nursing Process: Analysis
Client Needs: Physiological Integrity
Clinical Area: Medical Nursing

25. (2) The first action would be to sit the
client up in order to ventilate his lungs.
Then the nurse might give O2 and subse-
quently administer the order for Lasix. The
diuretic will return the overhydrated body
to homeostasis. The IV will be decreased
but not turned off. There must be a patent
IV for drug administration.

Nursing Process: Implementation
Client Needs: Safe, Effective Care Environment
Clinical Area: Medical Nursing

26. (2) KCl is lost because Lasix is a loop
diuretic. If the potassium level goes below
3.5–4.5 mEq/l, the normal range, it must be
replaced to prevent cardiac complications.

Nursing Process: Evaluation
Client Needs: Physiological Integrity
Clinical Area: Medical Nursing

27.　(2)　Normal changes in pregnancy are affected by diabetes, usually causing an alteration in insulin requirements. Carbohydrate metabolism is affected early in pregnancy by a rise in serum levels of estrogen and progesterone. During the second half of pregnancy, there is a resistance to insulin, possibly due to elevated hormones. Insulin changes include requiring less insulin during the first trimester and requirements that can be doubled or quadrupled by the end of pregnancy.

Nursing Process: Implementation
Client Needs: Physiological Integrity
Clinical Area: Maternity Nursing

28.　(4)　All statements are fairly accurate, but (4) is the best choice because it provides baseline information of the client's knowledge and expectations which is extremely important before dealing with the issue of diabetes and pregnancy.

Nursing Process: Implementation
Client Needs: Psychosocial Integrity
Clinical Area: Maternity Nursing

29.　(1)　Insulin levels are increased in these infants because the mother's glucose readily crosses the placenta and stimulates the fetal pancreas to secrete increased levels of insulin. The fetal insulin does not cross the placenta.

Nursing Process: Assessment
Client Needs: Health Promotion and Maintenance
Clinical Area: Maternity Nursing

30.　(2)　The client appears to be despondent and depressed; therefore, it is vital that the nurse assess her suicide potential. The client also may attempt to harm herself to manipulate the staff. Saying she messed up does not necessarily mean she will be able to verbalize or work on her feelings. There is no indication she will turn the depression into anger.

Nursing Process: Planning
Client Needs: Safe, Effective Care Environment
Clinical Area: Psychiatric Nursing

31.　(3)　High-Fowler's position ensures maximal utilization of accessory muscles in the respiratory process and allows for maximal lung expansion. In addition, high concentrations of oxygen are never recommended for obstructive respiratory disorders

Nursing Process: Planning
Client Needs: Safe, Effective Care Environment
Clinical Area: Pediatric Nursing

because oxygen interferes with the chemoreceptor feedback mechanism and may decrease or eliminate the stimulus for breathing. Steroids may be given via an inhaler; however, the effectiveness of the drug is delayed for as long as six hours.

32.   (1)   Unless the nurse accepts the symptoms as real, she will be focusing totally on the emotional aspect of the disease. While a nursing care plan would include the other three answer alternatives, the first priority is to treat the "total" person.

Nursing Process: Planning
Client Needs: Safe, Effective Care Environment
Clinical Area: Pediatric Nursing

33.   (4)   The Doppler ultrasound flow meter is an external device used to determine blood flow in large vessels. The Trendelenburg's test is a retrograde filling test done to demonstrate varicose veins. Dye injection studies can be done after the initial Doppler studies.

Nursing Process: Assessment
Client Needs: Physiological Integrity
Clinical Area: Medical Nursing

34.   (1)   Due to increased venous pressure in the leg veins, fluid leaks into the interstitial spaces causing edema. Arterial circulation is not compromised, so the extremity is still warm. Movement of the extremity does not increase the pain. Pallor is due to arterial rather than venous circulatory problems.

Nursing Process: Assessment
Client Needs: Physiological Integrity
Clinical Area: Medical Nursing

35.   (4)   Drug therapy is the treatment of choice for Raynaud's disease; therefore, instructions in the side effects of these agents is paramount. Buerger-Allen exercises improve peripheral arterial circulation and are used in the treatment of Buerger's disease.

Nursing Process: Planning
Client Needs: Safe, Effective Care Environment
Clinical Area: Medical Nursing

36.   (2)   Each state has regulations regarding the prophylactic treatment of newborn's eyes against gonococcal infection. Silver nitrate and erythromycin are the two medications most commonly used.

Nursing Process: Implementation
Client Needs: Physiological Integrity
Clinical Area: Maternity Nursing

37. (3) Engagement occurs when the biparietal diameter of the infant's head passes the inlet. All of the other answers are incorrect.

Nursing Process: Analysis
Client Needs: Health Promotion and Maintenance
Clinical Area: Maternity Nursing

38. (4) Pain occurs two to four hours after eating fatty foods and is located either in the epigastric region or in the upper right quadrant of the abdomen.

Nursing Process: Assessment
Client Needs: Safe, Effective Care Environment
Clinical Area: Surgical Nursing

39. (3) In biliary obstruction urobilinogen is decreased, the normal is 0 to 4 mg/24 hours. Urine bilirubin is increased with an obstruction; normally none is found in the urine.

Nursing Process: Evaluation
Client Needs: Physiological Integrity
Clinical Area: Medical Nursing

40. (3) The first action would be to stop the transfusion to avoid administering any additional incompatible cells. The incompatible cells can lead to agglutination, oliguric renal failure, pulmonary emboli, and death if administered in large quantities. Some resources state that as little as 50 ml of incompatible blood can lead to severe complications and death.

Nursing Process: Implementation
Client Needs: Safe, Effective Care Environment
Clinical Area: Medical Nursing

41. (4) Fever and chills are the usual first symptoms of a hemolytic reaction. Urticaria is an early symptom of an allergic reaction. If the client is cyanotic, he probably has other complications associated with his illness, such as respiratory involvement. If the transfusion is greatly advanced, it may cause laryngeal edema or perhaps even a blood clot to the lung if a hemolytic reaction has occurred. Hematuria is not an initial symptom.

Nursing Process: Assessment
Client Needs: Physiological Integrity
Clinical Area: Medical Nursing

42. (4) Legg-Perthes disease affects the femoral epiphysis in which aseptic necrosis occurs. Pressure on the necrotic femur can cause permanent damage.

Nursing Process: Planning
Client Needs: Physiological Integrity
Clinical Area: Pediatric Nursing

43.   (2)   Fantasy is very active in this stage of development. Telling stories with puppets will allow for expression of feelings. Also, this activity is more active than TV or books and involves the nurse or parent with the child, providing a positive way of establishing or maintaining a relationship.

Nursing Process: Planning
Client Needs: Health Promotion and Maintenance
Clinical Area: Pediatric Nursing

44.   (2)   Brown dialysate indicates that stool is present in the dialysate and is the result of a perforated bowel. The initial outflow returns may be bloody due to the insertion of the peritoneal catheter. If there is no return, you would initially turn the client side to side to facilitate drainage.

Nursing Process: Assessment
Client Needs: Physiological Integrity
Clinical Area: Medical Nursing

45.   (2)   Peritonitis is the most common complication with peritoneal dialysis. Muscle cramps may occur with rapid shifts of electrolytes; however, this does not usually occur with peritoneal dialysis. Respiratory distress is caused by pressure of the dialysate on the diaphragm, resulting in decreased chest excursion which leads to ineffective gas exchange (O_2–CO_2).

Nursing Process: Assessment
Client Needs: Physiological Integrity
Clinical Area: Medical Nursing

46.   (1)   Prednisone, a corticosteroid, is the usual drug of choice. The other medication classifications are not used in the routine care of transplant clients.

Nursing Process: Planning
Client Needs: Health Promotion and Maintenance
Clinical Area: Surgical Nursing

47.   (1)   The nurse is matter-of-factly dealing with the client's inappropriate attire without rejecting her. Answers (2) and (3) are incorrect because they avoid the problem. (4) is incorrect in that it offers false reassurance.

Nursing Process: Implementation
Client Needs: Psychosocial Integrity
Clinical Area: Psychiatric Nursing

48.   (2)   Tremors and hyperactivity are common symptoms of Valium detoxification. Although blood pressure should be monitored, it generally does not decrease.

Nursing Process: Evaluation
Client Needs: Physiological Integrity
Clinical Area: Psychiatric Nursing

Increased appetite and grandiosity are not symptoms of detoxification.

49. (2) The nurse must be direct and firm with a potentially manipulative client. The client must be reminded about her agreement to obey unit rules immediately after she breaks them. The nurse will need to report the incident to the psychiatrist and other staff so they may all observe the client for illicit drug reactions and other similar behavior, but initially she needs to deal directly with the client.

Nursing Process: Implementation
Client Needs: Psychosocial Integrity
Clinical Area: Psychiatric Nursing

50. (3) Headache is a very common complication and is the result of nonsealing of the dura mater after the needle is removed. There is a leak of cerebral spinal fluid into the epidural space. The headache can last several days. Numbness and no urge to void are usual results of spinal anesthesia unless the symptoms continue for several hours. The complication of hiccoughs can be associated with abdominal surgery, but not in relation to spinal anesthesia.

Nursing Process: Assessment
Client Needs: Physiological Integrity
Clinical Area: Surgical Nursing

51. (3) Iron intake must be increased during pregnancy and, because sufficient amounts cannot be ingested, it is supplemented. Protein should include both animal and vegetable, but probably will not have to be increased.

Nursing Process: Implementation
Client Needs: Health Promotion and Maintenance
Clinical Area: Maternity Nursing

52. (2) The emphysemic client's drive to breathe is hypoxia. When the client was given FIO2 to return his arterial pO2 level to above normal, the peripheral chemoreceptors no longer could respond to hypoxia. The center chemoreceptors had been dulled over the years by the constant increased CO2 level so they did not respond to an increasing pCO2 level.

Nursing Process: Evaluation
Client Needs: Physiological Integrity
Clinical Area: Medical Nursing

Hypercarbia (increased pCO2) exhibits symptoms of somnolence and coma in the acute situation.

53. (3) There is a normal dip in blood pressure in the second trimester with a return to the baseline in the third trimester.

Nursing Process: Evaluation
Client Needs: Physiological Integrity
Clinical Area: Maternity Nursing

54. (2) Women with PIH are put on 75–80 gram protein diets. Weight gain restriction may lead to low birth weight infants or fetal compromise. Sodium restriction and diuretic therapy may lead to decreased blood volume and decreased placental perfusion.

Nursing Process: Planning
Client Needs: Physiological Integrity
Clinical Area: Maternity Nursing

55. (4) The most appropriate method of handling manipulative behavior is to set firm, clear limits. Labeling the behavior or confronting the client with the fact that he manipulates is not as therapeutic. By staying and talking with him, the nurse is telling him that he can get positive attention without resorting to manipulation.

Nursing Process: Analysis
Client Needs: Psychosocial Integrity
Clinical Area: Psychiatric Nursing

56. (3) This client is experiencing side effects to the phenothiazine, but it is not life-threatening. The symptoms should be brought to the attention of the physician soon so that he can order an antiparkinson drug. (4) is incorrect. Thorazine is effective at certain blood levels, and holding the drug would lower the blood level. If possible, it is preferable to check with the physician before holding a drug.

Nursing Process: Implementation
Client Needs: Safe, Effective Care Environment
Clinical Area: Psychiatric Nursing

57. (1) Cogentin is a drug that reduces the extrapyramidal side effects—other medications that might be prescribed are Artane and Benadryl. Niamid and Ritalin are antidepressant drugs and Atarax is classified as an antianxiety drug.

Nursing Process: Analysis
Client Needs: Physiological Integrity
Clinical Area: Psychiatric Nursing

58. (4) A Class I pap smear is normal. A Class II smear shows atypical cells, but no malignancy. A Class III contains cytology suggestive of malignancy, a Class IV contains cytology strongly suggestive of malignancy, and a Class V is conclusive for malignancy.

Nursing Process: Implementation
Client Needs: Health Promotion and Maintenance
Clinical Area: Maternity Nursing

59. (1) Things that go into the room will have to be disinfected before they are removed, so they should be washable or disposable.

Nursing Process: Planning
Client Needs: Safe, Effective Care Environment
Clinical Area: Pediatric Nursing

60. (3) It is the nurse's responsibility to tell the head nurse or supervisor what is observed. Stealing drugs is obviously illegal but the administration should handle reporting it to the authorities.

Nursing Process: Implementation
Client Needs: Safe, Effective Care Environment
Clinical Area: Psychiatric Nursing

61. (3) Contact either the poison control center or the emergency department at a local hospital. The child will most likely be given water to dilute the ferrous sulfate tablets and syrup of ipecac to induce vomiting.

Nursing Process: Implementation
Client Needs: Safe, Effective Care Environment
Clinical Area: Pediatric Nursing

62. (2) A regular diet with moderate sodium is suggested for children who are in acute glomerulonephritis. If the client's condition progresses to renal failure, sodium, potassium and protein are restricted.

Nursing Process: Planning
Client Needs: Physiological Integrity
Clinical Area: Pediatric Nursing

63. (1) Hydrops fetalis occurs when large quantities of the Rh positive antibodies attach to the fetal hemoglobin and massive hemolysis results. If the infant is delivered alive, it will require an exchange transfusion.

Nursing Process: Implementation
Client Needs: Physiological Integrity
Clinical Area: Maternity Nursing

64. (2) Nausea, vomiting and twitching are indicative of disequilibrium syndrome. They occur as a result of the rapid shift of fluids, pH and osmolarity between fluid and blood that occurs during the dialysis

Nursing Process: Evaluation
Client Needs: Physiological Integrity
Clinical Area: Medical Nursing

treatment. In addition, it is thought that a rapid decrease in BUN levels during hemodialysis causes cerebral edema which leads to increased intracranial pressure.

65. (1) High creatinine levels will be decreased. Anemia is a result of decreased production of erythropoietin by the kidney and is not affected by hemodialysis (2). Hyperkalemia and high base bicarbonate levels are present in renal failure clients.

Nursing Process: Evaluation
Client Needs: Physiological Integrity
Clinical Area: Medical Nursing

66. (2) Infants with pyloric stenosis seem normal the first few weeks of life and then begin regurgitating after feedings with progression to forceful, projectile vomiting. The chronic loss of food results in weight loss, with extreme hunger following the vomiting episode. Infants eagerly eat following the vomiting. There is no visible evidence of pain with this condition.

Nursing Process: Assessment
Client Needs: Physiological Integrity
Clinical Area: Pediatric Nursing

67. (3) Many infants are fed in a semi-Fowler's or Fowler's position with either thick formula or small frequent feedings. They are best maintained in a Fowler's position or lying on their right side to facilitate gastric emptying following feeding.

Nursing Process: Implementation
Client Needs: Safe, Effective Care Environment
Clinical Area: Pediatric Nursing

68. (2) Conversion disorder symptoms are unconsciously triggered by the client as a way of dealing with high levels of anxiety. The client's aphasia may be (but is not always) symbolic of a basic problem. The level of affect the client displays is not relevant to this disorder.

Nursing Process: Analysis
Client Needs: Psychosocial Integrity
Clinical Area: Psychiatric Nursing

69. (2) The family needs to be given honest information in words they can understand. Above all, they need to know the nurse is aware of them and will keep them in mind. Answer (1) gives conflicting messages. Answer (3) may also be true but it is very

Nursing Process: Implementation
Client Needs: Psychosocial Integrity
Clinical Area: Medical Nursing

clinical and will frighten the family more than necessary. Answer (4) is a statement made without sufficient knowledge.

70. (3) Reacting to each client as an individual and spending time with him shows that the nurse is aware of the client's personal situation and will do her best to support him.

Nursing Process: Evaluation
Client Needs: Psychosocial Integrity
Clinical Area: Medical Nursing

71. (2) Myxedema, or hypothyroidism, is caused by a decrease in thyroid hormone production. Symptoms are related to a generalized decrease in the metabolic rate. Hypothermia and constipation are associated with a decreased metabolic rate. Bradycardia, constipation and cold intolerance are additional symptoms associated with myxedema.

Nursing Process: Assessment
Client Needs: Physiological Integrity
Clinical Area: Medical Nursing

72. (2) The increased pulse rate and increased cardiac output caused by thyroid compounds can cause angina, arrhythmias, or in extreme cases, heart failure. The older the client, the more compromised the cardiovascular system may become.

Nursing Process: Evaluation
Client Needs: Physiological Integrity
Clinical Area: Medical Nursing

73. (4) Before the nurse can implement any care plan that might include setting limits or integrating the child into the group, the nurse would need to establish a relationship, either through verbal or nonverbal communication. After establishing a relationship, the nurse will assess each child.

Nursing Process: Planning
Client Needs: Safe, Effective Care Environment
Clinical Area: Psychiatric Nursing

74. (4) This unusually clear communication should be restated back to the child so that he will feel accepted and supported for expressing his feelings of fear. Restatement also opens up communication Reassuring and questioning may be used later in the interaction.

Nursing Process: Implementation
Client Needs: Psychosocial Integrity
Clinical Area: Psychiatric Nursing

75. (2) Thigh-high elastic hose apply pressure on the venous walls which promotes venous blood return to the heart. Venous pooling is prevented as well. Thigh-high, rather than knee-high, hose should be worn as more emboli result from thigh thrombi than calf thrombi. Elevation of the legs promotes venous circulation to avoid venous stasis and more clot formation. Placing a pillow under the limb could bend the groin and cause decreased circulation. The client must be kept on bedrest until the danger of emboli passes (4–7 days).

Nursing Process: Implementation
Client Needs: Safe, Effective Care Environment
Clinical Area: Surgical Nursing

76. (3) If the bladder is full, it will push the uterus up out of the pelvis above the umbilicus. The uterus will not contract sufficiently which could lead to increased bleeding.

Nursing Process: Analysis
Client Needs: Physiological Integrity
Clinical Area: Maternity Nursing

77. (4) Bryant's traction is a form of skin traction and, therefore, does not require a pin insertion. Moleskin is frequently used as the stabilizing material for traction application. The child's hips are flexed at a 90-degree angle with the legs suspended by pulleys and weights. The weights must hang freely from the crib to maintain alignment and decrease the fracture. This type of traction is used for children under two.

Nursing Process: Evaluation
Client Needs: Safe, Effective Care Environment
Clinical Area: Pediatric Nursing

78. (2) All of the client's signs and symptoms are found in both cardiac tamponade and hypovolemic shock except the urinary output and CVP. In shock, urinary output decreases to less than 30 ml/hour and the CVP would be below 5 cm H_2O pressure; thus, these symptoms would distinguish hypovolemic shock from cardiac tamponade. The client would be likely to also exhibit tachycardia, hypertension and restlessness.

Nursing Process: Analysis
Client Needs: Physiological Integrity
Clinical Area: Medical Nursing

79. (3) Hypoxia is defined as inadequate oxygenation of the tissues. The quantity of oxygen delivered to the tissues depends upon the flow of blood to the tissues and the oxygen content of the blood. Mucosal cyanosis is an indication of hypoxia. The client would be likely to also exhibit tachycardia, hypertension and restlessness.

Nursing Process: Analysis
Client Needs: Physiological Integrity
Clinical Area: Medical Nursing

80. (2) The client has indicated a need to talk and explore her feelings. Sitting with her and following her cues is the most therapeutic response. This action will assist in developing a relationship.

Nursing Process: Implementation
Client Needs: Psychosocial Integrity
Clinical Area: Maternity Nursing

81. (2) A prolonged uterine contraction of over 90 seconds or a resting phase of less than 30 seconds is dangerous and the safety intervention is to turn off the Pitocin drip. Sixty seconds is an acceptable resting phase between contractions.

Nursing Process: Evaluation
Client Needs: Physiological Integrity
Clinical Area: Maternity Nursing

82. (2) Denial is a normal reaction when a client is suddenly faced with a life-threatening illness. Anger may occur later. The nurse should determine if she is shy and afraid to ask questions, as this can happen.

Nursing Process: Analysis
Client Needs: Psychosocial Integrity
Clinical Area: Psychiatric Nursing

83. (3) Successful teaching can best be shown when the client is able to repeat the information. A description of the surgery is irrelevant and application of the bag will be done later.

Nursing Process: Evaluation
Client Needs: Health Promotion and Maintenance
Clinical Area: Surgical Nursing

84. (1) Assuming responsibility for one's behavior includes acknowledging the behavior and may include a statement of one's current status. It does not include making excuses, focusing outside of one's self, or blaming another.

Nursing Process: Implementation
Client Needs: Psychosocial Integrity
Clinical Area: Psychiatric Nursing

85. (4) The client has all the signs of thrombophlebitis. To massage the area might cause a blood clot to become dislodged.

Nursing Process: Implementation
Client Needs: Safe, Effective Care Environment
Clinical Area: Maternity Nursing

The other actions would be included in the treatment plan.

86.   (4)   It is important to start immunizations at two to three months and have them completed on schedule. Breast feeding does not influence the immunization schedule.

Nursing Process: Implementation
Client Needs: Health Promotion and Maintenance
Clinical Area: Maternity Nursing

87.   (1)   Even before pneumonia, atelectasis may occur as a result of the alveoli not being expanded. This leads to an alteration in gas exchange. Paralytic ileus could result from any surgery, especially if the client ingests food before the bowel is functioning properly.

Nursing Process: Analysis
Client Needs: Physiological Integrity
Clinical Area: Surgical Nursing

88.   (3)   If a client has shallow respirations or splinting, the pain will interfere with ventilating the lungs. The most important priority is for this client to deep breathe, hyperventilate, and cough to prevent complications such as atelectasis or pneumonia; thus, the nurse would medicate him prior to the exercises.

Nursing Process: Implementation
Client Needs: Safe, Effective Care Environment
Clinical Area: Surgical Nursing

89.   (2)   An amniocentesis indicates congenital anomalies, such as Down's syndrome, and is important for women over the age of 35, when the incidence of the disorder increases. Amniocentesis also indicates fetal lung maturity, Rh status, and the sex of the infant.

Nursing Process: Implementation
Client Needs: Health Promotion and Maintenance
Clinical Area: Maternity Nursing

90.   (2)   In this instance, it would be most beneficial to strengthen the client's arm muscles to help him when walking with the crutches.

Nursing Process: Implementation
Client Needs: Safe, Effective Care Environment
Clinical Area: Surgical Nursing

Comprehensive Test 4

1. A male client with the diagnosis of generalized tonic-clonic seizures has physician's orders for Tegretol. Included in his discharge teaching will be instructions to report adverse side effects of the drug which would be

   1. Drowsiness, anorexia and constipation.
   2. Rash, pruritus and nausea.
   3. Mouth ulcerations, gastritis, vomiting.
   4. Vertigo, blurred vision and diplopia.

2. A postoperative cataract extraction client is instructed in the use of eye drops before discharge. The nurse will know he understands these instructions if he says that he will

   1. "Look down as I instill the drop in the center of the lower eyelid."
   2. "Look down and drop the medication in the lower eyelid near the nose."
   3. "Look up and drop the medication in the center of the lower eyelid."
   4. "Look up as I instill the drop on the lens."

3. A client has just returned from a myelogram when he complains of itching and dyspnea and the nurse observes that his face is flushed. The initial nursing intervention would be to

   1. Place him in low-Fowler's position.
   2. Administer oxygen at 6 L/min as ordered.
   3. Call the physician.
   4. Start an IV with normal saline as ordered.

4. The client has an order to be log rolled following his laminectomy. The most appropriate method to turn the client is to use

   1. One nurse positioned at his back.
   2. Two nurses, one in front and one in back.
   3. Three nurses, two in front and one in back.
   4. Four nurses, two on each side.

5. A 48-year-old male client has just been diagnosed with Insulin-Dependent Diabetes Mellitus, type I (IDDM). While completing his admission history, he will most likely describe which of the following symptoms?

   1. Headache, weight loss, muscle cramps.
   2. Blurred vision, nausea, vomiting, acetone breath.
   3. Polydipsia, fatigue, CNS manifestations.
   4. Slow wound healing, weight gain, polyuria.

6. A male client had a transurethral resection (TUR) done 36 hours ago. The physician has ordered that the indwelling catheter be removed. The nurse instructs the client that following removal of the catheter, he should expect

1. Urinary retention for up to eight hours.
2. Blood-tinged urine for at least four hours.
3. Urinary incontinence for several days.
4. Urgency, frequency and painful urination for 24 hours.

7. The nurse is preparing to teach a women's health care seminar to a group of young- to middle-age women. It should include information that a Pap smear is recommended

   1. Yearly if the woman is sexually active.
   2. Every three years if the woman abstains from sexual activity.
   3. Yearly if the woman is in a high risk category.
   4. Every five years if the previous smear was negative.

8. The nurse will counsel a client with a Cesium implant that expected side effects would include

   1. Increased temperature, anorexia and increased urinary output.
   2. Nausea, vomiting and profuse discharge.
   3. Dry skin, loss of pubic hair and nausea.
   4. Vaginal itching, constipation and abdominal cramping.

9. The nurse is teaching a class on testicular self-examination to a group of college freshmen. Instructions include telling them when to perform the exam, which would be

   1. Yearly until age 30 then monthly thereafter.
   2. Monthly, at the same time of day.
   3. Monthly, following a warm bath or shower.
   4. If they detect discomfort or pain.

10. Caring for a client following a lumbar puncture, the nurse will assess for the most common complication, which is

    1. Infection at the puncture site.
    2. Headache.
    3. Slight pain at the puncture site.
    4. Slight bleeding at the puncture site.

11. Postoperative instructions for a client having an orchiectomy for testicular cancer should include the information to expect

    1. An increased temperature above 101° F immediately following surgery.
    2. Little or no pain after 48 hours.
    3. Insertion of a drain into the scrotum and slight drainage.
    4. The application of hot packs for 24 hours.

12. Which one of the following instructions would *not* be included in client teaching for an individual with Systemic Lupus Erythematosus (SLE)?

    1. Apply sunscreen before going into the sun.
    2. Perform regular range-of-motion exercises.
    3. Encourage discussion of altered body image changes.
    4. Dietary restriction of foods high in purine.

13. Assessing a client with gout would reveal which of the following clinical manifestations?

    1. Erythema and tenderness of a joint.
    2. Sensitivity of extremities to cold.
    3. Changes in pigmentation of the skin.
    4. Cloudy urine in scant amounts.

14. The major difference between osteoarthritis and rheumatoid arthritis which has implications for a thorough nursing assessment is

    1. Rheumatoid arthritis is a condition that affects older women more than men.
    2. Rheumatoid arthritis is a systemic disease, whereas osteoarthritis affects only one, two or several joints.
    3. Osteoarthritis clients require surgical intervention of the affected joint to control pain.
    4. Osteoarthritis has a genetic component as an indicator for predisposition to the disease and rheumatoid does not.

15. A young male client has come to the clinic because he is afraid he might have contracted gonorrhea. The initial assessment question should focus on

    1. Pain in the pelvic area.
    2. Urethral discharge.
    3. Pain with intercourse.
    4. Difficulty urinating.

16. The nurse is working in a community clinic where sexually transmitted diseases are prevalent. Which one of the following groups have the greatest risk of contracting these diseases?

    1. Teenagers.
    2. Young adults.
    3. Middle-aged singles.
    4. Any single person regardless of age.

17. A client is being discharged in the morning to an extended care nursing facility. He asks the nurse why he has to go to that place. The best response is

    1. "The physician has determined that this is the best place for you right now."
    2. "You will need to ask the physician that question when he comes in to see you."
    3. "Did the physician or anyone else talk to you about going to the nursing home?"
    4. "Your family can't take care of you at home so you will need to go there."

18. Which of the following changes is *not* considered a normal process of aging?

    1. Renal function diminishes.
    2. Short-term memory diminishes.
    3. Intelligence diminishes.
    4. Secretions decrease or change in composition.

19. The most critical safety intervention for clients with a tracheostomy is to

    1. Suction through the tracheostomy at least every four hours.
    2. Maintain sterile technique during the suctioning procedure.
    3. Keep a sterile tracheostomy set at the bedside.
    4. Clean around the tracheostomy at least every four hours.

20. Alopecia may be minimized in clients undergoing chemotherapy by instructing them to use

    1. An alkaline-based shampoo to prevent a build-up of oil.
    2. Hair spray to decrease the need for frequent combing.
    3. Hair clips to prevent pulling on hair follicles with long hair.
    4. Satin pillows to minimize friction rubbing of the hair.

21. Cardiopulmonary resuscitation may be discontinued if

 1. The rescuer is tired.
 2. An emergency medical team cannot be notified.
 3. CPR has been in progress for more than 30 minutes.
 4. A faint palpable pulse returns.

22. In preparing a client teaching program on hypertension, it is important to discuss ways in which blood pressure can be reduced without the aid of medications. Which one of the following methods would be most beneficial?

 1. Decrease sodium level to less than 6 gm per day.
 2. Walk once or twice each week.
 3. Limit alcohol to one glass of wine each day.
 4. Increase intake of fish oil supplements.

23. A client received a cervical spinal cord injury in an automobile accident and a Halo traction device was used to support the neck and prevent flexion or extension. Which of the following safety measures will be carried out following application of the Halo traction?

 1. Continued monitoring of Halo device and vest.
 2. Maintaining bedrest during application of traction device.
 3. Secure an Allen wrench to vest or keep at bedside.
 4. Keep an endotracheal tray at the bedside.

24. A 68-year-old client comes to the clinic with complaints of pain in her joints. She is given the diagnosis of rheumatoid arthritis and the physician orders ASA therapy, 20 tabs/day. Before discharge, the nurse teaches the client that possible side effects of ASA therapy are

 1. Bleeding, nausea, constipation.
 2. Gastritis, nausea and vomiting, bleeding.
 3. Blurred vision, nausea and vomiting.
 4. Blurred vision, tinnitus.

25. As the nurse develops a care plan for a client who sustained an intertrochanteric fracture of the left hip, she knows that initial care includes

 1. Abductor splints in place until edema is reduced.
 2. Pelvic traction until edema is reduced.
 3. Buck's extension until edema is reduced.
 4. Balanced suspension traction until edema is reduced.

26. Following surgery for a total hip replacement, the client will be positioned

 1. On her back with knees supported by pillows.
 2. On her left side with pillows to prevent adduction.
 3. On either side with pillows to prevent adduction.
 4. In low-Fowler's with bed gatched for knee support.

27. One day postdelivery, a client complains of pain. An appropriate nursing intervention for postpartum episiotomy pain is to

 1. Gently swab the suture line with A&D ointment.

2. Suggest a tampon be used instead of a perineal pad.
3. Apply hot packs the first 24 hours.
4. Apply ice packs the first 24 hours.

28. A new mother expresses concern about her day-old daughter's edematous labia. The nurse informs the mother that this condition is the result of

1. Birth trauma.
2. Maternal hormones.
3. Diaper irritation.
4. Normal development.

29. A newborn is found to be slightly hypoglycemic. The intervention to prevent low blood sugar is to

1. Give early feedings of glucose.
2. Give only water until the mother's milk comes in.
3. Start formula as soon as possible.
4. Administer IV therapy.

30. Before a new mother is discharged, she discusses her situation at home with her first child who is 2½ years old. She says she fears her child will resent the new baby. The best nursing response is

1. "That's a common feeling. Give the child some time."
2. "Maybe you'd better talk with the pediatrician about this."
3. "Had you planned this pregnancy or was it a surprise?"
4. "If you act as though there is a problem, the child may respond to the new baby as a problem."

31. A male client, 58 years of age, has been complaining of a hacking cough, shortness of breath, and chest pain. He has smoked for years. His admitting diagnosis is suspected cancer of the lung. The symptoms that he has been experiencing are typical of what type of lung cancer?

1. Oat cell.
2. Adenocarcinoma.
3. Alveolar.
4. Metastatic.

32. A client is admitted to the hospital and scheduled for a pneumonectomy. The main purpose of pulmonary function tests prior to this surgery is to determine the

1. Amount of tidal volume that will most likely remain after surgery.
2. Extent of the lung tissue involved in the disease process.
3. Amount of functioning lung tissue that will most likely remain after surgery.
4. Oxygen saturation level of the lung tissue.

33. Following a pneumonectomy, the client is returned to the surgical unit. The nurse will position him in

1. Semi-Fowler's, turned on the unaffected side.
2. Sims' position on the unaffected side.
3. Semi-Fowler's, turned on the affected side.
4. High-Fowler's position.

34. A 3-year-old child has been admitted to the pediatric unit with a history of poor weight gain and repeated upper respiratory infections. She recently has had large, foul smelling, bulky stools. The physician has

made the tentative diagnosis of cystic fibrosis. Cystic fibrosis is characterized by

1. Excessive mucus secretion from the exocrine glands.
2. Abnormal sodium retention in the glomeruli.
3. Inadequate neurological innervation of the large bowel.
4. Bronchial spasms as a result of mucus secretions.

35. The most essential medication for a child with cystic fibrosis will be

1. Neo-Synephrine aerosol.
2. Pancreatic enzymes.
3. Fat-soluble vitamins.
4. Water-soluble vitamins.

36. After receiving a diagnosis of cystic fibrosis, the nurse knows that much of the nursing care will be oriented toward

1. Providing the child with appropriate physical care.
2. Teaching the child's parents a home care regimen.
3. Helping the family adjust to new life styles imposed by the child's special needs.
4. Explaining the progression of the disease to the child's parents.

37. A 21 year old is admitted to a locked psychiatric unit. She is withdrawn, talks and laughs to herself, is suspicious of everyone, and is hearing voices telling her to hurt herself. The admitting orders are as follows: Thorazine 200 mg bid PO. If refused, give IM. The nurse finds the client screaming and banging her hands on the wall. She refuses

oral medication. The best nursing action in this situation is to

1. Stay with her and get assistance to give her the IM injection.
2. Obtain assistance to put her in restraints.
3. Tell her firmly to stop hitting her hands or she will hurt herself further.
4. Assign an attendant to stay with her in the day room.

38. A schizophrenic client just sits, staring out the window, and laughs inappropriately. The nurse's analysis of this situation is that the client is probably

1. Seeing a funny scene.
2. Hallucinating.
3. Laughing instead of crying about her situation.
4. Getting ready to "act out" again.

39. The most common defense mechanism suspicious clients use is

1. Projection.
2. Integration.
3. Sublimation.
4. Rationalization.

40. Teaching a client about the effects of Parkinsonism when he has just learned that he has this diagnosis, the nurse would include information encouraging him to

1. Maintain employment as long as possible.
2. Retire and take part in limited social activities.
3. Work only when he feels up to it.
4. Decrease his work schedule immediately.

41. A client with a suspected small bowel obstruction is admitted to the hospital. As the nurse assists the client into bed, the nursing priority is to

    1. Have him sign an operative permit.
    2. Have him describe his symptoms completely.
    3. Explain to him that he will be on complete bedrest.
    4. Determine that he has completed the hospital paperwork.

42. The physician orders a nasogastric (NG) tube insertion for a client. As the nurse prepares to insert the NG tube, the client begins to cry silently. The best way to respond to this behavior is to say

    1. "The insertion of the tube will not be painful."
    2. "It is all right to cry."
    3. "Can you talk about why you are crying?"
    4. "Don't worry. I will give you pain medicine if you need it."

43. A client complains of discomfort from the nasogastric (NG) tube. The intervention that will provide the most comfort for a client with an NG tube is to

    1. Provide oral hygiene.
    2. Tape the tube so it doesn't move.
    3. Apply a cream to the lips and nares.
    4. Use a prn decongestant spray.

44. Following surgery, the client complains of pain and asks for medication. The first action is to

1. Determine the location and severity of the pain.
2. Administer the medication that is ordered.
3. Tell him it is too soon following the anesthetic for more medication.
4. Give him half the ordered dosage.

45. In planning postoperative care, the nurse will assess for the major complication occurring from abdominal surgery which is

    1. Hemorrhage.
    2. Stress ulcer.
    3. Infection.
    4. Fluid and electrolyte imbalance.

46. A client admitted to the labor room is a 28-year-old primipara in early labor. She tells the nurse that her water has broken. All of the following are appropriate nursing actions. The *first* nursing assessment that needs to be completed is to

    1. Check the fetal heart rate.
    2. Check for a prolapsed cord.
    3. Attach the external fetal monitor.
    4. Check color and quantity of fluid.

47. The nurse checks a pregnant client in the labor room, finds that the client is 6 cm dilated and having contractions every 3 to 4 minutes, lasting 40 to 50 seconds. She asks for medication to ease the pain. The most appropriate response is to say

    1. "It would be better to wait awhile as it will be more difficult later."
    2. "It's too early to give medication now. It would slow things down too much."

3. "It shouldn't be too much longer now until the baby is born. Are you sure you want something?"
4. "Let me check the physician's orders to see if you can have some medication now."

48. A 28-year-old client gives birth to a baby girl weighing 7 lbs, 6 oz. The baby has a bilirubin concentration of 14 mg/100 ml blood and the physician decides to order phototherapy. The nurse knows that the care of the infant receiving phototherapy includes

1. Clothing the infant to prevent chilling.
2. Covering the infant's eyes to prevent retinal damage.
3. Removing the infant from under the bili light for 15 minutes every hour to prevent overexposure.
4. Restricting fluids to prevent edema.

49. A male, age 32, is seen in the ER following an accident in which his 6-year-old daughter was seriously injured. The admitting nurse realizes after several minutes that the father cannot give any personal information and he seems not to be able to recall anything since shortly before the accident. In assessing the father, it is important that the nurse not only investigate his physical status but also consider that he may be experiencing

1. A schizophrenic episode.
2. Psychogenic localized amnesia.
3. Psychogenic fugue.
4. Affective disorder.

50. The physician orders a stat dose of Valium 10 mg PO to be given to an anxious client. Valium is classified as a/an

1. Narcoleptic.
2. Antianxiety drug.
3. Mood elevator.
4. Antibiotic.

51. A 48-year-old male client was admitted two days ago and is undergoing treatment of a recurrent episode of acute interstitial pancreatitis. The initial assessment will most likely reveal which of the following symptoms?

1. Nausea, vomiting, epigastric tenderness.
2. Diarrhea, generalized abdominal pain.
3. Abdominal and back pain, diarrhea.
4. Back pain, nausea and vomiting, tenderness across the upper abdominal quadrants.

52. The most common cause of chronic pancreatitis is

1. Chronic alcoholism.
2. Chronic biliary disease.
3. Pancreatic fibrosis.
4. Cancer of the pancreas.

53. The nurse will assess for the most common and fatal complication of severe acute pancreatitis. The condition is

1. Infection.
2. Hypovolemia.
3. Electrolyte imbalance.
4. Severe hyperglycemia.

54. The nurse will counsel the client that the measure to promote the most comfort during a herpes simplex virus, type 2 (HSV-2) outbreak is to

1. Keep lesions clean and dry.
2. Provide sitz baths three to four times a day.
3. Administer local anesthetic or systemic analgesia.
4. Apply Acyclovir.

55. A client who is in respiratory distress is admitted to the hospital. He is semicomatose, dyspneic and weak. His admitting diagnosis is AIDS-related Pneumocystis carinii. The statement that best describes the source of this disease is a/an

    1. Virus that invades the immune system.
    2. Retrovirus that attaches to the helper T-cells.
    3. Mutated virus that kills helper T-cells.
    4. Autoimmune disease that is caused by the release of an antigen.

56. The nurse is responsible to check that the nursing assistant is aware of universal precaution isolation techniques. If the nursing assistant understands these techniques, she will say that she must wear

    1. Gloves at all times when in contact with any clients, regardless of the diagnosis.
    2. Gloves and gown when in contact with blood or body fluids.
    3. Sterile gloves, gown and mask at all times when caring for identified AIDS clients.
    4. Mask and gloves at all times when caring for diagnosed AIDS clients.

57. A young client, age 12, is admitted in a comatose condition to the emergency room. There is no history of trauma, falls or recent headaches. Diabetes is a tentative diagnosis.

All of the following interventions will be carried out according to orders. The initial intervention will most likely be to

1. Administer intermediate acting insulin.
2. Insert an IV and infuse normal saline solution.
3. Administer IV potassium chloride.
4. Insert an indwelling catheter.

58. A 13 year old has just received the diagnosis of Insulin-Dependent Diabetes Mellitus, type I (IDDM), and is ready for discharge. In evaluating his understanding of the discharge instructions, the nurse knows he understands if he tells her that he will

    1. Avoid sports, as the erratic episodes of exercise can lead to premature complications.
    2. Tactfully refuse invitations to parties where eating and drinking will take place.
    3. Monitor his blood glucose levels at least qid for the first month he is at home.
    4. Vary his dietary intake but keep track of the calories.

59. A 53-year-old client is demonstrating catatonic excitement with extreme psychomotor agitation. She constantly jumps up and down in one spot, shouting, "Down the tubes! Down the tubes!" After all day, with little rest or nourishment, it is important to intervene. The nurse's most therapeutic approach to this client is to say

    1. "Stop this craziness right now!"
    2. "You must be getting tired of this one spot. Let's go outside and you can run in the grass."

3. "If you'll stop and eat something, I'll fix your favorite dish."
4. "I'm concerned about your physical condition. I'm going to help you control your behavior."

60. A male client, age 55, came to the emergency room complaining of severe pain in his left big toe. A diagnosis of gout is made. The nurse will explain to the client that the medication for treatment of this condition will be

1. ASA.
2. Colchicine.
3. Oruval.
4. Percodan.

61. Before a client who suffered an attack of gout is discharged from the hospital, it is important to evaluate his knowledge of dietary management. Which one of the following diet choices would indicate to the nurse that he understands his dietary restrictions?

1. Liver, potato and spinach.
2. Crab cakes, rice and peas.
3. Antipasto salad, beans, rice, and asparagus.
4. Steak, baked potato and green salad.

62. A 3-year-old child is who is semiconscious with a low-grade fever brought to the emergency room. The physician suspects a severe case of lead poisoning. The nurse expects that the child will be treated with

1. Calcium disodium edetate (EDTA).
2. Erythromycin.
3. Activated charcoal.
4. Syrup of ipecac.

63. In evaluating a child's condition who has been treated for lead poisoning, the nurse will assess for the complication of

1. Glomerulonephritis.
2. Reye's syndrome.
3. Multiple sclerosis.
4. Tetany.

64. A female client has been hospitalized for two days with chronic congestive heart failure. Her physician has written orders that include Lasix IV and oxygen. The client suddenly complains of breathing difficulty. The immediate assessment indicates that she has bi-basilar rales, increased pulse and blood pressure, and a frequent moist cough. The first nursing intervention is to

1. Give Lasix IV push according to standing orders.
2. Apply rotating tourniquets according to standing orders.
3. Place the client in high-Fowler's position.
4. Call the physician and inform him of the change in her condition.

65. When caring for a client diagnosed with pulmonary edema who is receiving oxygen, the nurse observes that she frequently removes her oxygen mask even though she is dyspneic. The appropriate nursing intervention is to

1. Change from O_2 mask to O_2 cannula.
2. Increase the liter flow of O_2 to 10 L/min.
3. Tighten the strap on the O_2 mask.
4. Change O_2 administration to a Venturi mask.

66. When a cardiac client is brought to the emergency room, the drug of choice administered for a ventricular arrhythmia is

1. Digoxin.
2. Inderal.
3. Lidocaine.
4. Morphine sulfate.

67. The nurse explains to a client with a duodenal ulcer that his ulcer diet will most likely include

    1. Six small feedings of regular food.
    2. Milk or cream every two hours.
    3. A regular diet without milk.
    4. A high-fiber diet without spices.

68. A client with an ulcer is placed on an antacid regimen consisting of 15 ml of Riopan one hour after meals and at bedtime. The nurse explains to the client that the reason this particular antacid is given is that it prevents

    1. Electrolyte imbalance.
    2. Hemorrhage.
    3. Vomiting.
    4. Diarrhea.

69. A client is diagnosed as schizophrenic, catatonic type and has been in the hospital for three weeks. The client has just been told that her father was in a bad automobile accident and is critically ill in the hospital. Her response is to smile and ask what time lunch is served. This is an example of

    1. Lack of affect.
    2. Inappropriate affect.
    3. Disturbed association of ideas.
    4. Primary disturbance.

70. The appropriate nursing response to a client's question asking when lunch will be served after the nurse tells her that a family member is in the hospital, critically ill, would be

    1. "Did you hear what I said?"
    2. "Your father is critically ill. Don't you want to talk about it?"
    3. "You are blocking, and I think you need to talk about your feelings."
    4. "I told you your father was critically ill, and you asked what time lunch would be served."

71. A client has been diagnosed as having early stage cancer of the transverse colon. The physician has explained to her that she needs to have part of her colon removed (partial colectomy). Knowing this, the nurse would tell the client that postoperatively the elimination process will be done through

    1. An ileostomy for elimination.
    2. Normal elimination.
    3. A temporary colostomy for elimination.
    4. A permanent colostomy for elimination.

72. A client with a partial colectomy was returned to the unit at 1:30 P.M. During a 6:00 P.M. assessment, the nurse observes the following data. Which sign or symptom would require the earliest intervention?

    1. Dressing that is moderately saturated with serosanguineous drainage.
    2. Warm and reddened area on the client's left calf.
    3. Distended bladder that is firm to palpation.
    4. Decrease in breath sounds on the right side.

73. A new client is being accompanied by a nurse from Admissions to the medical unit.

When they approach the elevator to go up to the unit, the client says intensely, "No! Don't make me go in there!" The nurse's most appropriate response is to say

1. "You need to confront your fear. Let's get on the elevator."
2. "Let's sit here in the lobby and talk about your fear of the elevator."
3. "Your fear is a symbolic way of dealing with anxiety. It's not rational, you know."
4. "It may take us a little longer, but I think you'd be more comfortable if we take the stairs."

74. A 24-year-old female client has come to the clinic for some information about contraceptive methods and asks the nurse how the pill actually works. The nurse explains that it combines estrogen and progesterone to provide contraception primarily by

1. Preventing ovulation.
2. Maintaining thick cervical mucus.
3. Altering the maturation of the endometrium.
4. Preventing fertilization in the fallopian tubes.

75. A client is in her 35th week of pregnancy and the physician decides to complete a lecithin/sphingomyelin (L/S) ratio test. The nurse explains to the client that the purpose of this test is to

1. Determine status of the fetus.
2. Test for fetal maturity.
3. Measure fetal baseline heart rate.
4. Measure the creatinine level.

76. A 3-month-old infant has unrepaired tetralogy of Fallot. Which of the following signs and symptoms would the nurse expect the infant to exhibit?

1. Circumoral cyanosis, hypoxic spells, feeding fatigue.
2. Tachycardia, hypertension, decreased femoral pulses.
3. Hypotension, bradycardia, dyspnea.
4. Cyanosis, tachypnea, hypertension in upper extremities.

77. A client's physician orders Aminophylline IV infusion at 2 mg per minute. A safety intervention for administering this medication is to

1. Use an IV controller.
2. Protect the IV bottle from sunlight.
3. Give the client a test dose of Aminophylline first.
4. Run the IV at 1 mg per minute for one hour before increasing dose.

78. Charting is one of the nurse's most important functions. Which of the following statements identifies the most important purpose of charting?

1. To communicate to other members of the client's health care team.
2. To evaluate the staff's performance.
3. To provide information for a nursing audit.
4. To enable physicians to monitor nursing care.

79. When moving the client up in bed, the nurse would remove the pillow and place it at the head of the bed. The rationale for this action is to

1. Get it out of the way.
2. Prevent the patient from striking his head.
3. Facilitate completing the procedure.
4. Enable the client to push from his knees.

80. Which of the following nursing actions would do the most to assist a client to cope with severe anxiety?

    1. Remaining with the client while she is anxious.
    2. Providing an activity to get the client's mind off feeling anxious.
    3. Encouraging the client to identify, discuss and find the cause of her anxiety.
    4. Establishing a nurse-client relationship.

81. A medication order is for one fluid dram of liquid. The medication cup is measured in ml's. How many ml's will be administered?

    1. 1 ml.
    2. 4 ml.
    3. 8 ml.
    4. 30 ml.

82. An elderly client on bedrest has developed a pressure ulcer. The nursing diagnosis pertinent to the care of this client requiring wound care is

    1. Health Maintenance, alteration in.
    2. Tissue Perfusion, alteration in.
    3. Grieving, dysfunctional.
    4. Self-care deficit.

83. Client teaching for home care should include which one of the following concepts?

    1. Good household cleaning practices will prevent the spread of infection.
    2. Any equipment that comes in contact with blood or body fluids needs to be disinfected for 24 hours.
    3. AIDS clients should not be responsible for food preparation.
    4. Soiled dressings should be burned, not placed in a trash container.

84. Percussion, vibration and postural drainage are ordered for a 15 year old client hospitalized for pneumonia. Prior to providing this intervention, the priority action is to

    1. Instruct the client in diaphragmatic breathing.
    2. Assess vital signs.
    3. Auscultate lung fields.
    4. Assess characteristics of her sputum.

85. When measuring a client for knee-high elastic hose, the nurse would measure

    1. Leg length from heel to buttocks and calf circumference while he is standing.
    2. Ankle and calf circumference while he is standing.
    3. Leg length to the knee when he is lying down.
    4. Calf circumference and leg length from bottom of heel to bend of knee.

86. When assessing a client for possible dehydration, which of the following clinical manifestations would indicate this state?

    1. Taut, shiny skin.
    2. Firm eyeballs.
    3. Bounding pulse.
    4. Dry, flaking skin.

87. During the first 10 minutes of a blood transfusion, the nurse will infuse the blood at how many drops per minute?

   1. 10 gtts/min.
   2. 20 gtts/min.
   3. 40 gtts/min.
   4. According to physician's orders.

88. The nurse explains to the client that the major difference between a plaster of Paris and a synthetic cast is that the

   1. Drying time is prolonged with a synthetic cast.
   2. Synthetic cast is less restrictive.
   3. Plaster cast requires expensive equipment for application.
   4. Synthetic cast is more effective for immobilizing severely displaced bones.

89. If a client developed atelectasis, a major postoperative complication, which of the following findings would be most conclusive?

   1. Bradycardia.
   2. Temperature of 102° F.
   3. Dullness to breath sound percussion.
   4. Restlessness.

90. A normal EKG strip can be identified when the

   1. P-R interval falls before the QRS complex on the strip.
   2. T-wave should be in the inverted position on the strip.
   3. P-R interval should be no longer than .12 seconds.
   4. QRS interval should be no longer than .20 seconds.

Comprehensive Test 4
Answers with Rationale

1. (4)   The symptoms indicate the adverse side effects associated with the use of Tegretol. The symptoms in answer (3) are adverse effects of Phenytoin. The other symptoms are not relevant to this class of drugs.

    Nursing Process: Implementation
    Client Needs: Health Promotion and Maintenance
    Clinical Area: Medical Nursing

2. (3)   The client is instructed to look up while the drop is placed in the center of the lower eyelid. In order to accomplish this, the client needs to keep the eye open and be careful not to touch the lid. Contamination of the eyedropper will occur if it touches the lid.

    Nursing Process: Evaluation
    Client Needs: Health Promotion and Maintenance
    Clinical Area: Surgical Nursing

3. (1)   Low-Fowler's position promotes optimal cerebral perfusion and promotes adequate ventilatory exchange. Oxygen administration is important and would be the second nursing intervention carried out.

    Nursing Process: Implementation
    Client Needs: Safe, Effective Care Environment
    Clinical Area: Medical Nursing

4. (3)   Two nurses, positioned in the front, will receive the client as he is turned. The nurse in back maintains the client's alignment during the turning process.

    Nursing Process: Planning
    Client Needs: Safe, Effective Care Environment
    Clinical Area: Surgical Nursing

5. (4)   These symptoms are indicative of type I diabetes. In addition to those listed in answer (4), blurred vision, fatigue, weakness, peripheral neuropathy, and polydipsia are common symptoms.

    Nursing Process: Assessment
    Client Needs: Physiological Integrity
    Clinical Area: Medical Nursing

6. (3)   Urinary incontinence is a usual occurrence as a result of impaired sphincter tone following surgical intervention. Practicing

    Nursing Process: Implementation
    Client Needs: Health Promotion and Maintenance
    Clinical Area: Surgical Nursing

Kegel's exercises before and after surgery (ten times each hour) will decrease the time that dribbling will occur.

7. (3) If the client is in a high risk category or over age 40, yearly smears are recommended by the American Cancer Society. Women between ages 20 and 40 who are not in the high-risk category and have had negative results for three previous tests should have Pap smears every three years.

Nursing Process: Planning
Client Needs: Health Promotion and Maintenance
Clinical Area: Maternity Nursing

8. (2) In addition to nausea, vomiting and discharge, clients may experience diarrhea, anorexia, dry sloughing skin, and blistering.

Nursing Process: Implementation
Client Needs: Health Promotion and Maintenance
Clinical Area: Medical Nursing

9. (3) Following a warm bath the scrotal skin is more relaxed and abnormalities will be easier to detect. Testicular examinations should be performed monthly after age 15. The same day of the month should be used for consistency in evaluation of findings.

Nursing Process: Implementation
Client Needs: Health Promotion and Maintenance
Clinical Area: Medical Nursing

10. (2) Headache occurs as a result of removal of the cerebrospinal fluid from the subarachnoid space. If the client does not have signs of increased intracranial pressure, fluids can be increased after the procedure. Cerebrospinal fluid is manufactured quickly as a result and the headache will improve.

Nursing Process: Assessment
Client Needs: Physiological Integrity
Clinical Area: Surgical Nursing

11. (2) Surgical pain lasts from 24 to 48 hours. Adequate scrotal support and positioning will decrease postoperative pain and edema. Ice packs can be used to decrease edema; hot packs will intensify the pain and, therefore, are not used. A temperature of 101° F should not occur postoperatively unless an infection is present.

Nursing Process: Implementation
Client Needs: Health Promotion and Maintenance
Clinical Area: Surgical Nursing

12.   (4)   Purine restriction is indicated for clients with gout. It does not have any significance in SLE. The other three answers contain interventions that are encouraged for clients with SLE.

Nursing Process: Implementation
Client Needs: Health Promotion and Maintenance
Clinical Area: Medical Nursing

13.   (1)   In addition to erythema and tenderness of the affected joint, the client experiences severe pain. Edema and limitation of motion are also symptoms frequently found in clients.

Nursing Process: Assessment
Client Needs: Physiological Integrity
Clinical Area: Medical Nursing

14.   (2)   Rheumatoid arthritis is a systemic disease which not only affects symmetrical joints but also can lead to pericarditis and pulmonary fibrosis. These conditions require acute assessment skills, not just assessing for joint involvement. Rheumatoid arthritis affects individuals between 25 and 55 years of age and there is a familial tendency with the disease. Surgical intervention may be required for both conditions to assist in pain control as well as mobility.

Nursing Process: Assessment
Client Needs: Safe, Effective Care Environment
Clinical Area: Medical Nursing

15.   (2)   The two most common presenting symptoms for a client with gonorrhea are urethral discharge (which is purulent) and dysuria.

Nursing Process: Assessment
Client Needs: Safe, Effective Care Environment
Clinical Area: Medical Nursing

16.   (1)   Reported cases of sexually transmitted diseases have increased dramatically for teenagers. The most common reason is perhaps the change in society's altered ethical and moral values related to sexual activity.

Nursing Process: Planning
Client Needs: Health Promotion and Maintenance
Clinical Area: Medical Nursing

17.   (3)   Answer (3) is the most appropriate response. It is important to identify what the client thinks he has heard about his discharge. Clarification of information can proceed after this. The other answers do not allow the client to verbalize his fears or concerns.

Nursing Process: Implementation
Client Needs: Psychosocial Integrity
Clinical Area: Medical Nursing

18. (3) Intelligence is not affected. Long-term memory usually is not affected. Short- or intermediate- memory changes are affected by the aging process.

Nursing Process: Analysis
Client Needs: Physiological Integrity
Clinical Area: Medical Nursing

19. (3) Keeping a sterile set at the bedside is the most critical aspect of client care. If the tube is dislodged accidentally, a new tube must be inserted immediately to maintain a patent airway. While the other interventions are essential, they are not the most critical.

Nursing Process: Implementation
Client Needs: Safe, Effective Care Environment
Clinical Area: Surgical Nursing

20. (4) Minimizing friction will help to protect the hair. A protein-based shampoo should be used to nourish hair cells. Sprays, dyes, hair dryers, and clips or elastic bands should not be used as they can damage or pull out hair.

Nursing Process: Implementation
Client Needs: Safe, Effective Care Environment
Clinical Area: Medical Nursing

21. (4) CPR must be continued unless a physician orders it to be discontinued, the rescuer is too exhausted to continue, an emergency medical team takes over, or pulse and respirations return.

Nursing Process: Planning
Client Needs: Safe, Effective Care Environment
Clinical Area: Medical Nursing

22. (1) The most effective method will be to reduce sodium intake. The other activities will also assist in decreasing blood pressure. Fish oil supplements do not affect blood pressure.

Nursing Process: Planning
Client Needs: Health Promotion and Maintenance
Clinical Area: Medical Nursing

23. (3) Important safety measures are to keep an Allen wrench in close proximity for emergency removal of screws from the vest if CPR has to be performed. A tracheostomy tray is kept at the bedside because endotracheal intubation is contraindicated in these clients. The client does not have to remain on bedrest.

Nursing Process: Implementation
Clinical Area: Safe, Effective Care Environment
Client Needs: Surgical Nursing

24. (2) Gastritis, nausea, vomiting, and bleeding are the most common side effects of ASA therapy. Blurred vision is not a side

Nursing Process: Implementation
Client Needs: Safe, Effective Care Environment
Clinical Area: Medical Nursing

effect of ASA therapy, and tinnitus would indicate that the toxic level of the drug had been reached.

25. (4) The client is usually placed in balanced suspension traction until surgery can be completed. This type of traction allows the client to move up and down in bed without interfering with the alignment of the bones. It also prevents muscle spasms. The surgical intervention is done early in elderly clients to prevent complications of immobilization.

Nursing Process: Planning
Client Needs: Safe, Effective Care Environment
Clinical Area: Surgical Nursing

26. (3) Following total hip replacement, most clients can be turned to either side, using pillows between the legs to prevent adduction. Following a partial hip replacement, clients normally are not to be turned to the operative side due to the possibility of subluxation (displacement) of the prosthesis.

Nursing Process: Implementation
Client Needs: Safe, Effective Care Environment
Clinical Area: Surgical Nursing

27. (4) In the first 24 hours, ice helps prevent edema and thus decreases pain. Swabbing the perineum with A&D would not be helpful, and tampons are not advised until at least 2–6 weeks postpartum. Hot compresses are not used, although sitz baths after 24 hours help reduce swelling and thereby decrease discomfort.

Nursing Process: Implementation
Client Needs: Safe, Effective Care Environment
Clinical Area: Maternity Nursing

28. (2) Maternal hormones may produce genital edema in both girls and boys. It is a normal occurrence and subsides spontaneously.

Nursing Process: Analysis
Client Needs: Health Promotion and Maintenance
Clinical Area: Maternity Nursing

29. (1) Early glucose feedings will prevent low blood sugar and are also the treatment for the hypoglycemic infant. The first feeding will be water followed by glucose feedings. Oral feedings are preferred to IV therapy if the infant can tolerate them.

Nursing Process: Implementation
Client Needs: Safe, Effective Care Environment
Clinical Area: Maternity Nursing

30. (4) This is the best response, as sibling rivalry can be a problem. If the mother discusses it and learns how to handle it before going home, she can do much to prevent its severity. The conversation can be continued and explored to deal with her concerns and rivalry problems.

Nursing Process: Implementation
Client Needs: Psychosocial Integrity
Clinical Area: Pediatric Nursing

31. (1) Oat cell and squamous cell carcinoma have the same symptomatology. In addition to the symptoms experienced by the client, hemoptysis and wheezing are frequently manifested.

Nursing Process: Analysis
Client Needs: Physiological Integrity
Clinical Area: Medical Nursing

32. (3) Pulmonary function tests assist in determining the amount of functioning lung tissue that will be available for O_2–CO_2 exchange following surgery. The tidal volume will determine the amount of air inhaled and exhaled with each normal respiration. Tidal volume is generally measured as one parameter of the pulmonary function tests. The extent of the disease process is not identified with pulmonary function tests.

Nursing Process: Analysis
Client Needs: Physiological Integrity
Clinical Area: Surgical Nursing

33. (3) Semi-Fowler's position, turned on the affected side, will allow the fluid in the thoracic cavity to accumulate and serous exudate to consolidate. This will prevent an extensive mediastinal shift of the other lung and the heart.

Nursing Process: Implementation
Client Needs: Safe, Effective Care Environment
Clinical Area: Surgical Nursing

34. (1) Abnormal, tenacious secretions from the exocrine glands of the body are found in cystic fibrosis. Answer (2) refers to the kidney.

Nursing Process: Analysis
Client Needs: Physiological Integrity
Clinical Area: Pediatric Nursing

35. (2) Pancreatic enzymes are a digestive aid. Without the pancreatic enzymes, the essential vitamins will not be assimilated. Fats are not absorbed well by children with cystic fibrosis. Water-soluble vitamins must be provided.

Nursing Process: Planning
Client Needs: Health Promotion and Maintenance
Clinical Area: Pediatric Nursing

36.   (2)   Parent teaching is very important and should include all of the answers. Teaching a home care regimen should provide for continuation of care the child receives in the hospital and this answer will include all of the other answers. It is the most comprehensive.

Nursing Process: Planning
Client Needs: Health Promotion and Maintenance
Clinical Area: Pediatric Nursing

37.   (1)   The client requires the Thorazine and a decrease in the amount of external stimuli. The nurse must provide limits because the client cannot do so at this time, so remaining with her is important.

Nursing Process: Implementation
Client Needs: Safe, Effective Care Environment
Clinical Area: Psychiatric Nursing

38.   (2)   Inappropriate laughter in psychotic behavior is generally caused by visual or auditory hallucinations. The most appropriate nursing action is to involve the client in an activity. A reality-oriented activity will divert focus from the hallucination.

Nursing Process: Analysis
Client Needs: Psychosocial Integrity
Clinical Area: Psychiatric Nursing

39.   (1)   The client is unable to deal with her own internal feelings, so she projects them onto others. Answers (2), (3) and (4) are normal, healthy defense mechanisms.

Nursing Process: Analysis
Client Needs: Psychosocial Integrity
Clinical Area: Psychiatric Nursing

40.   (1)   It is very important to keep Parkinsonism clients actively involved in work and social situations. They experience altered body images and tend to withdraw from society. When this happens, the complications of immobility increase. As complications increase, they tend to decrease the client's life span.

Nursing Process: Implementation
Client Needs: Safe, Effective Care Environment
Clinical Area: Medical Nursing

41.   (2)   Details of his symptoms and their progression often help the physician diagnose the specific problem, and the client often will tell the nurse details that he felt were not important enough to tell the physician. It is too soon to sign an operative permit and he has no orders for bedrest. Answer (4) is not relevant.

Nursing Process: Assessment
Client Needs: Safe, Effective Care Environment
Clinical Area: Medical Nursing

42. (3) Crying is not a normal response to an NG tube insertion, so the nurse needs to find out what has occurred in the client's past to evoke such a response, or what he may be afraid of for the future.

Nursing Process: Implementation
Client Needs: Psychosocial Integrity
Clinical Area: Medical Nursing

43. (3) Providing oral hygiene and taping the tube firmly are important but preventing dryness to the lips and nares would provide the most comfort.

Nursing Process: Implementation
Client Needs: Safe, Effective Care Environment
Clinical Area: Medical Nursing

44. (1) The pain might be from his position on the operating table or the position of his arm with the IV. These can be relieved without medication by repositioning or giving him a back rub. The client should be medicated if he needs it, but medication should not be used in place of good nursing care. The first dose of narcotic following surgery may be only one half the ordered dose, but an assessment of the pain should be done first.

Nursing Process: Implementation
Client Needs: Safe, Effective Care Environment
Clinical Area: Surgical Nursing

45. (4) Fluid and electrolyte imbalance can occur when the NG tube removes intestinal fluids and electrolytes and there is often a fluid shift within the gut from the trauma of surgery.

Nursing Process: Planning
Client Needs: Physiological Integrity
Clinical Area: Surgical Nursing

46. (2) When the amniotic sac breaks, there is a possibility of prolapsed cord. This must be ruled out immediately, because if the cord is prolapsed, the baby is in jeopardy due to fetal hypoxia. The next intervention would be to check the fetal heart rate.

Nursing Process: Implementation
Client Needs: Safe, Effective Care Environment
Clinical Area: Maternity Nursing

47. (4) Her labor is well-established now, and she should be able to have medication. Generally, physician's orders are written to encompass parameters for medication administration during the stages of labor.

Nursing Process: Implementation
Client Needs: Safe, Effective Care Environment
Clinical Area: Maternity Nursing

48.   (2)   The infant receiving phototherapy should have its eyes covered to prevent retinal damage. The eyes should be uncovered during feedings, when the infant is out from under the light, to prevent irritation and to promote stimulation of the infant. Infants should not be clothed but fully exposed during phototherapy so that maximum benefit from the treatment will be received. Fluids are usually given between feedings and are not restricted to promote excretion of the broken down bilirubin.

Nursing Process: Planning
Client Needs: Safe, Effective Care Environment
Clinical Area: Pediatric Nursing

49   (2)   Psychogenic localized amnesia is characterized by nonorganic memory loss caused by a recent traumatic event. Answer (1) is incorrect because the client is reality oriented and is not experiencing a thought disturbance. Answer (3) is incorrect because fugue is characterized by physical flight. Answer (4) is incorrect because the client is not primarily experiencing disturbance of his affect or mood.

Nursing Process: Assessment
Client Needs: Psychosocial Integrity
Clinical Area: Psychiatric Nursing

50.   (2)   Valium is a minor tranquilizer which is prescribed to decrease high anxiety.

Nursing Process: Analysis
Client Needs: Psychosocial Integrity
Clinical Area: Psychiatric Nursing

51.   (4)   Symptoms of acute interstitial pancreatitis result when the pancreas becomes edematous and irritated as a result of the release of its enzymes into the surrounding tissue and peritoneal cavity.

Nursing Process: Assessment
Client Needs: Safe, Effective Care Environment
Clinical Area: Medical Nursing

52.   (1)   Chronic alcoholism is by far the most common etiology of chronic pancreatitis in the absence of documented biliary tract disease. The pancreas is destroyed by a resulting fibrosis which ultimately interferes with its role in the digestion of proteins and fats.

Nursing Process: Analysis
Client Needs: Physiological Integrity
Clinical Area: Medical Nursing

53. (2) Large amounts of serous fluid leak from the blood channels into the peritoneum and decrease intravascular volume causing hypovolemia. Enzyme release may also damage the walls of the blood vessels and precipitate hemorrhage.

Nursing Process: Evaluation
Client Needs: Physiological Integrity
Clinical Area: Medical Nursing

54. (4) Acyclovir applied to the lesion will provide earlier remission and also provide more comfort. There is no known antibiotic for the virus. Acyclovir applied to the lesions shortens the episode but does not cure it.

Nursing Process: Planning
Client Needs: Physiological Integrity
Clinical Area: Maternity Nursing

55. (2) AIDS is caused by a retrovirus with a different life cycle than a normal virus. It may be dormant for years before affecting the helper T-cells and causing immunosuppression.

Nursing Process: Analysis
Client Needs: Physiological Integrity
Clinical Area: Medical Nursing

56. (2) Universal precautions, a code advocated by the Centers for Disease Control (CDC), include protecting oneself when there is any possibility of being in contact with contaminated body fluids or blood. The nurse manager is responsible to determine if those on the team understand these precautions.

Nursing Process: Evaluation
Client Needs: Safe, Effective Care Environment
Clinical Area: Medical Nursing

57. (2) An IV infusion is the first intervention instituted. It is essential that the body cells are not crenated. Hydration of the cells must occur first for the insulin to be effective in moving glucose into the cell. In the initial stage of ketoacidosis, there will be hyperkalemia due to a hemoconcentration of the plasma; therefore, potassium chloride would not be administered at this time. A catheter will be inserted early in the treatment for accurate urine output data and to facilitate urine testing for sugar and acetone.

Nursing Process: Implementation
Client Needs: Physiological Integrity
Clinical Area: Medical Nursing

58. (3) Clients are usually regulated in the hospital routine and when they get home their exercise level alters, their dietary intake frequently alters, and it is, therefore, essential that they observe for alterations in their diabetic control. Blood glucose level can give an indication of how well-controlled they are. Many diabetics participate in sports; however, they need to monitor their condition more closely, as increased exercise has an insulin-like effect and hypoglycemia could result. Adolescents and teenagers should lead as normal a life as possible, so they should learn to adjust to all types of conditions.

Nursing Process: Evaluation
Client Needs: Health Promotion and Maintenance
Clinical Area: Medical Nursing

59. (4) This client needs a clear, direct statement of what the nurse intends to do. At the moment, she is unable to "stop this craziness," and moving outside probably will not stop the behavior. Bargaining is unlikely to be effective and may increase the client's anxiety.

Nursing Process: Implementation
Client Needs: Safe, Effective Care Environment
Clinical Area: Psychiatric Nursing

60. (2) The drug of choice to reduce inflammation is colchicine PO or even IV every hour for eight hours until pain subsides. Allopurinol is then given to decrease uric acid levels. An analgesic may also be given for pain.

Nursing Process: Planning
Client Needs: Physiological Integrity
Clinical Area: Medical Nursing

61. (4) Steak is the best choice because foods highest in purine are shellfish, liver, chicken, beans, and various vegetables. The appropriate diet will include high carbohydrates with calorie control.

Nursing Process: Evaluation
Client Needs: Safe, Effective Care Environment
Clinical Area: Medical Nursing

62. (1) Calcium disodium edetate, or EDTA, is a chelating agent which promotes the excretion of lead from the body by attaching to the lead and carrying it out through the kidneys.

Nursing Process: Planning
Client Needs: Physiological Integrity
Clinical Area: Pediatric Nursing

63. (4) Following therapy children can develop tetany because the chelating agent, EDTA, will take out calcium along with the lead. Therefore, the nurse will monitor for hypocalcemia.

Nursing Process: Assessment
Client Needs: Physiological Integrity
Clinical Area: Pediatric Nursing

64. (3) It is best to first do the nursing intervention that immediately helps the client's condition while the nurse is preparing more definitive therapy. High-Fowler's position decreases venous return to the heart. Lasix would then be given and the physician notified.

Nursing Process: Implementation
Client Needs: Safe, Effective Care Environment
Clinical Area: Medical Nursing

65. (1) Clients often feel that they cannot breathe when experiencing pulmonary edema. A mask may increase this feeling. A cannula is often better tolerated and thus should be used in this case.

Nursing Process: Implementation
Client Needs: Safe, Effective Care Environment
Clinical Area: Medical Nursing

66. (3) Lidocaine is the drug of choice because it depresses ventricular irritability. Inderal is contraindicated as it is a beta-adrenergic blocking agent. It also depresses cardiac function. For a client who already has a compromised cardiac status, this could be fatal. Morphine reduces anxiety, but will not prevent arrhythmias. Digoxin is used to strengthen ventricular contraction.

Nursing Process: Planning
Client Needs: Physiological Integrity
Clinical Area: Medical Nursing

67. (3) Most physicians now prescribe a regular three-meal routine, eliminating roughage, gas-forming foods, highly spiced foods, and gastric acid stimulants such as caffeine, alcohol and smoking. In the past, milk and cream were the mainstays of dietary ulcer therapy. They were taken every hour with antacids in between. Currently, it is believed that this regimen increases gastric acid secretion. A bland diet has no effect on peptic ulcer disease. Some physicians prescribe six small

Nursing Process: Planning
Client Needs: Health Promotion and Maintenance
Clinical Area: Medical Nursing

feedings of bland food to keep food in the stomach.

68. (4) Riopan consists of aluminum and magnesium hydroxide combined into one chemical. This antacid helps prevent diarrhea that is caused by pure magnesium antacids, such as milk of magnesia, and constipation that is caused by aluminum product antacids, such as Amphojel, Phosphaljel and Basaljel.

Nursing Process: Implementation
Client Needs: Physiological Integrity
Clinical Area: Medical Nursing

69. (2) The client's response is inappropriate to the situation and is an example of inappropriate affect. Lack of affect is when there is no response (including facial expression). Both are indicative of a schizophrenic reaction.

Nursing Process: Analysis
Client Needs: Psychosocial Integrity
Clinical Area: Psychiatric Nursing

70. (4) Simply restating the interaction is the best response so that the client may see the connection and her inappropriate reply. She may or may not choose to talk about her feelings. The nurse's restatement will give her an opportunity to respond, but will not force her to do so.

Nursing Process: Implementation
Client Needs: Safe, Effective Care Environment
Clinical Area: Psychiatric Nursing

71. (2) A partial colectomy is removal of a portion of the colon and reanastamosis of the remaining ends; therefore, elimination will occur normally.

Nursing Process: Implementation
Client Needs: Physiological Integrity
Clinical Area: Surgical Nursing

72. (3) Inability to void after surgery is a common problem. It is important to be aware of the client's output for several reasons: to ensure adequate intake, to detect renal problems, and to assess for blood pressure problems. Solution to this problem is catheterization with a physician's order. The dressing should be closely observed but is not presently a problem. The area on the calf is probably thrombophlebitis and should be reported to the

Nursing Process: Implementation
Client Needs: Safe, Effective Care Environment
Clinical Area: Surgical Nursing

physician immediately. The breath sounds are due to potential lung problems and can be improved by turning, coughing and deep breathing.

73. (4) It is not appropriate to force the person to confront the feared situation because the underlying dynamics are unconscious. This is a phobia and, while the client probably knows his fear is irrational, he is not ready to deal with it in a rational way.

Nursing Process: Implementation
Client Needs: Psychosocial Integrity
Clinical Area: Psychiatric Nursing

74. (1) Birth control pills block the pituitary release of LH which prevents ovulation. This action provides the primary source of contraception.

Nursing Process: Implementation
Client Needs: Health Promotion and Maintenance
Clinical Area: Maternity Nursing

75. (2) The L/S or lecithin/sphingomyelin ratio test determines fetal maturity by examining the amniotic fluid for the presence of surfactant. By the 35th week, lecithin is two or more times greater than sphingomyelin which indicates that fetal lungs are mature enough not to develop respiratory distress syndrome.

Nursing Process: Implementation
Client Needs: Health Promotion and Maintenance
Clinical Area: Maternity Nursing

76. (1) These are classic manifestations of cyanotic heart disease, where partially unoxygenated blood is sent back to the systemic circulation.

Nursing Process: Assessment
Client Needs: Physiological Integrity
Clinical Area: Pediatric Nursing

77. (1) The infusion of all IV drugs that affect the CNS should be carefully monitored and an IV controller is essential for accurate monitoring. Toxic levels of Aminophylline could cause arrhythmias or seizures.

Nursing Process: Implementation
Client Needs: Safe, Effective Care Environment
Clinical Area: Medical Nursing

78. (1) All the answers except (4) are purposes of charting. Answer (1) is the most inclusive and, therefore, the best answer.

Nursing Process: Analysis
Client Needs: Health Promotion and Maintenance
Clinical Area: Medical Nursing

79.   (2) With no cushion, the client may hit his head as he is moved up in bed. With the pillow there, his head will be protected.

Nursing Process: Analysis
Client Needs: Safe, Effective Care Environment
Clinical Area: Medical Nursing

80.   (1) Staying with a client is the most effective way to reduce anxiety. A nurse-client relationship is important, but it will take time to establish. The nurse should proceed at the client's pace and not push her to deal directly with the source of her anxiety.

Nursing Process: Implementation
Client Needs: Psychosocial Integrity
Clinical Area: Psychiatric Nursing

81.   (2) 4 ml is equal to one dram of fluid.

Nursing Process: Planning
Client Needs: Safe, Effective Care Environment
Clinical Area: Medical Nursing

82.   (2) Blood supply may be altered to the wound area leading to an alteration in tissue perfusion. While Health Maintenance and Self-care deficit are appropriate areas of concern, the highest priority nursing diagnosis would be alteration in tissue perfusion.

Nursing Process: Analysis
Client Needs: Safe, Effective Care Environment
Clinical Area: Medical Nursing

83.   (1) Clean surfaces including floors, showers, kitchens, etc., prevent contact with the HIV virus. Therefore, good cleaning practices will prevent the spread of viruses and bacteria. Equipment does not require being disinfected for 24 hours.

Nursing Process: Planning
Client Needs: Health Promotion and Maintenance
Clinical Area: Medical Nursing

84.   (3) Auscultating lung fields provides knowledge of which lung areas are most affected. These areas should be treated first, as many clients cannot tolerate a 30 minute procedure.

Nursing Process: Implementation
Client Needs: Safe, Effective Care Environment
Clinical Area: Medical Nursing

85.   (4) The client should be in dorsal recumbent position with the bed elevated. For knee-high hose, measurement is taken from the Achilles tendon to the popliteal fold and the mid-calf circumference.

Nursing Process: Implementation
Client Needs: Safe, Effective Care Environment
Clinical Area: Surgical Nursing

86. (4) Dry, flaking skin is present when a client is dehydrated. All of the other responses are indicative of an overhydrated state.

Nursing Process: Assessment
Client Needs: Physiological Integrity
Clinical Area: Medical Nursing

87. (2) Infusing blood at 20 gtts/minute allows adequate time to observe for possible transfusion reactions. A faster flow rate would allow too much blood into the system before noting the reaction.

Nursing Process: Implementation
Client Needs: Safe, Effective Care Environment
Clinical Area: Medical Nursing

88. (2) A synthetic cast is less restrictive, lighter in weight and requires less drying time than a plaster of Paris cast.

Nursing Process: Implementation
Client Needs: Health Promotion and Maintenance
Clinical Area: Surgical Nursing

89. (2) The temperature usually reaches 102° F within the first 48 hours postoperatively. Restlessness and dullness to percussion might be present but the increase in temperature is the most significant finding. Tachypnea, not bradycardia, occurs in atelectasis.

Nursing Process: Evaluation
Client Needs: Physiological Integrity
Clinical Area: Medical Nursing

90. (1) The P-R interval indicates atrial contraction; therefore, it should precede the QRS complex, which is indicative of ventricular contraction.

Nursing Process: Assessment
Client Needs: Physiological Integrity
Clinical Area: Medical Nursing

Comprehensive Test 5

1. A client has been admitted to the hospital after an automobile accident. He complains of a headache, an early sign of increased intracranial pressure. The most appropriate position for the nurse to place the client in is

   1. Supine.
   2. Trendelenburg's position with feet elevated.
   3. Semi-Fowler's.
   4. Flat in bed in Sims' position.

2. For a client with increased intracranial pressure, the nurse would expect the physician's treatment orders to include

   1. Fluids decreased to 2000 ml/day.
   2. Lasix IV.
   3. Plasma volume expanders.
   4. Decadron IV.

3. A depressed client told the nurse that she had no reason to live and could not understand why anybody wanted to be bothered with her. The best response by the nurse would be

   1. "Where did you ever get ideas like those?"
   2. "Let's go and sit in the day room."
   3. "Tell me about those people who do not care for you."
   4. "I care for you and I am concerned that you feel so uncomfortable."

4. A client newly admitted to the psychiatric unit will receive electroconvulsive therapy (ECT). ECT is considered most effective in treating

   1. Young clients with depressive reactions.
   2. Elderly clients with depressive reactions.
   3. Any age client with schizophrenia.
   4. Young clients with paranoid reactions.

5. A female client, age 56, is admitted to the oncology unit for implantation of a radium needle after diagnosis of a cervical tumor. The client asks if she can get out of bed to go to the bathroom. The appropriate reply is to say,

   1. "Yes, but I will help you go to the bathroom."
   2. "No, you must have a catheter inserted instead."
   3. "No, you must remain on bedrest, so I will bring you a bedpan."
   4. "Yes, but after you go to the bathroom, please stay in bed.

6. A client sustained burns of her right arm, right chest, face, and neck. She has just been admitted to the burn unit. Her weight on admission is 50 kg. Using the rules of nines, the estimate of the extent of burns is

   1. 27 percent.
   2. 31.5 percent.
   3. 36 percent.
   4. 15 percent.

7. After the first week of hospitalization for a burn client, the diet should be

    1. High protein, low sodium, low carbohydrate.
    2. Low fat, low sodium, high calorie.
    3. High protein, high carbohydrate.
    4. High protein, high vitamin B complex, low sodium.

8. A 16-year-old male client was struck by a car. When the paramedics arrived at the scene, they found him in a prone position. When an initial assessment was made, he stated that he did not have feeling or sensation in his lower extremities. Before transporting the client to the emergency room, the paramedics would most probably

    1. Place him on a spinal board in prone position.
    2. Place a neck collar on the client.
    3. Log-roll him to a supine position and place him on a spinal board.
    4. Place the client in a MAST suit.

9. While reading the physician's progress notes on a client admitted following a bad fall, the nurse finds that he is a quadriplegic. Quadriplegia indicates there is spinal cord damage

    1. Above C8.
    2. Below T1.
    3. At C3.
    4. At T10.

10. A young woman, age 16, is three months pregnant. She has just been informed that she has chlamydia. When discussing the test results with her, she says, "That's not possible. I've only slept with my boyfriend." The best response would be

    1. "Well, then, he has probably slept with someone else who infected him."
    2. "It's all right to tell me the truth. Our conversation is confidential."
    3. "Can you tell me what you know about chlamydia?"
    4. "How you got it doesn't really matter. What's important is that we treat it now."

11. To help a mother-to-be increase her protein intake, the nurse would suggest that she eat a snack of

    1. One-half cup peanuts.
    2. Two apples.
    3. Beef jerky stick.
    4. One cup milk.

12. A young mother, pregnant with her first child, asks the nurse how she can tell if she is going into true labor. The nurse teaches her that the characteristic that distinguishes true labor from false labor is

    1. Painful contractions.
    2. Regular contractions.
    3. Contractions that do not go away with walking.
    4. Lower backache.

13. When a client is experiencing a manic episode, which one of the following problems would the nurse anticipate?

    1. Not enough activities to keep him busy.
    2. Protection of the other clients from his erratic and unpredictable behavior.

3. A rapid and cyclical mood change from manic to depressive to manic.
4. Inability to provide him with enough stimulation.

14. A 54-year-old male client with a 15 year history of cirrhosis from alcohol abuse has had several hospital admissions for bleeding esophageal varices. He has just been readmitted. Assessing his condition, the nurse will observe for

1. Varicose veins and stasis ulcers.
2. Ascites and hemorrhoids.
3. Intermittent claudication and cool extremities.
4. Decreased peripheral pulses and jugular vein distention.

15. A client with bleeding esophageal varices is on bedrest in a semi-Fowler's position. The major objective for using this position is to

1. Lower portal pressure.
2. Allow for effective breathing.
3. Decrease blood pressure.
4. Decrease risk of aspiration from vomiting.

16. After the placement of the Sengstaken-Blakemore tube, the nurse will evaluate the client for

1. Gastrointestinal hemorrhage.
2. Advancing of the tube.
3. Dislodging of the gastric balloon.
4. Esophagitis.

17. For a couple who have requested genetic counseling, the nurse explains that the most common autosomal defect is

1. Tay-Sachs disease.
2. Cystic fibrosis.
3. Turner's syndrome.
4. Down's syndrome.

18. The nurse is counseling a young couple who learned they were going to have a baby. They ask the nurse which partner is responsible for sex determination and sex-linked defects. The nurse would respond that the

1. Sperm and ova have both XY sex chromosomes.
2. XY chromosomes are in the ova only.
3. XY chromosomes are determined after fertilization.
4. Sperm has the determining XY chromosome.

19. A young client, suspecting she is pregnant, comes to the prenatal clinic. She asks the nurse what is included in the initial physical exam. The most appropriate response is a

1. Pelvic exam and x-ray pelvimetry.
2. Direct Coombs test, urinalysis, and physical examination.
3. Complete medical history, including family history and pregnancy history.
4. X-ray pelvimetry and urinalysis.

20. A 25-year-old male client comes to the college mental health clinic and expresses his concern about his increasing fear of cars. He now rides the bus to school and wants to sell his car. The nurse should understand that this behavior most likely represents an attempt by the client to

1. Decrease his anxiety.
2. Relieve his ambivalent feelings about college.

3. Control his fear of cars.
4. Deal with his feelings of resentment of authority and power.

21. When a client experiences an irrational fear, he is using the defense mechanism of

    1. Rationalization.
    2. Displacement.
    3. Conversion.
    4. Sublimation.

22. A 54-year-old client has a long-standing history of angina pectoris and has just been admitted to the hospital. In taking a nursing history, the nurse determines that the client's first action at home should have been to

    1. Call the physician.
    2. Call the ambulance.
    3. Take a nitroglycerin tablet.
    4. Lie down on the sofa to rest.

23. A client just admitted with suspected myocardial infarction has orders for oxygen via nasal cannula. Standing orders for oxygen would mean that the nurse starts oxygen at

    1. 2 liters/minute.
    2. 6 liters/minute.
    3. 10 liters/minute.
    4. 15 liters/minute.

24. Which of the following diagnostic indicators will be used in the diagnosis of an acute MI?

    1. Cardiac enzymes, EKG, arteriogram.
    2. Arteriogram, duration of pain, EKG.

3. EKG, symptoms, cardiac enzymes.
4. Symptoms, stress EKG, cardiac enzymes.

25. A three year old has not been feeling well for several weeks. When his mother brings him to the hospital, a tentative diagnosis of nephrosis is made. Which of the following clinical profiles would substantiate the diagnosis of nephrosis?

    1. Edema, hyperlipidemia, hypertension, tachycardia.
    2. Hematuria, hypertension, proteinuria, glycosuria.
    3. Hyperlipidemia, proteinuria, hypoalbuminemia, edema.
    4. Proteinuria, polydipsia, polyuria, edema.

26. The nurse group therapist in a weekly therapy group begins the meeting by introducing herself and having the members introduce themselves. Her next responsibility as the leader would be to

    1. Assist the group in handling problems through acting as a resource person.
    2. Orient the group to its task and promote group cohesion.
    3. Manage conflicts and resistances within the group.
    4. Encourage the group members to express their feelings.

27. A young schizophrenic client is started on Trilafon 10 mg tid. The nurse knows that antipsychotic drugs have side effects so the nurse will be observing the client for

    1. Drowsiness and blurred vision.
    2. Headaches, confusion, and drowsiness.

3. Uncoordinated, jerky movements, and difficulty speaking.
4. Drooling, shuffling gait, and spasms.

28. After their baby was diagnosed with phenylketonuria (PKU), the parents are concerned about future children and ask how it occurs in a child. The nurse responds with the statement,

1. "It is transmitted by a defective gene."
2. "The disease is not inherited; it is a defect in metabolism."
3. "The defect can only come from the mother."
4. "Both parents must carry one defective gene."

29. A 62-year-old female client is worried about a cataract forming in her eyes. The nurse tells her that if this is happening, she will experience

1. A white halo when looking at lights.
2. Floating spots before her eyes.
3. Blurred vision.
4. Difficulty seeing at night.

30. Which one of the following drugs would the nurse expect to be ordered for a cataract patient?

1. Pilocarpine.
2. Diamox.
3. Belladonna.
4. Atropine sulfate.

31. A client who is gravida 1 para 0 and 3½ months pregnant is admitted to the emergency room. Due to heavy bleeding, the nurse suspects that she may be having a spontaneous abortion. The client appears apprehensive. What is the most appropriate nursing statement at this time?

1. "It will be over soon. Try not to worry so much."
2. "This is probably God's way of getting rid of a problem pregnancy."
3. "Don't be frightened. What do you think caused this to happen?"
4. "You seem frightened. I will stay right here with you."

32. Which of the following people would be the best candidate for use of the insulin pump?

1. A working mother of two young children.
2. An adolescent with brittle diabetes.
3. A 40-year-old business executive.
4. A 25-year-old Down's syndrome individual.

33. The nurse in the newborn observation nursery is unable to pass a nasogastric tube into a baby's stomach; she has met resistance with each attempt. Tracheoesophageal fistula with atresia is suspected. Other observations that validate this condition and are important for the nurse to chart during an assessment include

1. Excessive mucus, coughing and gagging, frequent crying.
2. Gradual onset of projectile vomiting, cyanosis, irritability.
3. Excessive drooling, choking and coughing during feeding.
4. Abdominal distention, visible peristaltic waves.

34. The best nursing response to parents who are concerned about their baby's congenital defect is to say,

1. "You should express your concern to the physician."
2. "Don't be concerned about your baby. He's going to be fine."
3. "Tell me how you are feeling concerned."
4. "There seems to be little permanently wrong with your child."

35. A 34-year-old male client with a diagnosis of schizophrenia, paranoid type, barges into the dayroom yelling, "The President is on my side. If you bother me, I'll send him after you!" The most therapeutic response is to say

1. "We do not allow threatening behavior here."
2. "You don't expect me to believe the President is a friend of yours!"
3. "I understand your concern. I will see that the others don't bother you right now."
4. "What do you think we're going to do to bother you?"

36. A female client is eclamptic and has been receiving magnesium sulfate IV. The nurse evaluating her condition knows that the symptom indicating it is unsafe to continue the drug is

1. Presence of deep tendon reflexes.
2. Respiratory rate of 10 per minute.
3. Urine output of 150 ml over the last four hours.
4. Complaints of back pain.

37. A client is ready to begin sharing personal concerns and feelings and says, "I want to tell you something, and I want you to promise not to tell anyone else, okay?" The appropriate nursing response is

1. "Okay. You can trust me."
2. "That depends on what your secret is."
3. "I don't keep secrets. It's not therapeutic."
4. "I can't promise that; I do share information with the staff."

38. High birth-weight infants, infants large for their gestational age, need to be assessed for

1. Hyperglycemia.
2. Hypercalcemia.
3. Hypoglycemia.
4. Hypocalcemia.

39. A 54-year-old male alcoholic is admitted to the unit for detoxification and treatment. Which of the following statements by him may be a barrier to the development of a therapeutic relationship?

1. "Nurse, you said I reminded you of your alcoholic father."
2. "You want to spend some time talking with me. Won't you just be wasting your time?"
3. "I bet you love to see us old drunks come in!"
4. "How many children do you have, nurse?"

40. A client has been given the diagnosis of Alzheimer's disease. The nurse observes that he has been incontinent and soiled his clothes for the second time on this shift. The most appropriate nursing intervention is to

1. Put the client in adult diapers to protect him from embarrassment.
2. Scold the client and tell him not to wet his pants again.
3. Tell the client you will change his pants and establish a two-hour schedule of taking him to the bathroom.
4. Tell the client to ask you for assistance the next time he has to go to the bathroom.

41. If a child is brought into the emergency room and a case of child abuse is suspected, the legal responsibility of the staff who evaluate the case is that

    1. The nurse is legally responsible for reporting a suspected child abuse.
    2. The physician, not the nurse, is legally responsible for reporting child abuse.
    3. Both the physician and the nurse are legally responsible for reporting child abuse.
    4. Neither the physician nor the nurse is legally responsible for reporting child abuse.

42. A 38-year-old client has just returned from ileostomy surgery after a long history of ulcerative colitis. The nurse will pay strict attention to the skin around the ileostomy stoma because

    1. Digestive enzymes may cause skin breakdown.
    2. The effluent is more solid than watery.
    3. It is very difficult to ensure proper fit of the appliance.
    4. It will take longer to heal than a colostomy stoma.

43. A client who has had spinal surgery is placed on a Nelson bed. The primary goal of using this equipment is to

    1. Prevent orthostatic hypotension when a client is on bedrest.
    2. Maintain stress on bone at intervals.
    3. Change positions from horizontal to vertical at intervals when a client is on bedrest.
    4. Maintain optimal functioning of body systems.

44. A client with a fractured leg has had a steel pin inserted and skeletal traction attached. The most important assessment following this procedure is to

    1. Check the pin site for local pain, redness or drainage.
    2. Observe for a change in color or temperature in leg that does not have traction applied.
    3. Examine all bony prominences.
    4. Check for normal range of motion in the extremity.

45. While instructing a client with the with the diagnosis of Insulin-Dependent Diabetes Mellitus, type I (IDDM) about his diet, which of the following items constitute one meat exchange on the ADA exchange diet?

    1. One cup of whole milk.
    2. Two ounces of cheddar cheese.
    3. One-fourth cup of tuna fish.
    4. Ten small nuts.

46. A child, age five, has been admitted to the pediatric unit. His diagnosis is suspected

hookworm infestation. Hookworms are most frequently transmitted by

1. Contact with contaminated feces.
2. Ingestion of poorly cooked food.
3. Walking barefoot in soil.
4. Poor housekeeping.

47. When a change in the fetal heart rate occurs with the administration of the oxytocin challenge test, the nursing intervention is to

1. Apply an external fetal monitor.
2. Auscultate the fetal heart rate.
3. Place the client in a supine position.
4. Place the client in a semi-Fowler's position.

48 While taking a client's history, she relates that she has leg pains that begin when she walks but cease when she stops walking. The condition the nurse will do further assessment on is

1. An acute obstruction in the vessels of the legs.
2. Peripheral vascular problems in both legs.
3. Diabetes.
4. Calcium deficiency.

49. The nurse is evaluating a client's renal function lab results and notes that her specific gravity is 1.020. The nurse understands that this number indicates that the client's kidneys

1. Are unable to concentrate urine.
2. Have lost the ability to dilute urine.
3. May be developing renal failure.
4. Are functioning within normal limits.

50. A client with the diagnosis of acute pancreatitis has orders for her to remain NPO. The nurse understands that the purpose of this order is to

1. Keep the stomach empty.
2. Avoid interference with the pain medication.
3. Eliminate the chief stimulus to enzyme release.
4. Avoid the use of an anticholinergic drug.

51. A neurological evaluation indicates that the client has a brain abscess. A priority on-going assessment is to observe for

1. Weight loss.
2. Fluid imbalance.
3. Increased temperature.
4. Neurological deficits.

52. A client is admitted to the hospital with a diagnosis of Meniere's syndrome. She complains of infrequent symptomatic episodes and difficulty walking. During the assessment, the nurse will assess for a common symptom associated with this syndrome which is

1. Nausea and vomiting.
2. Profound dizziness.
3. Vertigo.
4. Tinnitus.

53. A client has been admitted to the medical unit with a diagnosis of hepatitis type A. A primary nursing intervention with type A hepatitis is to

1. Eliminate all shellfish from the diet.
2. Change from rectal to oral temperatures.

3. Put the client on a low calorie diet immediately.
4. Isolate the client during the time he is jaundiced.

54. A client's admitting diagnosis is major depressive episode. In formulating a nursing care plan, the nurse will include as a priority goal

1. Establishing a nurse-client relationship.
2. Providing a structured schedule of activities.
3. Providing a safe milieu.
4. Building the client's self-esteem.

55. A 16 year old comes to the maternity clinic with her mother. She is three months pregnant, unmarried and lives in an economically deprived area of the city. Completing an initial assessment on this client, the nurse realizes that a pregnant adolescent has an increased risk of

1. Severe emotional problems.
2. Nutritional deficiency.
3. Pregnancy induced hypertension (PIH).
4. Diabetes.

56. A pregnant client is admitted to the maternity unit with a more severe form of PIH, eclampsia. She is hospitalized and magnesium sulfate is administered. Evaluating the effects of the medication, an important toxic sign to observe for is

1. Generalized edema.
2. Increased blood pressure.
3. Increased patellar reflex.
4. Extreme thirst.

57. A 35-year-old client just admitted to the psychiatric unit is experiencing a manic episode. The nursing diagnosis that is most appropriate for her condition is

1. Activity Intolerance; Comfort, Alterations in; and Sexual Dysfunction.
2. Self-Care Deficit: Feeding, Bathing, and Dressing; Thought Processes, Alterations in; and Social Interaction, Impaired.
3. Violence, Potential for; Home Maintenance Management, Impaired; and Activity Intolerance.
4. Coping, Ineffective Individual; Injury, Potential for; and Nutrition, Alterations in.

58. Lithium carbonate is ordered for a client in a manic episode. The nurse expects that the therapeutic blood level will be between

1. 0.8 and 1.2 mEq/liter of blood.
2. 1.5 and 2.0 mEq/liter of blood.
3. 1.5 mEq/liter of blood and any level up to 3.0.
4. 0.5 and 0.8 mEq/liter of blood.

59. A client's condition with cirrhosis and ascites deteriorates and he develops prehepatic encephalopathy. The care plan includes monitoring bile salts that have been administered. The nurse understands that the purpose of bile salts is to

1. Control hemorrhage.
2. Increase prothrombin time.
3. Improve absorption of vitamin K.
4. Enrich a diet lacking in vitamin K.

60. A client has been admitted to the hospital with a diagnosis of suspected bacterial

endocarditis. The complication that the nurse will constantly observe for is

1. Presence of a heart murmur.
2. Systemic emboli.
3. Fever.
4. Congestive heart failure.

61. A 25 year old has been admitted to the psychiatric unit with a diagnosis of acute schizophrenic disorder. He is unkempt and speaks in unclear sentences. In the first nurse-client interaction, the client says, "Yesternoon the sunmoon went over the rover to see the lawnmower." The nurse knows that the client is manifesting

    1. A delusion.
    2. Associative looseness.
    3. An hallucination.
    4. Disturbance of affect.

62. A client is to receive codeine for pain with her diagnosis of head injury. The nurse would also expect the physician to order a stool softener. The reason for this order is to

    1. Prevent paralytic ileus.
    2. Avoid straining during evacuation.
    3. Prevent bowel stasis.
    4. Prevent complications from the codeine.

63. A client was hospitalized briefly with an episode of urolithiasis until a stone was passed. She has now been readmitted with complaints of low back pain, nausea and diarrhea. Formulating a care plan for this client, the nurse knows that a priority goal is to

    1. Encourage fluids to 3000 ml per day.
    2. Record intake and output.

3. Provide appropriate diet therapy.
4. Limit fluid intake initially.

64. An 18 year old was hospitalized for anorexia nervosa. After one week of treatment, the nursing team met to evaluate the client's progress. An indication that she was improving would be when she

    1. Talked about going home.
    2. Attended all groups.
    3. Had gained four pounds.
    4. Expressed a desire to "get into shape" again.

65. A client with peptic ulcer disease has had a subtotal gastric resection. His postoperative pain can most effectively be controlled by

    1. Medicating for pain before the previous dose totally wears off.
    2. Medicating for pain at least every six hours.
    3. Waiting until the client requests pain medication.
    4. Alternating a maximum with a minimum dose.

66. An 18 year old is hospitalized after an accident where she lost the use of her legs. The nurse observes her when she is approached, sitting in a wheelchair crying and she says, "Go away; no one can help me." Your best response is to say

    1. "It will help to talk about it."
    2. "I'll go away, but I'll come back in half an hour and perhaps we can talk."
    3. "I'd like to help. Can you tell me about what's wrong?"
    4. "Crying doesn't help; perhaps talking will make you feel better."

67. A 52-year-old male client has an admitting diagnosis of rheumatoid arthritis. He is started on indomethacin, an anti-inflammatory medication. Part of the care plan is to assess effects of the drug. The nurse would expect

    1. Hypertension.
    2. GI disturbance.
    3. Tinnitus.
    4. Joint stiffness.

68. A six month old is admitted with a diagnosis of severe diarrhea. The most important nursing objective is to

    1. Make constant assessment of the child's dehydration level.
    2. Accurately record the number of the child's stools.
    3. Dispose of the stools in proper containers.
    4. Monitor the child's electrolyte lab results.

69. A young child with severe diarrhea is to be fed via intravenous hyperalimentation. A complication related to the implanted catheter that the nurse will assess for is

    1. Plugging or dislodging of the catheter.
    2. Air embolism.
    3. Insertion in the superior vena cava.
    4. Generalized infection.

70. A 15 year old has been admitted to the adolescent unit with scoliosis and will be having surgery for insertion of a Harrington rod. Considering the course of therapy with a Harrington rod insertion, the problem that she is most likely to exhibit is

    1. Identity crisis.
    2. Body image changes.

3. Feelings of displacement.
4. Loss of privacy.

71. During the hospitalization of a 14-month-old toddler, his parents tried to spend time at his bedside. One day, however, after his parents left his room and returned home, he began screaming and throwing things out of his crib. In this situation the most therapeutic nursing action is to

    1. Turn on TV as a distractor.
    2. Ignore the crying and wait until he wears himself out.
    3. Stay in his room, talking and trying to comfort him.
    4. Call his parents and have them return.

72. The severity of a burn is the combination of the depth of the burn and the extent of body surface area (BSA) involved. Which of the following factors is the first priority when assessing the severity of the burn?

    1. Age of the client.
    2. Associated medical problems.
    3. Location of the burn.
    4. Cause of the burn.

73. A female client is admitted to the hospital with an obstruction just proximal to her old ileostomy stoma. She has had the ileostomy for six months. For a client with an ileostomy which one of the following foods should be eliminated in the diet because it could cause obstruction?

    1. Cabbage.
    2. Corn.
    3. Red meat.
    4. Radishes.

74. One of the primary principles that guides therapy for a client in prehepatic coma is

    1. Maintaining protein intake at a moderate or normal level.
    2. Administering neomycin and lactulose to reduce bacterial production and ammonia.
    3. Maintaining a mildly sedative state to reduce stress.
    4. Offering the client adequate fluids by mouth to maintain fluid and electrolyte balance.

75. An important initial goal for a client just admitted to the psychiatric unit because he attacked a friend is to

    1. Establish a relationship and set the limits of the relationship.
    2. Explain to the client that his behavior was unacceptable and dangerous.
    3. Explore the truth of the client's statements.
    4. Set behavioral limits on the client.

76. A client has just returned from surgery for evacuation of a hematoma. Immediately after the evacuation, the nursing intervention considered a priority is

    1. Observing for CSF leaks around the evacuation site.
    2. Assessing for an increase in temperature indicating infection.
    3. Establishing and maintaining a patent airway.
    4. Observing for signs of increasing intracranial pressure.

77. The nurse is assisting a 9-year-old's mother to plan her care at home following discharge after an acute asthma attack. Which of Erikson's stages of growth and development would it be important to take into account in the discharge planning?

    1. Autonomy vs. shame and doubt.
    2. Initiative vs. guilt.
    3. Industry vs. inferiority.
    4. Identity vs. role confusion.

78. Assessing the urine of a client with suspected cholecystitis, the nurse expects that the color will most likely be

    1. Pale yellow.
    2. Greenish-brown.
    3. Red.
    4. Yellow-orange.

79. An 18 year old has been in a motorcycle accident and sustained a head injury. The nurse admitting him notices that his IV is infusing at 125 ml/hour. Until there are orders for the IV rate, the nurse will

    1. Slow the rate to 20 ml/hour.
    2. Continue the rate at 125 ml/hour.
    3. Slow the rate to 50 ml/hour.
    4. Increase the rate to 150 ml/hour.

80. An 11 year old with cystic fibrosis will take pancreatic enzymes three times a day. The nurse will know that her mother needs more education on the purpose and timing of these enzymes if she says

    1. "They should be taken at meal times, three times a day."
    2. "They should be given following breakfast, lunch and dinner."

3. "The purpose of the enzymes is to help digest the fat in foods."

4. "My daughter should take them prior to meals."

81. For a 38-year-old client with chronic lymphocytic leukemia, a priority nursing diagnosis is

1. Infection, Potential for.
2. Impairment of Skin Integrity.
3. Alteration in Tissue Perfusion.
4. Fluid Volume Deficit.

82. A client, age 60, has been admitted to the hospital with a diagnosis of right ventricular failure. With a central venous line in place, the nurse would expect that the CVP reading would be

1. 0–2 mmHg.
2. 5–10 cm H_2O.
3. 8–10 mmHg.
4. 15–20 cm H_2O.

83. A client is brought into the emergency room bleeding profusely from a deep laceration on his left lower forearm. After observing universal precautions, the initial nursing action should be to

1. Apply a tourniquet just below the elbow.
2. Apply pressure directly over the wound.
3. Cleanse the wound to determine the extent of damage.
4. Elevate the limb and apply ice to decrease blood flow.

84. A client is admitted to the psychiatric unit with a diagnosis of anxiety disorder.

Effective nursing measures to help this client cope with anxiety would include

1. Giving her some responsibility for manipulating the environment.
2. Removing all disturbing factors in the environment.
3. Encouraging her to read to provide distraction.
4. Remaining close by her and allowing her to express her feelings.

85. A client is brought into the emergency room with an admitting diagnosis of delirium tremens (DTs). After finding a private room for the client, the priority intervention is to

1. Administer the standing order of Valium.
2. Put up the siderails of the bed.
3. Attempt to get a history to validate if he really is experiencing DTs.
4. Keep the room very quiet with lights down to minimize stimulation.

86. A client is admitted to the labor room. She tells the nurse that contractions started two hours ago, and she has soaked a perineal pad with bright-red blood in the past ten minutes. The nurse suspects a placenta previa. The first nursing action is to

1. Perform a vaginal examination to determine cervical dilatation.
2. Notify the physician immediately.
3. Order blood to be typed and cross matched.
4. Apply an external fetal monitor.

87. A three year old is brought to the hospital by his mother who explains that the child has been sick for several days and has had a

"barklike" cough. The nurse assesses nasal flaring. The nursing action is to

1. Tell him to cough.
2. Give four back blows.
3. Ask him to speak.
4. Obtain an immediate order for oxygen.

88. If a child has impetigo contagiosa, to prevent further spread of the disease the nurse should instruct the mother to

1. Strictly isolate this child from others in his family.
2. Wash toys and other objects the child uses with soap and very hot water.
3. Take all other children in the family to the physician to be vaccinated for this disease.
4. Not take any special precautions.

89. A client is admitted to the maternity unit two weeks before her actual delivery date. She is there for evaluation because she is experiencing polyhydramnios. The nurse understands that this diagnosis means that

1. There is the normal amount of amniotic fluid, thinner in volume.
2. A less-than-normal amount of amniotic fluid is present.
3. An excessive amount of amniotic fluid is present.
4. A leak is causing fluid to accumulate outside the amniotic sac.

90. A client is unable to sleep. He is pacing the floor, head down, and wringing his hands. As the nurse recognizes that he is anxious, what is the most appropriate intervention?

1. Encourage him to talk about his behavior.
2. Give him his prn sleeping medication.
3. Let him know that the nurse is interested and willing to listen.
4. Explore with him the alternatives to pacing the floor.

Comprehensive Test 5
Answers with Rationale

1. (3) In the acute phase, the semi-Fowler's position allows for increased venous drainage from the brain. Trendelenburg's position should be avoided.

    Nursing Process: Implementation
    Client Needs: Safe, Effective Care Environment
    Clinical Area: Medical Nursing

2. (4) Steroids (Decadron) reduce the incidence and severity of cerebral edema by their anti-inflammatory effect. They act slowly, while the hypertonic solutions rapidly reduce pressure. Fluids would be limited to 1200 ml/day. Mannitol might also be given to provide diuretic action.

    Nursing Process: Planning
    Client Needs: Physiological Integrity
    Clinical Area: Medical Nursing

3. (4) It is important for the client to be aware that someone cares, and this response may be meaningful enough to interrupt ideas of suicide. The other responses do not relate directly to the underlying dynamics of depression.

    Nursing Process: Implementation
    Client Needs: Psychosocial Integrity
    Clinical Area: Psychiatric Nursing

4. (2) Depression is more successfully treated by ECT than are the other conditions listed. It is a treatment of choice for elderly clients who experience depression with vegetative aspects. A dramatic lift of the depression may be seen after only a few treatments. None of the other disorders have been found to be successfully treated with ECT.

    Nursing Process: Planning
    Client Needs: Psychosocial Integrity
    Clinical Area: Psychiatric Nursing

5. (3) Bedrest is important when a radiation source is in place, because restricted movement prevents dislodging. Often a teflon catheter is inserted to avoid the necessity of a bedpan while the radiation source is in

    Nursing Process: Implementation
    Client Needs: Physiological Integrity
    Clinical Area: Medical Nursing

place. (Teflon is used instead of rubber because radiation decomposes rubber.)

6.   (1)   Head = 9 percent (face and neck each equal 4 1/2 percent), arm = 9 percent, and chest = 9 percent for a total of 27 percent.

Nursing Process: Analysis
Client Needs: Physiological Integrity
Clinical Area: Medical Nursing

7.   (3)   A diet high in protein as well as carbohydrates is essential to allow the protein to be spared for tissue regeneration.

Nursing Process: Planning
Client Needs: Health Promotion and Maintenance
Clinical Area: Medical Nursing

8.   (1)   For transporting the client without additional injury to the spinal cord, he should be placed on a spinal board in the position in which he was found by the paramedics. An abnormal movement or twisting of the injured cord segment could extend the injury. There are no predisposing injuries which would prohibit a transfer to the spinal board. A MAST suit is used in shock states.

Nursing Process: Analysis
Client Needs: Physiological Integrity
Clinical Area: Medical Nursing

9.   (1)   Injury above C8 would involve motor and sensory activity of all four extremities. This is termed quadriplegia.

Nursing Process: Analysis
Client Needs: Physiological Integrity
Clinical Area: Medical Nursing

10.   (3)   This is a good opportunity for client teaching, and the first thing the nurse must do is ascertain the client's knowledge base.

Nursing Process: Assessment
Client Needs: Health Promotion and Maintenance
Clinical Area: Maternity Nursing

11.   (1)   One-half cup of peanuts has twice the protein as one cup of milk or the beef jerky. Apples contain very little protein.

Nursing Process: Implementation
Client Needs: Health Promotion and Maintenance
Clinical Area: Maternity Nursing

12.   (3)   False labor pains tend to go away with walking. Both may be painful and regular, and a lower backache may be present with both true and false labor.

Nursing Process: Analysis
Client Needs: Health Promotion and Maintenance
Clinical Area: Maternity Nursing

13.   (2) The other clients may have to be protected from the client. The nurse would not expect the course of illness to move rapidly through the manic-depressive-manic cycle,

Nursing Process: Planning
Client Needs: Psychosocial Integrity
Clinical Area: Psychiatric Nursing

although she should observe for signs of depression. The unit would probably provide too much, rather than too little, stimulation.

14. (2)   Along with ascites, another reflection of increased portal pressure is hemorrhoids. Varicose veins result from faulty superficial leg vein valves. Intermittent claudication results from decreased circulating blood to muscles. Decreased peripheral pulses occur as a result of arterial occlusion.

Nursing Process: Assessment
Client Needs: Physiological Integrity
Clinical Area: Medical Nursing

15. (2)   Any position that impedes respirations by the pressure of abdominal contents on the diaphragm should be avoided; therefore, the best position for the client is semi-Fowler's position, which allows for more effective breathing.

Nursing Process: Planning
Client Needs: Safe, Effective Care Environment
Clinical Area: Medical Nursing

16. (3)   Once the gastric balloon is inflated with 100–300 ml of air, the tube is pulled back slowly so that the balloon is held firmly against the cardioesophageal junction. The tube is secured to the nose to prevent necrosis of tissue. If the gastric balloon dislodges itself into the esophagus, the client will experience airway obstruction. The Sengstaken-Blakemore tube does not advance by gravity as does the Miller-Abbott tube, which contains mercury in its balloon. The tube is used to control esophageal hemorrhage. Esophagitis is not a complication of the Sengstaken-Blakemore tube.

Nursing Process: Evaluation
Client Needs: Physiological Integrity
Clinical Area: Medical Nursing

17. (4)   Down's syndrome is the most common autosomal defect which occurs most frequently in women over age 36; Tay-Sachs and cystic fibrosis occur less frequently; and Turner's syndrome is a sex chromosome defect.

Nursing Process: Analysis
Client Needs: Health Promotion and Maintenance
Clinical Area: Maternity Nursing

18. (4) Only the sperm has the determining XY chromosome. The ova only has the female XX chromosome.

Nursing Process: **Analysis**
Client Needs: **Health Promotion and Maintenance**
Clinical Area: **Maternity Nursing**

19. (3) The first physical exam should include a complete medical history, including past history, family history, and pregnancy history. It should also include a complete physical, blood work, and a urinalysis. X-ray pelvimetry early in pregnancy may cause fetal malformations and should only be done in the latter part of pregnancy if cephalopelvic disproportion is suspected. A direct Coombs test is a test of the umbilical cord blood to detect Rh sensitization of infants of Rh-negative mothers.

Nursing Process: **Analysis**
Client Needs: **Health Promotion and Maintenance**
Clinical Area: **Maternity Nursing**

20. (1) The client has unrealistic, irrational fears which would cause the nurse to suspect a phobia. Phobic reactions are an attempt to deal with a high level of anxiety.

Nursing Process: **Analysis**
Client Needs: **Psychosocial Integrity**
Clinical Area: **Psychiatric Nursing**

21. (2) In phobic reactions, the individual displaces his anxiety onto a symbolic objective that presents no actual fear or danger to him.

Nursing Process: **Analysis**
Client Needs: **Psychosocial Integrity**
Clinical Area: **Psychiatric Nursing**

22. (3) Recalling that the client has a past history of angina, he should have taken nitroglycerin and then lain down to rest. This client probably needs more instruction on his cardiac condition and the purpose of taking nitroglycerin.

Nursing Process: **Assessment**
Client Needs: **Health Promotion and Maintenance**
Clinical Area: **Medical Nursing**

23. (2) Six liters is usually sufficient to increase oxygen flow to 38–44 percent. If the client had a history of chronic pulmonary obstructive disease, the oxygen would be set at 2 liters/minute. High levels of oxygen will disrupt the CO_2 center.

Nursing Process: **Implementation**
Client Needs: **Physiological Integrity**
Clinical Area: **Medical Nursing**

24.   (3)   The cardiac enzymes LDH, CPK and SGOT are enzymes contained within the heart muscle cells. When injury occurs to myocardial cells, these enzymes are released in the bloodstream, and elevated levels are found in the serum. Usually, the pain of an MI begins spontaneously, persists for hours or days, and is not relieved by rest or nitrates. Often, the EKG reveals changes indicating the presence and location of the infarction.

Nursing Process: Assessment
Client Needs: Physiological Integrity
Clinical Area: Medical Nursing

25.   (3)   Hyperlipidemia, proteinuria, hypoalbuminemia, and edema are the four classic symptoms of childhood nephrosis. Tachycardia, hematuria and polyuria are not symptoms of nephrosis. Hypertension might be present, especially if there is fluid overload.

Nursing Process: Assessment
Client Needs: Physiological Integrity
Clinical Area: Pediatric Nursing

26.   (2)   The group is in the orientation phase, and it is the leader's responsibility to orient the group to its purpose and task. Later in the group process, the leader will perform the other tasks of group leader, such as assisting the members to handle conflict.

Nursing Process: Planning
Client Needs: Psychosocial Integrity
Clinical Area: Psychiatric Nursing

27.   (3)   Dystonia, uncoordinated jerky movements and difficulty speaking, may occur early (in one or two days) in the use of antipsychotics, whereas (4) symptoms occur with tardive dyskinesia, which tends to occur late. (1) are side effects of antianxiety drugs, and (2) are side effects of MAO inhibitor drugs.

Nursing Process: Assessment
Client Needs: Safe, Effective Care Environment
Clinical Area: Psychiatric Nursing

28.   (4)   PKU is transmitted by an autosomal recessive gene, and each parent must carry one defective gene. Answer (4) is more specific than answer (1). This condition occurs once in about 16,000 births in the United States.

Nursing Process: Implementation
Client Needs: Physiological Integrity
Clinical Area: Pediatric Nursing

29. (3) Blurred vision, peripheral visual loss, and an opacity are the symptoms associated with cataracts. Seeing white halos and floating spots are symptoms of a detached retina.

Nursing Process: Implementation
Client Needs: Safe, Effective Care Environment
Clinical Area: Medical Nursing

30. (4) Atropine sulfate is the drug used for mydriasis; the other drugs are used to treat glaucoma.

Nursing Process: Planning
Client Needs: Physiological Integrity
Clinical Area: Medical Nursing

31. (4) Acknowledging her apprehension lets the client know that the nurse is sensitive to what she's feeling. Reassuring her that she will not be alone is important. This statement is also open-ended and will allow her to talk about whatever might be on her mind.

Nursing Process: Implementation
Client Needs: Psychosocial Integrity
Clinical Area: Maternity Nursing

32. (3) The best candidate for use of the insulin pump is a bright, conscientious client who has the time and will take the time to learn pump use and follow through on the instructions. Therefore, the best candidate of those listed is the business executive.

Nursing Process: Assessment
Client Needs: Safe, Effective Care Environment
Clinical Area: Medical Nursing

33. (3) A tracheoesophageal (TE) fistula is a connection between the esophagus and trachea. Symptoms such as drooling, choking and coughing are caused by an overflow of liquid into the larynx and trachea.

Nursing Process: Assessment
Client Needs: Physiological Integrity
Clinical Area: Pediatric Nursing

34. (3) The parents should be given an opportunity to express their fears verbally. This response from the nurse would facilitate further communication and not invalidate the parents' fears concerning their child.

Nursing Process: Implementation
Client Needs: Psychosocial Integrity
Clinical Area: Pediatric Nursing

35. (3) The client's grandiose attacking statements probably reflect his feelings of fear and his anger at being afraid. His fear should be respected but not necessarily confronted since this might increase his

Nursing Process: Implementation
Client Needs: Safe, Effective Care Environment
Clinical Area: Psychiatric Nursing

anxiety. Confrontation would probably escalate his aggressiveness and add to his defensiveness. In his present state, a probing question would be threatening and inappropriate, although it might be useful later.

36. (2) The respiratory rate must be maintained at a rate of at least twelve per minute as a precaution against excessive depression of impulses at the myoneural junction. When deep tendon reflexes are absent and the urine output is decreased, the medication should be held to prevent complications of CNS depression.

Nursing Process: Evaluation
Client Needs: Safe, Effective Care Environment
Clinical Area: Maternity Nursing

37. (4) It is important for the nurse not to be manipulated into agreeing to keep a secret. This approach goes against a total team effort in caring for the client and results in the client feeling insecure. It is, however, important to discuss the confidentiality of what the client relates.

Nursing Process: Implementation
Client Needs: Psychosocial Integrity
Clinical Area: Psychiatric Nursing

38. (3) Infants who are large for their gestational age are frequently hypoglycemic and must be observed closely for signs of low blood-sugar levels. These infants are fed early and frequently.

Nursing Process: Assessment
Client Needs: Physiological Integrity
Clinical Area: Pediatric Nursing

39. (1) The nurse's unresolved attitudes and feelings toward her father may spill over and influence her relationship with the client. If the nurse is not aware of her attitudes, she may lose her objectivity and this would affect the relationship.

Nursing Process: Analysis
Client Needs: Psychosocial Integrity
Clinical Area: Psychiatric Nursing

40. (3) Even though the nurse may eventually have to place diapers on the client, this is not the first intervention. An every two-hour bathroom schedule may solve the problem because he will not remember to say when he needs to urinate.

Nursing Process: Implementation
Client Needs: Safe, Effective Care Environment
Clinical Area: Psychiatric Nursing

41.   (3)   Both the nurse and physician, independently, are legally responsible to report a suspected battered child to the proper authorities.

Nursing Process: Evaluation
Client Needs: Safe, Effective Care Environment
Clinical Area: Psychiatric Nursing

42.   (1)   The discharge from an ileostomy is watery and contains many digestive enzymes that have not been absorbed by the intestinal villi. These enzymes may cause skin breakdown. None of the other answers is accurate.

Nursing Process: Analysis
Client Needs: Physiological Integrity
Clinical Area: Surgical Nursing

43.   (2)   The Nelson bed provides position variation. The most important goal, although all of the answers meet objectives, is to maintain stress on bone to prevent loss of calcium with long-term bedrest.

Nursing Process: Planning
Client Needs: Physiological Integrity
Clinical Area: Surgical Nursing

44.   (1)   One of the most important nursing responsibilities is to assess and prevent complications at the pin site. Any observation of pain, redness, heat, or drainage at the pin site may indicate infection. While it is important to check bony prominences to prevent pressure ulcers and range of motion, pin site care is the priority assessment.

Nursing Process: Assessment
Client Needs: Safe, Effective Care Environment
Clinical Area: Surgical Nursing

45.   (3)   The correct exchange is one-fourth cup of tuna fish. Milk is from the milk exchange; one ounce, not two, of cheese is equivalent and nuts are from the fat exchange.

Nursing Process: Planning
Client Needs: Health Promotion and Maintenance
Clinical Area: Medical Nursing

46.   (3)   Hookworm is usually transmitted through soil contaminated with feces. Answer (1) is not as accurate as (3). Ingestion of inadequately cooked pork could result in spread of tapeworm. Poor housekeeping and hygiene may contribute to the spread of roundworms.

Nursing Process: Analysis
Client Needs: Physiological Integrity
Clinical Area: Pediatric Nursing

47. (4) A semi-Fowler's or lateral recumbent position will prevent or reverse the supine hypotensive syndrome. Supine position is not appropriate. Positioning the client is the intervention, but monitoring the fetal heart rate is also important.

Nursing Process: Implementation
Client Needs: Safe, Effective Care Environment
Clinical Area: Maternity Nursing

48. (2) Intermittent claudication is a condition that indicates vascular deficiencies in the peripheral vascular system. If an obstruction were present, the leg pain would persist when the client stops walking. Diabetes can result in vascular deficiency in the legs, but it is not the only cause. Low calcium level may cause leg cramps, but would not necessarily be related to walking.

Nursing Process: Assessment
Client Needs: Physiological Integrity
Clinical Area: Medical Nursing

49. (4) This is the correct answer. If specific gravity is 1.018 or greater, it indicates that the kidneys are functioning within normal limits and are able to concentrate urine.

Nursing Process: Evaluation
Client Needs: Physiological Integrity
Clinical Area: Medical Nursing

50. (3) Keeping the stomach empty is important to prevent release of the pancreatic enzymes. Answer (3) is correct because it is more specific. Pain medication (Demerol) will be given and will be effective regardless of food ingested. Anticholinergic drugs will probably be ordered to reduce pancreatic fluid.

Nursing Process: Analysis
Client Needs: Physiological Integrity
Clinical Area: Medical Nursing

51. (3) Spiking temperature will be caused by the infectious process and must be monitored. Weight loss may occur due to dehydration and should be assessed for, but it is not a priority assessment. Fluid imbalance may occur, but it will be primarily due to increased temperature. Deficits such as seizures and blurred vision may occur and should be assessed for, but they are not as high a priority as increased temperature.

Nursing Process: Assessment
Client Needs: Physiological Integrity
Clinical Area: Medical Nursing

52. (3) Vertigo results when vasospasm stimulates congestion and edema of the cochlear membranes and there is fluid pressure in the labyrinth. In vertigo, the individual complains that the room appears to spin around versus a lightheaded sensation associated with dizziness. Tinnitus may be present but is not a primary symptom.

Nursing Process: Assessment
Client Needs: Physiological Integrity
Clinical Area: Medical Nursing

53. (4) Isolate the client during the period of jaundice because this is the time he would be most susceptible to infections and still contagious to others. Type A hepatitis may have been transmitted through uncooked shellfish, but at this point it would not be eliminated from the diet. The route of transmission is fecal-oral, but this precaution is not indicated. Isolation, strict handwashing, and gloves are important. Diet should be high calorie and well balanced.

Nursing Process: Implementation
Client Needs: Health Promotion and Maintenance
Clinical Area: Medical Nursing

54. (3) Whenever a person is depressed there is a danger of suicide, so the priority goal is to provide a safe milieu to protect the client from self-injury. A nurse-client relationship is an important intervention for a depressed client, but safety takes priority. Structure is necessary to mobilize the client, but does not take priority over safety. Self-esteem is important, but the goals of safety, structure, and a one-to-one relationship take priority.

Nursing Process: Planning
Client Needs: Safe, Effective Care Environment
Clinical Area: Psychiatric Nursing

55. (3) Statistics show that adolescent pregnancy has an increased risk of prematurity and pregnancy induced hypertension. Emotional problems may be increased by the pregnancy, but studies do not reveal this fact. Nutritional deficiency occurs because of the diet, which could contribute to premature labor and PIH. Adolescence does not increase the risk of developing diabetes.

Nursing Process: Analysis
Client Needs: Physiological Integrity
Clinical Area: Maternity Nursing

56. (4) Extreme thirst is one of the first indications of magnesium toxicity. Increased blood pressure and edema are symptoms of PIH. A loss of patellar reflex, not an increase, is a symptom of toxicity.

Nursing Process: Evaluation
Client Needs: Safe, Effective Care Environment
Clinical Area: Maternity Nursing

57. (2) Self-care deficit, thought process, and social interaction impairment are the most relevant for a manic episode. While sexual dysfunction may occur, data was not given in the situation. Activity intolerance is not relevant. None of these three nursing diagnoses are pertinent, although manic episodes frequently manifest as violent behavior. Injury, potential for, is not relevant to manic episode.

Nursing Process: Analysis
Client Needs: Psychosocial Integrity
Clinical Area: Psychiatric Nursing

58. (1) The therapeutic range is 0.8-1.2; if it is a severe acute manic state, the level may be 1.2-1.5 mEq/liter of blood. Lithium toxicity may appear after the 1.5 level. Below 0.8 mEq/liter of blood would probably not be enough lithium to cause a change in behavior.

Nursing Process: Evaluation
Client Needs: Safe, Effective Care Environment
Clinical Area: Psychiatric Nursing

59. (3) The absorption of vitamin K in oily solutions is facilitated by bile and bile salts are necessary for breakdown of fats in the intestinal tract. Hemorrhage may be present with this condition and vitamin K is important to control bleeding, but (3) is a more direct answer. Vitamin K will reduce prothrombin time (which is prolonged with liver cell damage). Bile salts are important for the absorption of vitamin K, but they don't enrich a diet lacking in vitamin K.

Nursing Process: Analysis
Client Needs: Physiological Integrity
Clinical Area: Medical Nursing

60. (2) Emboli are the major problem; those arising in right heart chambers will terminate in the lungs and left chamber emboli may travel anywhere in the arteries. Heart murmurs, fever and night sweats may be present, but do not indicate a complication

Nursing Process: Assessment
Client Needs: Physiological Integrity
Clinical Area: Medical Nursing

of emboli. Congestive heart failure may result, but this is not as dangerous an outcome as emboli. Emboli may occur in the spleen, kidneys, brain, lungs and in the extremities.

61. (2) This is an example of disordered thought process where the ideas do not connect to each other and are expressed in garbled language. A delusion is a false belief. This example represents disturbed thoughts. A hallucination is an unwilled sensory perception with no basis in reality. Affect refers to feelings that are flat or inappropriate; a disturbance in this area is typical of this disorder.

Nursing Process: Assessment
Client Needs: Psychosocial Integrity
Clinical Area: Psychiatric Nursing

62. (2) Codeine is constipating and it is important to avoid straining during evacuation so that the ICP is not increased. Bowel stasis is not the issue. A complication of codeine ingestion is constipation and this may increase ICP, but answer (2) is more specific than (4).

Nursing Process: Analysis
Client Needs: Safe, Effective Care Environment
Clinical Area: Medical Nursing

63. (1) Fluids are essential to flush the kidneys and urinary system. The other goals such as intake and output are important, but not priority. Diet consultation will be a later goal to be implemented before discharge and after the chemical composition of the stones has been determined..

Nursing Process: Planning
Client Needs: Safe, Effective Care Environment
Clinical Area: Medical Nursing

64. (3) Gaining four pounds is concrete evaluation criteria for her positive progress. She may talk about going home and continue to not deal with her problem. The client may attend all groups and never deal with her problem. This answer is incorrect because it may indicate the client's continual obsession with her altered body image.

Nursing Process: Evaluation
Client Needs: Psychosocial Integrity
Clinical Area: Psychiatric Nursing

65.   (1)   Immediate postoperative pain can best be controlled by medicating before pain becomes severe—usually every four hours. Waiting until the effect of the medication wears off is not therapeutic; nor is alternating doses.

Nursing Process: Planning
Client Needs: Safe, Effective Care Environment
Clinical Area: Surgical Nursing

66.   (2)   The nurse is responding to the client's wishes, but coming back lets her know the nurse is concerned and open to talk about her feelings. Asking the client to talk right now is putting an extra demand on her. Telling her that crying doesn't help is denying her feelings.

Nursing Process: Implementation
Client Needs: Psychosocial Integrity
Clinical Area: Psychiatric Nursing

67.   (2)   An expected side effect of the anti-inflammatory medication, indomethacin, is GI disturbance. Hypertension is not an expected side effect of this drug. Tinnitus is a side effect of salicylates.

Nursing Process: Evaluation
Client Needs: Physiological Integrity
Clinical Area: Medical Nursing

68.   (1)   All objectives listed are important, but assessing for dehydration level and acidosis are most crucial, as this can be life-threatening. Answer (1) is more critical even though correct disposal of stools is also necessary because they don't know what is causing the diarrhea.

Nursing Process: Planning
Client Needs: Physiological Integrity
Clinical Area: Pediatric Nursing

69.   (1)   If the catheter becomes plugged or dislodged, it is a complication. Air embolism can occur during a tube change, not during infusion. A local skin infection, not generalized, may occur.

Nursing Process: Assessment
Client Needs: Physiological Integrity
Clinical Area: Pediatric Nursing

70.   (2)   A change in body image is the most likely problem. Identity crisis occurs in adolescence, but will probably not be related to the surgery. The body casting that follows the rod insertion creates some privacy problems; however, a changed body image will cause more difficulty.

Nursing Process: Analysis
Client Needs: Psychosocial Integrity
Clinical Area: Pediatric Nursing

71. (3) This will help promote a nurse-client relationship and provide the child with comfort. While the nurse cannot take the place of his parents, the nurse can be comforting, and the more time the nurse is with the child, the more trust develops.

Nursing Process: Implementation
Client Needs: Safe, Effective Care Environment
Clinical Area: Pediatric Nursing

72. (3) The location of the burn requires priority assessment as burns surrounding the face, neck, and upper extremities can lead to respiratory involvement.

Nursing Process: Assessment
Client Needs: Physiological Integrity
Clinical Area: Medical Nursing

73. (2) Corn can cause obstruction of the ileostomy and thus should be avoided. Answers (1) and (4) cause flatus and usually are avoided by clients as well.

Nursing Process: Evaluation
Client Needs: Health Promotion and Maintenance
Clinical Area: Surgical Nursing

74. (2) Neomycin exerts a powerful effect on intestinal bacterial and lactulose decreases ammonia by pulling ammonia into the bowel. Protein should be reduced in the diet, sedatives restricted and intravenous intake started to maintain fluid and electrolyte balance.

Nursing Process: Analysis
Client Needs: Physiological Integrity
Clinical Area: Medical Nursing

75. (1) Initiating a relationship that includes limit-setting is the first priority. To do any interacting with a client requires a beginning relationship before explaining, exploring the truth, or setting limits.

Nursing Process: Planning
Client Needs: Psychosocial Integrity
Clinical Area: Psychiatric Nursing

76. (3) All of the nursing interventions listed would be carried out for the client; however, the most important one is to prevent cerebral hypoxia, which contributes to cerebral edema. The acid-base imbalance and hypoxia are often mistaken for signs of increased intracranial pressure, leading to unnecessary surgical intervention. A patent airway will establish adequate oxygenation and prevent carbon dioxide build-up.

Nursing Process: Implementation
Client Needs: Safe, Effective Care Environment
Clinical Area: Surgical Nursing

77. (3)   According to Erikson's developmental stages, a school-age child is working on developing industry vs. inferiority. This is the stage where children need to engage in tasks and activities that they can carry through to completion.

Nursing Process: Analysis
Client Needs: Health Promotion and Maintenance
Clinical Area: Pediatric Nursing

78. (4)   The presence of bile in the urine would lead to a yellow-orange or brow-colored urine.

Nursing Process: Assessment
Client Needs: Safe, Effective Care Environment
Clinical Area: Medical Nursing

79. (3)   Because of the potential increased cerebral fluid, fluids will be given very sparingly at approximately 50 ml/hour before the nurse has a physician's order. 20 ml/hour is barely a "keep open" rate.

Nursing Process: Implementation
Client Needs: Safe, Effective Care Environment
Clinical Area: Medical Nursing

80. (2)   The purpose of the pancreatic enzymes is to replace the enzymes unavailable in the child's system that assist with the digestion of fats. Therefore, they should be taken at or prior to, not following, the ingestion of food.

Nursing Process: Evaluation
Client Needs: Health Promotion and Maintenance
Clinical Area: Pediatric Nursing

81. (1)   Immature white blood cells predispose the client to infections, so this nursing diagnosis is a priority. Fluid volume deficit may also be an important nursing diagnosis, because the client may be prone to bleeding. It does not, however, have as high a priority as (1).

Nursing Process: Analysis
Client Needs: Physiological Integrity
Clinical Area: Medical Nursing

82. (4)   An elevated central venous pressure is expected in this client due to the increased right atrial pressure. The normal reading is 5–10 cm of water pressure.

Nursing Process: Evaluation
Client Needs: Physiological Integrity
Clinical Area: Medical Nursing

83. (2)   The initial nursing action is to stop the bleeding with direct pressure over the wound unless there is glass in the wound. If that is not successful, the nurse then has the option of using elevation, pressure on

Nursing Process: Implementation
Client Needs: Safe, Effective Care Environment
Clinical Area: Surgical Nursing

the supplying arteries, and as a last resort, a tourniquet.

84. (4)   Once anxiety has risen to a high level, staying near the client and allowing her to ventilate will help decrease anxiety. If the client chooses to pace around the unit, the nurse might walk with her.

Nursing Process: Planning
Client Needs: Safe, Effective Care Environment
Clinical Area: Psychiatric Nursing

85. (2)   The first intervention is a safety issue. Because the client may respond to illusions or hallucinations or he may experience a seizure due to the DTs, siderails need to be in place. The lights should be on so that they do not create shadows on the walls. After these actions, an IV will be started and a tranquilizer administered.

Nursing Process: Implementation
Client Needs: Safe, Effective Care Environment
Clinical Area: Psychiatric Nursing

86. (2)   The nurse would first notify the physician so that he is present to prepare for an emergency cesarean section. Vaginal examinations are never performed when there is heavy vaginal bleeding and the possibility of a placenta previa. Massive hemorrhage can result when a placenta is touched by an examining finger.

Nursing Process: Implementation
Client Needs: Safe, Effective Care Environment
Clinical Area: Maternity Nursing

87. (4)   The child may be suffering from either croup or epiglottitis. From the symptoms, the nurse knows that he does not have a foreign object in his airway. Attempting to have him cough to open his airway could lead to laryngospasm. Administering high-flow O_2 and keeping him calm is the appropriate nursing care.

Nursing Process: Implementation
Client Needs: Physiological Integrity
Clinical Area: Pediatric Nursing

88. (2)   Impetigo is a bacterial infection. Washing with soap and hot water keeps the objects relatively free of streptococci and lessens the danger of spreading the disease.

Nursing Process: Implementation
Client Needs: Health Promotion and Maintenance
Clinical Area: Pediatric Nursing

89. (3) Polyhydramnios is a condition where an excessive amount of amniotic fluid is present. The normal amount is 500–1000 ml. While the actual cause of this condition is unknown, it occurs more frequently in mothers with diabetes and eclampsia.

Nursing Process: Analysis
Client Needs: Physiological Integrity
Clinical Area: Maternity Nursing

90. (3) This is the most comprehensive answer, although (1) and (4) are also appropriate. Sleeping medication should be avoided if at all possible or unless absolutely necessary, because it helps suppress the client's feelings only temporarily.

Nursing Process: Implementation
Client Needs: Safe, Effective Care Environment
Clinical Area: Psychiatric Nursing

IV

SELF-ASSESSMENT AND EVALUATION GRIDS

Self-Assessment and Evaluation Grids

Introduction

The purpose of this section—self-assessment and evaluation—is to assist you to direct your own review based on your individual needs. After you complete the comprehensive tests, you can utilize the following grids to determine your specific areas of competence as well as your areas of vulnerability. The self-study suggestions will assist you to correct your deficient areas. This process should increase your confidence regarding the NCLEX CAT.

The self-assessment grids explained on the following pages are designed to provide you with helpful feedback. If you have a short period of time to prepare for your licensure exam, it is important that you identify the areas that require review and further study promptly. These assessment and evaluation grids will enable you to assess weak areas and evaluate your strengths so that you will be able to focus your further review systematically and efficiently.

Use the grids as a tool to diagnose possible areas of weakness by assessing where you answered most questions incorrectly. If in reviewing those areas, you feel confident with your knowledge base, reread the questions you answered incorrectly, then read the rationale to determine why you choose the wrong answer. Perhaps you misunderstood the question or simply forgot something you once knew, such as the pharmacological action of a drug. *It is important to pinpoint your specific weaknesses so that you can design a study program and prioritize your learning objectives.*

After completing the assessment and evaluation grids and your self-study program, you can use the computer disk accompanying this book to further test your mastery of nursing content. This disk is designed to increase your confidence concerning computer testing. As you gain more experience with answering questions presented on screen and practice under simulated test conditions, your comfort level and, hence, confidence should increase. After taking the test on the disk, you can obtain a computer-generated Performance Summary. This feedback will include your results in terms of Nursing Process, Client Needs and Clinical Area. These results will indicate areas of relative weakness where you can focus further study and review.

General Directions for Using Self-Assessment Grids

1.   Complete Comprehensive Tests 1–3.
2.   Place the number of the questions answered incorrectly on Grids I and II.
3.   After you have recorded your incorrect answers, total them and enter the number in the Total Answers Wrong column on each grid.
4.   Now complete your self-assessment. You will be able to identify areas requiring additional review by following the directions later in this section (see *Prioritizing Topics for Further Review*).
5.   After you have studied material relating to your weak areas, complete Comprehensive Tests 4 and 5.
6.   Repeat steps #2–4.

The Comprehensive Tests cover all areas of nursing. In order for you to complete a self-assessment and identify your deficient areas of nursing knowledge, it is necessary to categorize the questions. Thus, the five areas of clinical practice are included in each grid: medical nursing, surgical nursing, pediatric nursing, maternity nursing, and psychiatric nursing. As you will note after completing all five Comprehensive Tests, the five clinical areas are quite evenly dispersed throughout.

Because the NCLEX Test Plan is essentially oriented around the Nursing Process and Client Needs, the self-assessment grids follow a similar focus. Grid I enables you to list the questions you missed in terms of Nursing Process and Clinical Area. To complete Grid II, you will record your missed questions in terms of Client Needs and Clinical Area.

Grid I Nursing Process/Clinical Area

The focus of this grid is to assess your ability to answer questions reflecting the nursing process. The questions are categorized according to the following steps.

Assessment: This phase in the nursing process requires skilled observation, reasoning, and a theoretical knowledge base to differentiate data, verify data, and document findings.

Analysis: This phase includes comprehension and interpretation of data collected during assessment. It also includes identification of client needs, formulation of client goals with priorities for goal achievement, and the nursing diagnoses.

Planning: This phase refers to the identification of nursing actions which are strategies to achieve the established goals. This phase also includes nursing measures for the delivery of care. Clients may be involved in the planning phase.

Implementation: This phase refers to the priority nursing action or interventions performed to accomplish a specified goal. Nursing actions center on implementing the plan of care (to achieve a goal).

Evaluation: Dependent on the previous steps of the nursing process, this phase determines the extent to which goals are accomplished. This step completes the Nursing Process and determines if the nursing action was appropriate and goals were achieved. If the goals were not achieved, an examination of the steps of nursing process is completed to determine at which phase there is a need for change.

Grid II Client Needs/Clinical Area

After filling out Grid II, you will be able to identify your areas of relative weakness in terms of Client Needs. The National Council of State Boards of Nursing has defined the entry level nurse's job tasks as providing four essential Client Needs: (1) Safe, effective care environment, (2) Physiological integrity, (3) Psychosocial integrity, and (4) Health promotion and maintenance. Additional description of Client Needs and their subcategories is contained on pages 10 and 11 in this book.

Prioritizing Topics for Further Review

1   After completing the grids, you will have a general indication of your deficient areas.

2   Identify weak areas by determining in which sections you have the most incorrect answers in descending order. List your weakest areas of knowledge first.

Grid I, Nursing Process   Grid I, Clinical Area   Grid II, Client Needs

_____   _____   _____

_____   _____   _____

_____   _____   _____

_____   _____   _____

_____   _____   _____

3. This is an overview of potentially vulnerable areas in which you may require further review.

4. Note any patterns you see developing. For example, do you have many incorrect answers in the implementation phase of the nursing process, the clinical discipline of medicine, the client needs of safe, effective care environment? If so, this pattern would direct you to begin your review in these areas: the client needs area of safe, effective care within the discipline of medicine, with a focus on implementation.

5. Now, prioritize and focus on these topics for further study and review.

6. The best resource to assist you to review in an efficient manner is an NCLEX review book in which the material is presented in a concise and comprehensive format. A recommended review book is *Sandra Smith's Review for NCLEX-RN,* also published by National Nursing Review. This book is organized by clinical area and nursing process.

7. After you have completed additional study and review, answer the questions in this book organized by subject area.
   a. Do you find that after further review, you now feel comfortable with the material?
   b. Did you score relatively high (between 60 and 70 percent correct) on the subject area exams?
   c. If your score was lower than 60 percent on any of the subject area tests, then it would be useful to do more review in that area.

8. Finally, you should complete the Comprehensive Test on the disk enclosed with this book. These questions were not included in the book, so you will be able to take a new test and obtain a detailed Performance Summary. Compare your results on the computer disk to your earlier grids. If your study and review sessions have been effective, your Performance Summary percentages should show your progress. If not, you may need further review. Find more practice questions in other NCLEX review books. Continue to identify your weak areas and review this material again until you feel confident.

Grid I Comprehensive Tests 1–3		Clinical Area					
		Medicine	Surgery	Pediatrics	Maternity	Psychiatry	Total Answers Wrong
Nursing Process	Assessment						
	Analysis						
	Planning						
	Implementation						
	Evaluation						
	Total Answers Wrong						

Grid I Comprehensive Tests 4 & 5	Clinical Area					
	Medicine	Surgery	Pediatrics	Maternity	Psychiatry	Total Answers Wrong
Assessment						
Analysis						
Planning						
Implementation						
Evaluation						
Total Answers Wrong						

Nursing Process

Grid II Comprehensive Tests 1–3		Clinical Area					
		Medicine	**Surgery**	**Pediatrics**	**Maternity**	**Psychiatry**	**Total Answers Wrong**
Client Needs	**Safe, Effective Care Environment**						
	Physiological Integrity						
	Psychosocial Integrity						
	Health Promotion and Maintenance						
Total Answers Wrong							

Grid II Comprehensive Tests 4 & 5	Clinical Area					
	Medicine	Surgery	Pediatrics	Maternity	Psychiatry	Total Answers Wrong
Safe, Effective Care Environment						
Physiological Integrity						
Psychosocial Integrity						
Health Promotion and Maintenance						
Total Answers Wrong						

Client Needs

V

CLINICAL AREA
QUESTIONS

Medical Nursing

1. For a client who has received a diagnosis of skin cancer, the type that has the poorest prognosis because it metastasizes so rapidly and extensively via the lymph system is

   1. Basal cell epithelioma.
   2. Squamous cell epithelioma.
   3. Malignant melanoma.
   4. Sebaceous cyst.

2. After the lungs, the kidneys work to maintain body pH. The best explanation of how the kidneys accomplish regulation of pH is that they

   1. Secrete hydrogen ions and sodium.
   2. Secrete ammonia.
   3. Exchange hydrogen and sodium in the kidneys tubules.
   4. Decrease sodium ions, hold on to hydrogen ions, and then secrete sodium bicarbonate.

3. A client, admitted to the emergency room following a car accident, complains of a severe headache and demonstrates nuchal rigidity and Kernig's sign. The nurse will assess for which complication?

   1. Subdural hemorrhage.
   2. Increased intracranial pressure.
   3. Shock.
   4. Subarachnoid hemorrhage.

4. Dyspnea associated with congestive heart failure is primarily due to

   1. Blockage of a pulmonary artery by an embolus.
   2. Accumulation of fluid in the interstitial spaces and alveoli of the lungs.
   3. Blockage of bronchi by mucous secretions.
   4. Compression of lungs by the dilated heart.

5. A male client, age 44, has recurring abscesses and recent weight loss despite a healthy appetite. What history will be most important to elicit from this client?

   1. Family history of blood disorders.
   2. Family history of Insulin-Dependent Diabetes Mellitus, type I.
   3. Presence of pruritus, muscle cramps.
   4. Presence of nocturia, excessive fatigue.

6. The nurse explains to a client who has just received the diagnosis of Noninsulin-Dependent Diabetes Mellitus (NIDDM) that sulfonylureas, one group of oral hypoglycemic agents, acts by

   1. Stimulating the pancreas to produce or release insulin.
   2. Making the insulin that is produced more available for use.
   3. Lowering the blood sugar by facilitating the uptake and utilization of glucose.
   4. Altering both fat and protein metabolism.

7. For a client diagnosed with epilepsy, of the following nursing actions, which one should receive priority during a tonic-clonic seizure?

 1. Place padding under and around the client's head.
 2. Restrain the client.
 3. Monitor respirations.
 4. Monitor pupillary reactions.

8. A client is experiencing tachycardia. The nurse's understanding of the physiological basis for this symptom is explained by which of the following statements?

 1. The demand for oxygen is decreased because of pleural involvement.
 2. The inflammatory process causes the body to demand more oxygen to meet its needs.
 3. The heart has to pump faster to meet the demand for oxygen when there is lowered arterial oxygen tension.
 4. Respirations are labored.

9. Myasthenic crisis and cholinergic crisis are the major complications of myasthenia gravis. Which of the following is essential nursing knowledge when caring for a client in crisis?

 1. Weakness and paralysis of the muscles for swallowing and breathing occur in either crisis.
 2. Cholinergic drugs should be administered to prevent further complications associated with the crisis.
 3. The clinical condition of the client usually improves after several days of treatment.
 4. Loss of body function creates high levels of anxiety and fear.

10. A client comes into the out-patient clinic and tells the nurse that he has leg pains that begin when he walks but that cease when he stops walking. Which of the following conditions would the nurse assess for?

 1. An acute obstruction in the vessels of the legs.
 2. Peripheral vascular problems in both legs.
 3. Diabetes.
 4. Calcium deficiency.

11. A female client with a tentative diagnosis of urinary tract infection has been admitted to the unit. The nurse knows that the most important factor influencing ascending infection is

 1. Not enough fluid intake.
 2. Obstruction of free urine flow.
 3. A change in pH.
 4. Presence of micro-organisms.

12. A 54-year-old client was put on Quinidine (a drug that decreases myocardial excitability) to prevent arterial fibrillation. He also has kidney disease. The nurse is aware that this drug, when given to a client with kidney disease, may

 1. Cause cardiac arrest.
 2. Cause hypotension.
 3. Produce mild bradycardia.
 4. Be very toxic even in small doses.

13. A client is about to be discharged on the drug bishydroxycoumarin (Dicumarol). Of the principles below, which one is the most important to teach the client before discharge?

1. He should be sure to take the medication before meals.
2. He should shave with an electric razor.
3. If he misses a dose, he should double the dose at the next scheduled time.
4. It is the responsibility of the physician to do the teaching for this medication.

14. Caring for a client with the diagnosis of acute pancreatitis, which of the following drugs would be contraindicated in the treatment of this condition?

    1. Opiates.
    2. Meperidine (Demerol).
    3. Antibiotics.
    4. Anticholinergics.

15. In an individual with the diagnosis of hypoparathyroidism, the nurse will assess for which primary symptom?

    1. Fatigue, muscular weakness.
    2. Cardiac arrhythmias.
    3. Tetany.
    4. Constipation.

16. A cyanotic client with an unknown diagnosis is admitted to the emergency room. In relation to oxygen, the first nursing action would be to

    1. Wait until the client's lab work is done.
    2. Not administer oxygen unless ordered by the physician.
    3. Administer two liters of oxygen.
    4. Administer ten liters of oxygen and check the client's nail beds.

17. A client is placed on ASA therapy. She tells the nurse that she is having a great deal of gastrointestinal distress. The therapeutic response would be to

    1. Inform the physician so he can change to another drug.
    2. Explain that this happens frequently and there is nothing to be concerned about.
    3. Ask the client when she takes the drug during the day.
    4. Tell the client to take an antacid with the drug.

18. A client with a diagnosis of gout will be taking colchicine and allopurinol bid to prevent recurrence. The most common early sign of colchicine toxicity that the nurse will assess for is

    1. Blurred vision.
    2. Anorexia.
    3. Diarrhea.
    4. Fever.

19. An employee at the local factory comes to the nurse's office with a large furuncle (boil) on his left upper arm. He has come to the office with this same complaint over the past six months. In addition to some specific care for the boil itself, the nursing intervention should include

    1. Advising the client to bathe more regularly.
    2. Doing nothing else, as furuncles are not related to any other disease process.
    3. Calling in all employees and checking them for furuncles.
    4. Encouraging the client to see his family physician as recurrent boils may be a sign of underlying disease.

20. A client has chronic dermatitis involving the neck, face and antecubital creases. She has a strong family history of varied allergy disorders. This type of dermatitis is probably best described as

1. Contact dermatitis.
2. Atopic dermatitis.
3. Eczema.
4. Dermatitis medicamentosa.

21. The importance of providing instructions to women on self-examination of the breast is best reflected in which of the following statements?

1. The majority of breast abnormalities are first discovered by women.
2. Once a lesion has been discovered, the informed client may monitor the progress of the abnormality themselves.
3. Breast cancer occurs much more often in women than men and is a major cause of death in women.
4. The high mortality rate of breast cancer can be most effectively reduced by early detection and adequate surgical treatment.

22. Which of the following complications of acute bacterial endocarditis would the nurse constantly observe for in an acutely ill client?

1. Presence of a heart murmur.
2. Emboli.
3. Fever.
4. Congestive heart failure.

23. Cancer is the second major cause of death in this country. What is the first step toward effective cancer control?

1. Increased government control of potential carcinogens.
2. Change in habits and customs predisposing the individual to cancer.
3. Conduction of more mass screening programs.
4. Education of public and professional people about cancer.

24. Alkylating drugs are used as chemotherapeutic agents in cancer therapy. The nurse understands that these drugs stop the cancer's growth by

1. Damaging DNA in the cell's nucleus.
2. Interrupting the production of necessary cellular metabolites.
3. Creating a hormonal imbalance.
4. Destroying messenger RNA.

25. Antineoplastic drugs are dangerous because they affect normal and cancer tissue alike. Normal cells that divide and proliferate rapidly are more at risk. Which of the following areas of the body are least at risk?

1. Bone marrow.
2. Nervous tissue.
3. Hair follicles.
4. Lining of the GI tract.

26. In order to educate clients, the nurse should understand that the most common site of cancer for a female is the

1. Uterine cervix.
2. Uterine body.
3. Vagina.
4. Fallopian tubes.

27. A female client complains of gnawing midepigastric pain for a few hours after meals. At

times, when the pain is severe, vomiting occurs. Specific tests are indicated to rule out

1. Cancer of the stomach.
2. Peptic ulcer disease.
3. Acute gastritis.
4. Pylorospasm.

28. A 60-year-old female client has received the diagnosis of hypertension. Her blood pressure is 160/100. Which of the following symptoms would the nurse find in the assessment?

1. Dizziness and flushed face.
2. Drowsiness and confusion.
3. Faintness when getting out of bed.
4. Ataxia and tachycardia.

29. A 50-year-old client has a tracheostomy and requires tracheal suctioning. The first intervention in completing this procedure would be to

1. Change the tracheostomy dressing.
2. Provide humidity with a trach mask.
3. Apply oral or nasal suction.
4. Deflate the tracheal cuff.

30. A 24-year-old client is admitted to the hospital following an automobile accident. She was brought in unconscious with the following vital signs: BP 130/76, P 100, R 16, T 98° F. The nurse observes bleeding from the client's nose. Which of the following interventions will assist in determining the presence of cerebrospinal fluid?

1. Obtain a culture of the specimen using sterile swabs and send to the laboratory.
2. Allow the drainage to drip on a sterile gauze and observe for a halo or ring around the blood.

3. Suction the nose gently with a bulb syringe and send specimen to the laboratory.
4. Insert sterile packing into the nares and remove in 24 hours.

31. An 18 year old has a known arteriovenous malformation of the middle cerebral artery. In talking to the nurse, she complains of a headache and stiff neck. The nurse would take which of the following actions?

1. Call her mother and have her pick up her daughter.
2. Send her home right away to rest.
3. Make preparations for emergency transfer to an acute care setting.
4. Have the client rest for two hours, then reevaluate the situation.

32. The nurse notices that a client on a medical unit is alone in his room and crying. The most therapeutic nursing approach would be to say

1. "Don't cry, you'll just feel worse."
2. "Cheer up now—crying can make you feel more sad."
3. "Spending so much time alone makes one feel lonely—let's go out on the unit."
4. "I'll get a tissue then come back and sit with you."

33. Following surgery, a client has developed superficial vein thrombophlebitis. The nursing assessment would reveal

1. Bluish discoloration along the vein.
2. Severe pain and tenderness.
3. Varicosities.
4. Surrounding area is cool to the touch.

34. A client with an admitting diagnosis of head injury has a Glasgow Coma Score of 3 - 5 - 4. The nurse's understanding of this test is that the client

   1. Can follow simple commands.
   2. Will make no attempt to vocalize.
   3. Is unconscious.
   4. Is able to open his eyes when spoken to.

35. A 24-year-old male is admitted with a possible head injury. His arterial blood gases show that his pH is less than 7.3, his $PaCO_2$ is elevated above 60 mmHg, and his PaO_2 is less than 45 mmHg. Evaluating this ABG panel, the nurse would conclude that

   1. Edema has resulted from a low pH state.
   2. Acidosis has caused vasoconstriction of cerebral arterioles.
   3. Cerebral edema has resulted from a low oxygen state.
   4. Cerebral blood flow has decreased.

36. Part of a plan of care for a client with increased intracranial pressure is to maintain an adequate airway and to promote gas exchange. To accomplish these goals, an effective nursing action is to

   1. Encourage the client to cough vigorously.
   2. Avoid hypercapnia in the client.
   3. Suction the client nasotracheally at frequent intervals.
   4. Pack gauze in the nares when there is drainage from the nose.

37. A client is admitted to the trauma unit with a suspected arterial bleed in his head following an injury. He is experiencing periods of confusion and lucidity. As the nurse assesses his status, she suspects

   1. Subdural hematoma.
   2. Increased intracranial pressure.
   3. Epidural hematoma.
   4. Increased blood pressure.

38. Based on nursing knowledge, the nurse is aware that an epidural hematoma is characterized by

   1. A long period of unconsciousness followed by complete lucidity.
   2. A short period of unconsciousness followed by a lucid period, followed by rapid deterioration.
   3. Slowly developing signs of increasing intracranial pressure.
   4. No complaints of headaches.

39. A client is admitted with suspected acute subdural hematoma. The nurse will assess for

   1. Headache, drowsiness, hemiparesis, and contralateral pupil dilatation.
   2. Headache, ipsilateral pupil dilation, and slow cerebration.
   3. Drowsiness, slow cerebration, confusion, and ipsilateral pupil dilatation.
   4. Drowsiness, confusion, hemiparesis, and contralateral pupil dilatation.

40. A client is admitted following an automobile accident in which he sustained a contusion. The nurse knows that the significance of a contusion is

   1. It is reversible.
   2. Amnesia will occur.
   3. Loss of consciousness may be transient.
   4. Laceration of the brain may occur.

41. The major rationale for the use of acetylsalicylic acid (aspirin) in the treatment of rheumatoid arthritis is to

1. Reduce fever.
2. Reduce inflammation of the joints.
3. Assist the client in range-of-motion activities without pain.
4. Prevent extension of the disease process.

42. A client with tuberculosis is given the drug pyrazinamide (Pyrazinamide). Which one of the following diagnostic tests would be inaccurate if the client is receiving the drug?

1. Liver function test.
2. Gall bladder studies.
3. Thyroid function studies.
4. Blood glucose.

43. Lactulose is ordered for a 68-year-old client hospitalized with hepatic failure. The nurse knows that the primary action of this drug is to

1. Prevent constipation.
2. Decrease the blood ammonia level.
3. Increase intestinal peristalsis.
4. Prevent portal hypertension.

44. The major goal of therapy when Dexamethasone (Decadron) is ordered for a client is to

1. Replace adrenocorticoids in clients following adrenalectomy.
2. Decrease inflammation in cerebral edema.
3. Reverse signs and symptoms of septic shock.
4. Delay complications of hepatic coma in cirrhosis clients.

45. In developing a nursing care plan for a client with multiple sclerosis, the nurse would *not* include

1. Preventative measures for falls.
2. Interventions to promote bowel elimination.
3. Instructions on moderate activities.
4. Techniques to promote safe swallowing.

46. Which one of the following conditions could lead to an inaccurate pulse oximetry reading if the sensor is attached to the client's ear?

1. Artificial nails.
2. Vasodilation.
3. Hypothermia.
4. Movement of extremity.

47. A client has physician's orders to take chemotherapeutic hormonal agents. The nurse would prepare the client to anticipate which of the following side effects?

1. Stomatitis, diarrhea, dermatitis.
2. Fluid retention, mood changes, anxiety.
3. Epistaxis, fever, ototoxicity.
4. Anorexia, nausea, rashes.

48. Thrombolytic therapy would be appropriate for which of the following conditions?

1. Continual blood pressure above 200/120.
2. History of diabetic retinopathy.
3. History of significant kidney disease.
4. Myocardial infarction.

49. While on a camping trip, a friend sustains a snake bite from a poisonous snake. The most effective initial intervention would be to

1. Place a restrictive band above the snake bite.
2. Elevate the bite area above level of the heart.
3. Position the client in a supine position.
4. Immobilize the limb.

50. Which one of the following rules for charting narrative notes does *not* fit into acceptable charting procedures?

    1. Each entry should be signed with the nurse's name and professional status.
    2. Objective facts are more relevant than nursing interpretation.
    3. Behaviors rather than feelings should be charted.
    4. Use of the word "client" or "patient" is important to designate particular entries.

51. There is a physician's order to irrigate a client's bladder. Which one of the following nursing measures will ensure patency?

    1. Use a solution of sterile water for the irrigation.
    2. Apply a small amount of pressure to push the mucus out of the catheter tip if the tube is not patent.
    3. Carefully insert about 100 ml of aqueous Zephiran into the bladder, allow it to remain for one hour, and then siphon it out.
    4. Irrigate with 20 ml's of normal saline to establish patency.

52. When assessing an EKG, the nurse knows that the P-R interval represents the time it takes for the

    1. Impulse to begin atrial contraction.

2. Impulse to traverse the atria to the AV node.
3. SA node to discharge the impulse to begin atrial depolarization.
4. Impulse to travel to the ventricles.

53. When a client has suffered severe burns all over his body, the most effective method of monitoring the cardiovascular system is

    1. Cuff blood pressure.
    2. Arterial pressure.
    3. Central venous pressure.
    4. Pulmonary artery pressure.

54. A female client has orders for an oral cholecystogram. Prior to the test, the nursing intervention would be to

    1. Provide a high fat diet for dinner, then NPO.
    2. Explain that diarrhea may result from the dye tablets.
    3. Administer the dye tablets following a regular diet for dinner.
    4. Administer enemas until clear.

55. The physician has just completed a liver biopsy. Immediately following the procedure, the nurse will position the client

    1. On his right side to promote hemostasis.
    2. In Fowler's position to facilitate ventilation.
    3. Supine to maintain blood pressure.
    4. In Sims' position to prevent aspiration.

56. Knowing that a client has the diagnosis of congestive heart failure (CHF), what symptoms would the nurse most likely expect to find during an assessment?

1. Crackles, bradycardia, arrhythmias.
2. Cyanosis, crackles, gallop rhythm.
3. Anxiety, bronchospasm, pedal edema.
4. Diaphoresis, orthopnea, sensorium changes.

57. The primary symptoms associated with cholinergic crisis that the nurse would assess for are

    1. Muscle weakness, increased pulse rate, dry mouth.
    2. Decreased pulse rate, respiratory difficulty, dysphagia.
    3. Muscle fasciculations, dry mouth, increased pulse rate.
    4. Dilated pupils, decreased pulse rate, muscle weakness.

58. When a client has peptic ulcer disease, the nurse would expect a priority intervention to be

    1. Assisting in inserting a Miller-Abbott tube.
    2. Assisting in inserting an arterial pressure line.
    3. Inserting a nasogastric tube.
    4. Inserting an IV.

59. A client with myxedema has been in the hospital for three days. The nursing assessment reveals the following clinical manifestations: respiratory rate 8 per minute, diminished breath sounds in the right lower lobe, rales in left lower lobe. The most appropriate nursing intervention is to

    1. Increase the use of ROM, turning and deep breathing exercises.
    2. Increase the frequency of rest periods.

3. Initiate postural drainage.
4. Continue with routine nursing care.

60. The nurse is assigned to draw blood from a suspected AIDS client. Universal precautions dictates that she should use

    1. Gown, clean gloves, and mask.
    2. Gown, sterile gloves.
    3. Gown, clean gloves.
    4. Sterile gloves.

61. When the nurse is completing an assessment of a burned client, second-degree burns would appear as

    1. Full thickness with extension to underlying muscle and bone.
    2. Partial thickness with erythema and often edema, but no vesicles.
    3. Partial thickness with involvement of epidermis and dermis, showing edema and vesicles.
    4. Full thickness with dry, waxy, or leathery appearance without vesicles.

62. A 45-year-old male client with leg ulcers and arterial insufficiency is admitted to the hospital. The nurse understands that leg ulcers of this nature are usually caused by

    1. Decreased arterial blood flow secondary to vasoconstriction.
    2. Decreased arterial blood flow leading to hyperemia.
    3. Atherosclerotic obstruction of arteries.
    4. Trauma to the lower extremities.

63. In preparation for discharge of a client with arterial insufficiency and Raynaud's disease, client teaching instructions should include

1. Walking several times each day as part of an exercise routine.
2. Keeping the heat up so that the environment is warm.
3. Wearing TED hose during the day.
4. Using hydrotherapy for increasing oxygenation.

64. Assessing the urine of a client with suspected cholecystitis, the nurse expects that the color will most likely be

   1. Pale yellow.
   2. Greenish-brown.
   3. Red.
   4. Yellow-orange.

65. In order to formulate a care plan for a client receiving dialysis, the nurse understands that the physiological mechanism associated with peritoneal dialysis is that the

   1. Peritoneum allows solutes in the dialysate to pass into the intravascular system.
   2. Peritoneum acts as a semipermeable membrane through which solutes move via diffusion and osmosis.
   3. Presence of excess metabolites causes increased permeability of the peritoneum and allows excess fluid to drain.
   4. Peritoneum permits diffusion of metabolites only from intravascular to interstitial spaces.

66. The treatment prescribed for the burned area of skin before skin grafting can take place will include

   1. Silver nitrate soaks for 24 hours.
   2. Burn irrigations with Sulfamylon.

3. Warm soaks with sterile water.
4. Germicidal soap scrubs to the affected area.

67. When a client asks the nurse why the physician says he "thinks" he has tuberculosis, the nurse explains to him that diagnosis of tuberculosis can take several weeks to confirm. Which of the following statements supports this answer?

   1. A positive reaction to a tuberculosis skin test indicates that the client has active tuberculosis, even if one negative sputum is obtained.
   2. A positive sputum culture takes at least three weeks, due to the slow reproduction of the bacillus.
   3. Because small lesions are hard to detect on chest x-rays, x-rays usually need to be repeated during several consecutive weeks.
   4. A client with a positive smear will have to have a positive culture to confirm the diagnosis.

68. The nurse is counseling a client with the diagnosis of glaucoma. She explains that if left untreated, this condition leads to

   1. Blindness.
   2. Myopia.
   3. Retrolental fibroplasia.
   4. Uveitis.

69. A young client hit by a car was fortunate because the level of his injury did not interrupt his respiratory function. The cord segments involved with maintaining respiratory function are

   1. Thoracic level 5 and 6.

2. Thoracic level 2 and 3.
3. Cervical level 7 and 8.
4. Cervical level 3 and 4.

70. The most important pathophysiologic factor contributing to the formation of esophageal varices is

1. Decreased prothrombin formation.
2. Decreased albumin formation by the liver.
3. Portal hypertension.
4. Increased central venous pressure.

71. When a client has lung cancer that has been classified as Stage 1 T_1, NO, MO, the nurse knows that this indicates that the client has a tumor

1. With metastasis to the lymph nodes.
2. That has invaded the visceral pleura.
3. With distant metastasis to the scalene nodes.
4. Without distant metastasis.

72. Following a car accident, a newly admitted client seems concerned about his sudden loss of memory. He seeks out the nurse for an explanation. Before responding to the client, the nurse needs to consider that

1. Her answer should be reassuring and brief, as the client is still very anxious.
2. She needs to wait until all the test results are in before responding.
3. The client's amnesia is a result of his guilt.
4. The client's anxious behavior would be best dealt with by having the physician order a tranquilizer.

73. A nursing assessment for initial signs of hypoglycemia will include

1. Pallor, blurred vision, weakness, behavioral changes.
2. Frequent urination, flushed face, pleural friction rub.
3. Abdominal pain, diminished deep tendon reflexes, double vision.
4. Weakness, lassitude, irregular pulse, dilated pupils.

74. While planning the nursing care of a client with an ulcer, the nurse would keep in mind that a major goal of therapy is to help the client

1. Talk about the recent stressful situations in her life which may have contributed to the ulcer formation.
2. Understand the pathogenesis of the ulcer.
3. Accept that she is under stress and needs rest.
4. Discover what foods caused pain.

75. The physician has ordered a 24-hour urine specimen. After explaining the procedure to the client, the nurse collects the first specimen. This specimen is then

1. Discarded, then the collection begins.
2. Saved as part of the 24-hour collection.
3. Tested, then discarded.
4. Placed in a separate container and later added to the collection.

76. A client admitted with the diagnosis of cardiac disease tells the nurse he is afraid of dying from a heart attack. The most therapeutic response is
1. "Perhaps you should discuss this with your physician."
2. "Of course you aren't going to die."

3. "What makes you think you will die?"
4. "Tell me more about these fears of dying from a heart attack."

77. An elderly client is in a long-term care facility. She had a left-sided CVA four weeks ago and has been bedridden since that time. A sign or symptom indicating a possible complication of immobility is

1. A reddened area over the sacrum.
2. Stiffness in the left leg.
3. Difficulty moving her left arm.
4. Difficulty hearing low voices.

78. A 20-year-old male client sustained a head injury in an automobile accident. He is admitted to a medical-surgical unit. During the initial assessment, the nurse observes fluid draining from the client's left ear. The nurse will immediately position the client with the head of his bed

1. Elevated and his head turned to the left.
2. Flat and his head turned to the right.
3. Flat and his head turned to the left.
4. Elevated and his head turned to the right.

79. Following an accident, a client is admitted with a head injury and concurrent cervical spine injury. The physician will use Crutchfield tongs. The purpose of these tongs is to

1. Hypoextend the vertebral column.
2. Hyperextend the vertebral column.
3. Decompress the spinal nerves.
4. Allow the client to sit up and move without twisting his spine.

80. As the nurse is completing evening care for a client, he observes that the client is upset, quiet and withdrawn. The nurse knows that the client is scheduled for diagnostic tests the following day. An important assessment question to ask the client is

1. "Would you like to go to the dayroom to watch TV?"
2. "Are you prepared for the test tomorrow?"
3. "Have you talked with anyone about the test tomorrow?"
4. "Have you asked your physician to give you a sleeping pill tonight?"

81. The nurse knows that the most informative measurement for determining cardiogenic shock is

1. Arterial blood pressure.
2. Central venous pressure.
3. Pulmonary artery pressure.
4. Cardiac index.

82. A client is scheduled for a voiding cystogram. Which nursing intervention would be essential to carry out several hours before the test?

1. Maintain NPO status.
2. Medicate with urinary antiseptics.
3. Administer bowel preparation.
4. Force fluids.

83. Assessing a client's shunt for patency by using a stethoscope and the nurse's hand, the nurse would expect to hear

1. A loud bruit and feel the area cool to touch.

2. The sound of rushing blood and feel the area warm to touch.
3. No sound, but feel the area warm to touch.
4. A regular heartbeat and feel the area cool to touch.

84. A client has orders for a Sengstaken-Blakemore tube to be inserted. The purpose of this procedure is to

   1. Apply direct pressure to bleeding ulcers.
   2. Apply indirect pressure to bleeding ulcers via the esophagus.
   3. Decrease the blood supply to the cardiac sphincter of the stomach.
   4. Apply direct pressure to the esophagus and cardiac sphincter.

85. A male client complaining of persistent lower back pain for several months has been admitted for a work-up prior to a laminectomy. After a myelogram, which uses a water soluble dye, the nurse will position him in a

   1. Side-lying position.
   2. Supine position with the head of the bed elevated.
   3. Dorsal recumbent position with the head flat.
   4. Prone position.

86. The most appropriate nursing intervention for a client requiring a finger probe pulse oximeter is to

   1. Apply the sensor probe over a finger and cover lightly with gauze to prevent skin breakdown
   2. Set alarms on the oximeter to at least 100 percent.

3. Identify if the client has had a recent diagnostic test using intravenous dye.
4. Remove the sensor between oxygen saturation readings.

87. A female client is admitted with a diagnosis of seizure disorder. A priority in protecting the client against injury during a seizure is to

   1. Restrain her arms so that she won't hit herself.
   2. Use a padded tongue blade so that she won't injure her tongue.
   3. Keep her on her back so that she can breathe.
   4. Position her on her side to facilitate drainage.

88. A client being treated for esophageal varices has a Sengstaken-Blakemore tube inserted to control the bleeding. The most important assessment is for the nurse to

   1. Check that a hemostat is at the bedside.
   2. Monitor IV fluids for the shift.
   3. Regularly assess respiratory status.
   4. Check that the balloon is deflated on a regular basis.

89. A client with a long-standing history of alcoholic cirrhosis with ascites is admitted to the hospital. His diagnosis is acute bleeding from esophageal varices secondary to cirrhosis with portal hypertension. Which of the following laboratory findings indicates that blood is being digested and absorbed by the GI tract?

   1. Elevated BUN.
   2. Elevated serum ammonia.

3. Decreased hemoglobin.
4. Elevated bilirubin.

90. When a client is in liver failure, which of the following behavioral changes is the most important assessment to report?

1. Shortness of breath.
2. Lethargy.
3. Fatigue.
4. Nausea.

91. A 55-year-old client with severe epigastric pain due to acute pancreatitis has been admitted to the hospital. The client's activity at this time should be

1. Ambulation as desired.
2. Bedrest in supine position.
3. Up ad lib and right side-lying position in bed.
4. Bedrest in Fowler's position.

92. Peritoneal reaction to acute pancreatitis results in a shift of fluid from the vascular space into the peritoneal cavity. If this occurs, the nurse would evaluate for

1. Decreased serum albumin.
2. Abdominal pain.
3. Oliguria.
4. Peritonitis.

93. A client, age 25 with a lower urinary tract infection, is admitted to the hospital. Her history indicates she has suffered from repeated infections. The initial assessment will most likely reveal

1. Frequency and dysuria.

2. Fever and chills.
3. Malodorous, cloudy urine.
4. Leukocytosis and back pain.

94. The most common cause of bladder infection in the client with a retention catheter is contamination

1. Due to insertion technique.
2. At the time of catheter removal.
3. Of the urethral/catheter interface.
4. Of the internal lumen of the catheter.

95. The nurse will know a client with lupus erythematosus understands principles of self-care when she can discuss

1. Drying agents.
2. Moisturizing agents.
3. Antifungal creams.
4. Solar protection.

96. Of the following blood gas values, the one the nurse would expect to see in the client with acute renal failure is

1. pH 7.49, HCO_3 24, PCO_2 46.
2. pH 7.49, HCO_3 14, PCO_2 30.
3. pH 7.26, HCO_3 24, PCO_2 46.
4. pH 7.26, HCO_3 14, PCO_2 30.

97. A client in acute renal failure receives an IV infusion of 10% dextrose in water with 20 units of regular insulin. The nurse understands that the rationale for this therapy is to

1. Correct the hyperglycemia that occurs with acute renal failure.
2. Facilitate the intracellular movement of potassium.

3. Provide calories to prevent tissue catabolism and azotemia.
4. Force potassium into the cells to prevent arrhythmias.

98. A client in the early stages of progressive renal failure is admitted to the hospital. The initial assessment will probably reveal

    1. Oliguria, nausea, high urine specific gravity.
    2. Anuria, weight gain, hypertension.
    3. Polyuria, low urine specific gravity, polydipsia.
    4. Hematuria, proteinuria, oliguria.

99. The client who is well managed with intermittent hemodialysis would have a clear understanding that

1. Diet and fluid adherence between sessions will help control the development of complications.
2. His blood pressure will be adequately controlled by the hemodialysis treatments.
3. His energy level will be greatly increased following each session.
4. There will be no urine output between procedures and excess fluid will be removed during hemodialysis.

100. The nurse will evaluate for the most significant complication in clients undergoing chronic peritoneal dialysis, which is

    1. Pulmonary embolism.
    2. Hypotension.
    3. Dyspnea.
    4. Peritonitis.

Medical Nursing
Answers with Rationale

1.   (3)   Basal cell epithelioma and squamous cell epithelioma are both superficial, easily excised, slow-growing tumors. A sebaceous cyst is a benign (nonmalignant) growth.

    Nursing Process: Analysis
    Client Needs: Health Promotion and Maintenance
    Clinical Area: Medical Nursing

2.   (4)   By decreasing NA+ ions, holding onto hydrogen ions, and secreting sodium bicarbonate, the kidneys can regulate pH. Therefore, this is the most complete answer, and while this buffer system is slowest, it can completely compensate for acid-base imbalance.

    Nursing Process: Analysis
    Client Needs: Physiological Integrity
    Clinical Area: Medical Nursing

3.   (4)   Blood in the CSF, within the brain, ventricles or subarachnoid space, is irritating to the meninges and causes headache and nuchal rigidity.

    Nursing Process: Assessment
    Client Needs: Physiological Integrity
    Clinical Area: Medical Nursing

4.   (2)   Failure of the left ventricle to pump effectively causes damming of blood back into the pulmonary circuit, increasing pressure, and causing extravasation of fluid into interstitial spaces and alveoli.

    Nursing Process: Analysis
    Client Needs: Physiological Integrity
    Clinical Area: Medical Nursing

5.   (2)   The onset of Insulin-Dependent Diabetes Mellitus, type I is often insidious, becoming manifest only after some metabolic stress, such as infection.

    Nursing Process: Assessment
    Client Needs: Safe, Effective Care Environment
    Clinical Area: Medical Nursing

6.   (1)   Sulfonylurea drugs, Orinase for example, lowers the blood sugar by stimulating the beta cells of the pancreas to synthesize and release insulin.

    Nursing Process: Implementation
    Client Needs: Health Promotion and Maintenance
    Clinical Area: Medical Nursing

7. (1)   The primary nursing goal during a seizure is to protect the client from physical injury and to maintain a patent airway, if possible. Clients should not be restrained during seizure activity, as both soft tissue damage and fractures could occur.

Nursing Process: Implementation
Client Needs: Safe, Effective Care Environment
Clinical Area: Medical Nursing

8. (3)   The arterial oxygen supply is lowered and the demand for oxygen is increased, which results in the heart having to beat faster to meet body needs for oxygen.

Nursing Process: Analysis
Client Needs: Physiological Integrity
Clinical Area: Medical Nursing

9. (1)   The client cannot handle his own secretions, and respiratory arrest may be imminent. Atropine may be administered to prevent crisis. Anticholinergic drugs are administered to increase the levels of acetylcholine at the myoneural junction. Cholinergic drugs mimic the actions of the parasympathetic nervous system and would not be used.

Nursing Process: Analysis
Client Needs: Physiological Integrity
Clinical Area: Medical Nursing

10. (2)   Intermittent claudication is a condition that indicates vascular deficiencies in the peripheral vascular system. If an obstruction were present, the leg pain would persist when the client stops walking. Low calcium level may cause leg cramps but would not necessarily be related to walking.

Nursing Process: Assessment
Client Needs: Safe, Effective Care Environment
Clinical Area: Medical Nursing

11. (2)   Free flow of urine together with large urine output and pH are antibacterial defenses. If free flow is obstructed, the infection will most likely ascend up the tract.

Nursing Process: Analysis
Client Needs: Physiological Integrity
Clinical Area: Medical Nursing

12. (1)   Kidney disease interferes with metabolism and excretion of Quinidine, resulting in higher drug concentrations in the body. Quinidine can depress myocardial excitability enough to cause cardiac arrest.

Nursing Process: Evaluation
Client Needs: Safe, Effective Care Environment
Clinical Area: Medical Nursing

13.   (2)   Dicumarol is an anticoagulant drug and one of the dangers involved is bleeding. Using a safety razor can lead to bleeding through cuts. The drug should be given at the same time daily but not related to meals. Due to danger of bleeding, missed doses should not be made up.

Nursing Process: Planning
Client Needs: Health Promotion and Maintenance
Clinical Area: Medical Nursing

14.   (1)   Opiates are contraindicated, as they may produce spasm of the biliary-pancreatic ducts. Synthetic narcotics (Demerol) are the drugs of choice for pain control.

Nursing Process: Planning
Client Needs: Safe, Effective Care Environment
Clinical Area: Medical Nursing

15.   (3)   Tetany occurs mainly in the distal extremities, manifested by flexion of the fingers, hands and toes (carpopedal spasms). Increased mechanical irritability exists especially with attempts at voluntary movements. Laryngeal spasms, convulsions and death will result if the tetany is not treated promptly.

Nursing Process: Assessment
Client Needs: Safe, Effective Care Environment
Clinical Area: Medical Nursing

16.   (3)   Administer two liters of oxygen and no more, for if the client is emphysemic and receives too high a level of oxygen, he will develop CO_2 narcosis and the respiratory system will cease to function.

Nursing Process: Implementation
Client Needs: Safe, Effective Care Environment
Clinical Area: Medical Nursing

17.   (3)   It is important to find out whether the drug is taken on a full or empty stomach. Gastric irritation is a common side effect of ASA therapy. It can be decreased by taking the drug with meals. An antacid can be given with the drug at bedtime; however, the nurse cannot arbitrarily tell the client to do so as it takes a physician's order.

Nursing Process: Assessment
Client Needs: Health Promotion and Maintenance
Clinical Area: Medical Nursing

18.   (3)   Diarrhea is by far the most common. When given in the acute phase of gout, the dose of colchicine is usually 0.6 mg (PO) q hr (not to exceed 10 tablets) until pain is relieved or gastrointestinal symptoms ensue.

Nursing Process: Assessment
Client Needs: Safe, Effective Care Environment
Clinical Area: Medical Nursing

19. (4) Sometimes recurrent boils are symptoms of an underlying disease process such as glycosuria. Bathing will not influence the course of the boils and they are not communicable.

Nursing Process: Implementation
Client Needs: Health Promotion and Maintenance
Clinical Area: Medical Nursing

20. (2) Atopic dermatitis is chronic, pruritic and allergic in nature. Typically it has a longer course than contact dermatitis and is aggravated by commercial face or body lotions, emotional stress, and, in some instances, particular foods.

Nursing Process: Analysis
Client Needs: Physiological Integrity
Clinical Area: Medical Nursing

21. (4) Health professionals have the responsibility to provide clear guidelines focused on the prevention and early treatment of breast cancer. Self-examinations following menstruation coupled with annual screening examination by the physician is very effective in detecting early breast cancer.

Nursing Process: Analysis
Client Needs: Health Promotion and Maintenance
Clinical Area: Medical Nursing

22. (2) While all of the answers may be relevant, the characteristic problem with this condition is the problem of emboli. If the emboli arise in the right heart chambers, they will terminate in the lungs; left chamber emboli may travel anywhere in the arterial tree.

Nursing Process: Assessment
Client Needs: Safe, Effective Care Environment
Clinical Area: Medical Nursing

23. (4) The most important step in controlling cancer is education of the public about cancer and its warning signs. Education will have an effect on early diagnosis and treatment.

Nursing Process: Planning
Client Needs: Health Promotion and Maintenance
Clinical Area: Medical Nursing

24. (1) Alkylating agents affect production of DNA which, in turn, disrupts cell growth and division.

Nursing Process: Analysis
Client Needs: Physiological Integrity
Clinical Area: Medical Nursing

25. (2) Nervous tissue is least at risk. (1), (3) and (4) are the cells that are most vulnerable because they have rapid cell division and proliferation similar to cancer cells.

Nursing Process: Analysis
Client Needs: Physiological Integrity
Clinical Area: Medical Nursing

The nervous tissue cells do not have rapid cell division.

26. (1) Cervical cancer is the most common site and squamous cell CA is the most common cell type.

Nursing Process: Planning
Client Needs: Health Promotion and Maintenance
Clinical Area: Medical Nursing

27. (2) Peptic ulcer disease is characteristically gnawing epigastric pain that may radiate to the back. Vomiting usually reflects pyloric spasm from muscular spasm or obstruction.

Nursing Process: Assessment
Client Needs: Physiological Integrity
Clinical Area: Medical Nursing

28. (1) Cardinal symptoms are dizziness and flushed face as well as headache, tinnitus and epistaxis. Drowsiness and confusion occur in hypertensive crisis and faintness would occur in hypotension.

Nursing Process: Assessment
Client Needs: Physiological Integrity
Clinical Area: Medical Nursing

29. (3) Before deflating the tracheal cuff, the nurse will apply oral or nasal suction to the airway to prevent secretions from falling into the lung. Dressing change and humidity do not relate to suctioning.

Nursing Process: Implementation
Client Needs: Safe, Effective Care Environment
Clinical Area: Medical Nursing

30. (2) The halo or "bull's eye" sign seen when drainage from the nose or ear of a head-injured client is collected on a sterile gauze is indicative of CSF in the drainage. The collection of a culture specimen using any type of swab or suction would be contraindicated because brain tissue may be inadvertently removed at the same time or other tissue damage may result.

Nursing Process: Implementation
Client Needs: Physiological Integrity
Clinical Area: Medical Nursing

31. (3) The client's complaints are consistent with meningeal irritation from bleeding into the subarachnoid space; therefore, she needs immediate transfer to an acute care setting.

Nursing Process: Implementation
Client Needs: Safe, Effective Care Environment
Clinical Area: Medical Nursing

32. (4) The most therapeutic response is to acknowledge that the client is upset and offer the opportunity to discuss these

Nursing Process: Implementation
Client Needs: Psychosocial Integrity
Clinical Area: Medical Nursing

feelings. The other responses close off communication.

33.   (2)   Superficial thrombophlebitis will present with pain, redness, tenderness, and be warm to the touch. There could be palpable "cord" present, but it will not be bluish in color.

Nursing Process: Assessment
Client Needs: Physiological Integrity
Clinical Area: Medical Nursing

34.   (4)   A Glasgow Coma Score of 3 - 5 - 4 means that the client is able to open his eyes when spoken to and can localize pain, attempting to remove noxious stimuli when motor function is tested. He is not able to follow commands. He is able to vocalize, but is confused. Verbal response is usually tested by asking the client to state who he is, where he is, or the date.

Nursing Process: Analysis
Client Needs: Physiological Integrity
Clinical Area: Medical Nursing

35.   (3)   Hypoxic states may cause cerebral edema. Hypoxia also causes cerebral vasodilatation particularly in response to a decrease in the PaO_2 below 60 mmHg.

Nursing Process: Analysis
Client Needs: Physiological Integrity
Clinical Area: Medical Nursing

36.   (2)   Hypercapnia leads to vasodilation, thus increasing cerebral blood flow and increasing intracranial pressure. The client should not be encouraged to cough vigorously, as this will also raise the intracranial pressure. An intact autoregulation mechanism provides for sharp fluctuation in intracranial pressure, as might occur during coughing or sneezing in the client without increased intracranial pressure; however, clients with increased intracranial pressure have compromised autoregulation.

Nursing Process: Planning
Client Needs: Physiological Integrity
Clinical Area: Medical Nursing

37.   (3)   Epidural hematomas usually form quickly within six hours after injury, as a result of an arterial bleed. They usually cause periods of confusion and lucidity, and may or may not cause loss of consciousness. While epidural hematomas if

Nursing Process: Assessment
Client Needs: Physiological Integrity
Clinical Area: Medical Nursing

left untreated are fatal; in fact, subdural hematomas, not epidural hematomas, have the highest mortality of all head injuries (60 to 90 percent).

38. (2) Epidural hematomas classically present with a brief period of unconsciousness, followed by a lucid interval of varying duration, and finally followed by rapid deterioration of the level of consciousness accompanied by complaints of a severe headache.

Nursing Process: Analysis
Client Needs: Physiological Integrity
Clinical Area: Medical Nursing

39. (3) The most common signs of acute subdural hematoma include headache, drowsiness, some agitation, and confusion. Dilation of the ipsilateral pupil occurs and eventually becomes fixed. A late finding is hemiparesis.

Nursing Process: Assessment
Client Needs: Physiological Integrity
Clinical Area: Medical Nursing

40. (4) Laceration, a more severe consequence of closed head injury, occurs as the brain tissue moves across the uneven base of the skull in a contusion. Contusion causes cerebral dysfunction which results in bruising of the brain. A concussion causes transient loss of consciousness, retrograde amnesia, and is generally reversible.

Nursing Process: Analysis
Client Needs: Physiological Integrity
Clinical Area: Medical Nursing

41. (2) Aspirin acts as an anti-inflammatory drug and, thus, reduces the inflammation of the joint. In doing so, it also relieves pain. Aspirin does not prevent extension of the disease. While aspirin reduces fever, this is not the major reason for its use in the treatment of rheumatoid arthritis.

Nursing Process: Analysis
Client Needs: Physiological Integrity
Clinical Area: Medical Nursing

42. (1) Liver function tests can be elevated in clients taking pyrazinamide. This drug is used when primary and secondary antitubercular drugs are not effective. Urate levels may be increased and there is a chemical interference with urine ketone levels if

Nursing Process: Evaluation
Client Needs: Physiological Integrity
Clinical Area: Medical Nursing

these tests are done while the client is on the drug.

43.   (2)   Lactulose decreases blood ammonia levels in clients with hepatic coma. It is thought to decrease the colon pH through bacterial degradation.

Nursing Process: Analysis
Client Needs: Physiological Integrity
Clinical Area: Medical Nursing

44.   (2)   Decadron decreases inflammation by stabilizing leukocyte lysosomal membranes. It also suppresses the immune response so is contraindicated in clients with infection, cirrhosis and debilitating disease.

Nursing Process: Planning
Client Needs: Physiological Integrity
Clinical Area: Medical Nursing

45.   (4)   Clients with multiple sclerosis do not usually have difficulty swallowing; therefore, techniques to promote safe swallowing would not be included on a care plan. The three other responses are important aspects in client care and should be included in the care plan.

Nursing Process: Planning
Client Needs: Health Promotion and Maintenance
Clinical Area: Medical Nursing

46.   (3)   Hypothermia or fever may lead to an inaccurate reading. Artificial nails may distort a reading if a finger probe is used. Vasoconstriction can cause an inaccurate reading of oxygen saturation. Arterial saturations have a close correlation with the reading from the pulse oximeter as long as the arterial saturation is above 70 percent.

Nursing Process: Analysis
Client Needs: Safe, Effective Care Environment
Clinical Area: Medical Nursing

47.   (2)   These common side effects are a direct result of using androgens or estrogens as chemotherapeutic agents.

Nursing Process: Planning
Client Needs: Health Promotion and Maintenance
Clinical Area: Medical Nursing

48.   (4)   For clients with an MI, thrombolytic therapy minimizes the infarct size through lyses of the clot in the occluded coronary artery. The patent artery then promotes perfusion of the heart muscle. The other three responses are all contraindications for the use of thrombolytic agents.

Nursing Process: Analysis
Client Needs: Physiological Integrity
Clinical Area: Medical Nursing

49. (1) A restrictive band 2 to 4 inches above the snake bite is most effective in containing the venom and minimizing lymphatic and superficial venous return. Elevation of the limb or immobilization would not be effective interventions.

Nursing Process: Implementation
Client Needs: Safe, Effective Care Environment
Clinical Area: Medical Nursing

50. (4) The word "patient" or "client" should not be used, as the chart belongs to the client; thus, adding it to the chart is redundant.

Nursing Process: Planning
Client Needs: Safe, Effective Care Environment
Clinical Area: Medical Nursing

51. (4) It is never advisable to force fluids into a tubing to check for patency. Sterile water and aqueous Zephiran will affect the pH of the bladder as well as cause irritation. Normal saline is the fluid of choice for irrigation.

Nursing Process: Planning
Client Needs: Safe, Effective Care Environment
Clinical Area: Medical Nursing

52. (4) The P-R interval is measured on the EKG strip from the beginning of the P wave to the beginning of the QRS complex. It is the time it takes for the impulse to travel to the ventricle.

Nursing Process: Assessment
Client Needs: Physiological Integrity
Clinical Area: Medical Nursing

53. (4) Pulmonary artery pressure is the most effective method. Clients with a large percentage of body surface burned often do not have an area where a cuff can be applied. Cuff blood pressures are also affected more by peripheral vascular changes. Pulse monitoring is not accurate enough to detect subtle changes in the system. Central venous pressures are less than optimal because changes in left heart pressure (sign of pulmonary edema) are often not reflected in the right heart pressures.

Nursing Process: Assessment
Client Needs: Safe, Effective Care Environment
Clinical Area: Medical Nursing

54. (2) Diarrhea is a very common response to the dye tablets. A dinner of tea and toast is usually given to the client. Each dye tablet is given at five minute intervals, usually with one glass of water following each

Nursing Process: Implementation
Client Needs: Safe, Effective Care Environment
Clinical Area: Medical Nursing

tablet. The number of tablets prescribed will vary, because it is based on the weight of the client.

55. (1) Placing the client on his right side will allow pressure to be placed on the puncture site, thus promoting hemostasis and preventing hemorrhage. The other positions will not be effective in achieving these goals.

Nursing Process: Implementation
Client Needs: Safe, Effective Care Environment
Clinical Area: Medical Nursing

56. (2) Cyanosis is a result of impaired oxygen-carbon dioxide exchange at the alveolar level. Advent of the gallop (S_3, S_4) rhythm indicates that the client is in CHF. Cerebral/mental changes often occur but they are due to hypoxia rather than edema. Changes in the lungs occur because of increased fluid that expands in the interstitial spaces and decreased oxygen transport, not because of airway changes.

Nursing Process: Assessment
Client Needs: Physiological Integrity
Clinical Area: Medical Nursing

57. (2) Cholinergic crisis is the result of an excessive dose of a anticholinesterase drug that the client took. In addition to the symptoms listed, the client will experience muscle tightness and fasciculations, decreased blood pressure, and constricted pupils.

Nursing Process: Assessment
Client Needs: Health Promotion and Maintenance
Clinical Area: Medical Nursing

58. (3) An NG tube insertion is the most appropriate intervention because it will determine the presence of active gastrointestinal bleeding. A Miller-Abbott tube is a weighted, mercury-filled ballooned tube used to resolve bowel obstructions. There is no evidence of shock or fluid overload in the client; therefore, an arterial line is not appropriate at this time.

Nursing Process: Implementation
Client Needs: Safe, Effective Care Environment
Clinical Area: Medical Nursing

59. (1) Clients with myxedema often experience a decreased respiratory rate and chest excursion, so they require extra care to pre-

Nursing Process: Implementation
Client Needs: Safe, Effective Care Environment
Clinical Area: Medical Nursing

vent atelectasis. Encouraging moving, turning and coughing exercises will open the alveoli, thus decreasing the risk of atelectasis. Postural drainage will not prevent atelectasis because the treatment does not expand the alveoli.

60. (3) The most important protection for the nurse is clean gloves. She may wear a gown to protect herself if the client is not alert. A mask is advised if the client is coughing.

Nursing Process: Implementation
Client Needs: Safe, Effective Care Environment
Clinical Area: Medical Nursing

61. (3) A second-degree burn involves the epidermis and dermis. (1) is the definition of a fourth-degree burn, (2) is characteristic of a first-degree burn, and (4) is the definition of a third-degree burn.

Nursing Process: Assessment
Client Needs: Physiological Integrity
Clinical Area: Medical Nursing

62. (1) Decreased arterial flow is a result of vasospasm. The etiology is unknown. It is more problematic in colder climates or when the person is under stress. Hyperemia occurs when the vasospasm is relieved.

Nursing Process: Analysis
Client Needs: Physiological Integrity
Clinical Area: Medical Nursing

63. (2) The client's instructions should include keeping the environment warm to prevent vasoconstriction. Wearing gloves, warm clothes, and socks will also be useful in preventing vasoconstriction, but TED hose will not be therapeutic. Walking will most likely increase his pain.

Nursing Process: Implementation
Client Needs: Health Promotion and Maintenance
Clinical Area: Medical Nursing

64. (4) The presence of bile in the urine would lead to a yellow-orange or brown-colored urine.

Nursing Process: Assessment
Client Needs: Safe, Effective Care Environment
Clinical Area: Medical Nursing

65. (2) The dialysate contains small amounts or none of the substances that are to be removed from the body. The peritoneum acts as a semipermeable membrane across which the substances move by osmosis

Nursing Process: Planning
Client Needs: Physiological Integrity
Clinical Area: Medical Nursing

from an area of high concentration (the blood) to an area of lower concentration (the dialysate). This process takes 48–72 hours to be effective, and this time frame must be considered in planning for care.

66. (4)   In addition to the germicidal soap scrubs, systemic antibiotics are administered to prevent infection of the wound. Silver nitrate is not a common treatment today.

Nursing Process: Planning
Client Needs: Safe, Effective Care Environment
Clinical Area: Medical Nursing

67. (2)   Answer (2) is correct because the culture takes three weeks to grow. Usually even very small lesions can be seen on x-rays due to the natural contrast of the air in the lungs; therefore, chest x-rays do not need to be repeated frequently (3). Clients may have positive smears but negative cultures if they have been on medication (4). A positive skin test indicates the person only has been infected with tuberculosis but may not necessarily have active disease (1).

Nursing Process: Analysis
Client Needs: Physiological Integrity
Clinical Area: Medical Nursing

68. (1)   The increase in intraocular pressure causes atrophy of the retinal ganglion cells and the optic nerve, and leads eventually to blindness.

Nursing Process: Analysis
Client Needs: Physiological Integrity
Clinical Area: Medical Nursing

69. (4)   Nervous control for the diaphragm (phrenic nerve) exists at C3 or C4. Quadriplegia involves cervical injuries C1–C8.

Nursing Process: Analysis
Client Needs: Physiological Integrity
Clinical Area: Medical Nursing

70. (3)   As the liver cells become fatty and degenerate, they are no longer able to accommodate the large amount of blood necessary for homeostasis. The pressure in the liver increases and causes increased pressure in the venous system. As the portal pressure increases, fluid exudes into the abdominal cavity. This is called ascites.

Nursing Process: Analysis
Client Needs: Physiological Integrity
Clinical Area: Medical Nursing

71.   (4) "T_1" means the tumor is less than 3 cm in diameter without invasion proximal to a lobar bronchus. "NO" means there is no demonstrable metastasis to regional lymph nodes and "MO" indicates no distant metastasis.

Nursing Process: Analysis
Client Needs: Physiological Integrity
Clinical Area: Medical Nursing

72.   (1) The client is very anxious and his ability to comprehend and process information is extremely limited. A quiet, reassuring manner with a brief, concrete response will be most helpful at this point. Interventions to decrease the client's anxiety is priority whether the cause is guilt feelings or not.

Nursing Process: Planning
Client Needs: Psychosocial Integrity
Clinical Area: Medical Nursing

73.   (1) Weakness, fainting, blurred vision, pallor, and perspiration are all common symptoms when there is too much insulin or too little food—hypoglycemia. The signs and symptoms in answers (2) and (3) are indicative of hyperglycemia.

Nursing Process: Assessment
Client Needs: Physiological Integrity
Clinical Area: Medical Nursing

74.   (3) Physical and psychosocial assessments are most important in dealing with ulcer clients. The nursing goal is to promote physical rest and psychological relief. Discussing stressful situations may cause the client to become anxious and delay ulcer healing. Discussing the pathogenesis of ulcer disease will not help the client to relax. Identification of substances that cause pain will assist in planning for teaching. Dietary teaching needs to include incorporating the client's food preferences into such a regimen.

Nursing Process: Planning
Client Needs: Psychosocial Integrity
Clinical Area: Medical Nursing

75.   (1) The first specimen is discarded because it is considered "old urine" or urine that was in the bladder before the test began. After the first discarded specimen, urine is collected for 24 hours.

Nursing Process: Implementation
Client Need: Safe, Effective Care Environment
Clinical Area: Medical Nursing

76. (4) This response opens up communication to allow the client to discuss his fears of dying. (1) Referring to his physician is nontherapeutic, as is answer (2), which is giving him false reassurance. (3) questions his feelings and does not encourage him to express them.

Nursing Process: Implementation
Client Needs: Psychosocial Integrity
Clinical Area: Medical Nursing

77. (1) A reddened area over the sacrum may be the first sign of a pressure ulcer. If it is recognized at this stage and nursing actions taken to avoid additional pressure (frequent turning, massaging the skin, etc.), the ulcer may be avoided. Answer (2) and (3) can be expected with left-sided CVA and (4) is probably expected with an elderly person.

Nursing Process: Assessment
Client Needs: Physiological Integrity
Clinical Area: Medical Nursing

78. (1) It is important to decrease intracranial pressure (head of bed elevated) and to allow for drainage (head turned to left). All of the other responses are incorrect because the position would not facilitate cerebral drainage or ear drainage.

Nursing Process: Implementation
Client Needs: Safe, Effective Care Environment
Clinical Area: Medical Nursing

79. (2) The purpose of the tongs is to decompress the vertebral column through hyperextending it. Both (1) and (3) are incorrect because they might cause further damage. (4) is incorrect because the client cannot sit up with the tongs in place; only the head of the bed can be elevated.

Nursing Process: Analysis
Client Needs: Physiological Integrity
Clinical Area: Medical Nursing

80. (3) An important assessment question is to find out how the client feels about the tests to be performed. Learning if he has talked with anyone about his concerns or fears will help the nurse assess the client's resources for emotional support and whether the client needs to talk about his fears or feelings.

Nursing Process: Assessment
Client Needs: Physiological Integrity
Clinical Area: Medical Nursing

81.   (4)   The cardiac output is that amount of blood pumped by the left ventricle each minute. It is a good indicator of left ventricular function. As the left ventricle fails, the pressure in the chamber rises. Then the arterial blood pressure falls. The CVP would increase later when peripheral flow is impeded into the right atrium due to pulmonary congestion.

Nursing Process: Analysis
Client Needs: Physiological Integrity
Clinical Area: Medical Nursing

82.   (4)   Forcing fluids ensures a continuous flow of urine to provide adequate urine output for specimen collection. High fluid intake also prevents multiplication of bacteria that may have been introduced during the procedure.

Nursing Process: Implementation
Client Needs: Safe, Effective Care Environment
Clinical Area: Medical Nursing

83.   (2)   If the shunt is patent, it will feel warm to the touch and the nurse will hear the sound of rushing blood and a loud bruit. The nurse can also feel the thrill by palpating over the fistula site.

Nursing Process: Assessment
Client Needs: Safe, Effective Care Environment
Clinical Area: Medical Nursing

84.   (4)   The gastric balloon of the Sengstaken-Blakemore tube reduces the amount of blood going to the esophagus and cardiac sphincter by direct tamponade. It does not affect gastric or duodenal ulcers, as the pressure is only in the esophagus and cardiac sphincter.

Nursing Process: Analysis
Client Needs: Physiological Integrity
Clinical Area: Medical Nursing

85.   (2)   Clients must have the head of the bed elevated to prevent the contrast medium from irritating cervical nerve roots and cranial structures. Clients may sit up in a chair following the procedure if they are comfortable.

Nursing Process: Implementation
Client Needs: Safe, Effective Care Environment
Clinical Area: Medical Nursing

86.   (3)   Clients may experience inaccurate readings if dye has been used for a diagnostic test. Dyes use colors that tint the blood which leads to inaccurate readings.

Nursing Process: Implementation
Client Needs: Safe, Effective Care Environment
Clinical Area: Medical Nursing

87.   (4)   The major goal in protecting the seizure client against injury is to always maintain an adequate airway. Placing the client in a side position assists in preventing aspiration. Current treatment of seizures no longer advocates the use of a padded tongue blade during a seizure because of possible injury to teeth. Restraints may also cause injury.

Nursing Process: Implementation
Client Needs: Safe, Effective Care Environment
Clinical Area: Medical Nursing

88.   (3)   The respiratory system can become occluded if the balloon slips and moves up the esophagus, putting pressure on the trachea. This would result in respiratory distress and should be assessed frequently. Scissors should be kept at the bedside to cut the tube if distress occurs. This is a safety intervention.

Nursing Process: Assessment
Client Needs: Safe, Effective Care Environment
Clinical Area: Medical Nursing

89.   (1)   As blood is digested, the blood urea nitrogen rises rapidly. A result of bleeding may also be a lowered hemoglobin, but this does not indicate digestion and absorption of blood nitrogen. An elevation of serum ammonia may ensue if the liver is unable to handle the protein load of digested blood.

Nursing Process: Analysis
Client Needs: Physiological Integrity
Clinical Area: Medical Nursing

90.   (2)   Lethargy may indicate impending encephalopathy and dictate the need for client safety measures. Fatigue is expected due to anemia, shortness of breath due to ascites, and nausea due to GI vascular congestion, but these are not as grave as lethargy.

Nursing Process: Assessment
Client Needs: Physiological Integrity
Clinical Area: Medical Nursing

91.   (4)   The pain of pancreatitis is made worse by walking and supine positioning. The client is more comfortable sitting up and leaning forward.

Nursing Process: Implementation
Client Needs: Safe, Effective Care Environment
Clinical Area: Medical Nursing

92.   (3)   Oliguria, with accompanying hypovolemic shock, is a dangerous complication from acute pancreatitis. This condition

Nursing Process: Evaluation
Client Needs: Physiological Integrity
Clinical Area: Medical Nursing

may necessitate large volumes of parenteral fluids to maintain vascular volume; a CVP catheter is often inserted for monitoring fluid needs.

93. (1) Frequency and dysuria are most specific symptoms of lower urinary tract infection while (2) and (3) are more indicative of upper urinary tract infection. Cloudy urine may indicate microscopic hematuria, while odor may be related to diet.

Nursing Process: Assessment
Client Needs: Physiological Integrity
Clinical Area: Medical Nursing

94. (4) Infection due to catheter presence is most commonly associated with migration to the bladder along the internal lumen of the catheter after contamination. Keeping the collection bag dependent of the tubing is important to prevent reflux and contamination. The other distractors are potential, but not as common, causes of infection.

Nursing Process: Analysis
Client Needs: Safe, Effective Care Environment
Clinical Area: Medical Nursing

95. (4) It is most important that the client with lupus protects herself from sun exposure with large brimmed hats, long sleeves, and sunscreen cream. Keeping the skin moist and clean are also important, but lesions are best prevented by sun protection.

Nursing Process: Evaluation
Client Needs: Health Promotion and Maintenance
Clinical Area: Medical Nursing

96. (4) The client with acute renal failure would be expected to have metabolic acidosis (low HCO_3) resulting in acid blood pH (acidemia) and respiratory alkalosis (lowered PCO_2) as a compensating mechanism. Normal values are pH 7.35 to 7.45; HCO_3 23 to 27 mEg; and PCO_2 35 to 45 mmHg.

Nursing Process: Assessment
Client Needs: Physiological Integrity
Clinical Area: Medical Nursing

97. (2) Dextrose with insulin helps move potassium into cells and is immediate management therapy for hyperkalemia due to acute renal failure. An exchange resin may also be employed. This type of

Nursing Process: Analysis
Client Needs: Physiological Integrity
Clinical Area: Medical Nursing

infusion is also administered sometimes before cardiac surgery to stabilize irritable cells and prevent arrhythmias, but in this case KCl is also added to the infusion.

98. (3) Early in progressive (chronic) renal failure, the tubules lose ability to concentrate urine so there is increased urinary output with urine of low specific gravity and concomitant increase in fluid intake. This stage goes unnoticed by most clients.

Nursing Process: Assessment
Client Needs: Physiological Integrity
Clinical Area: Medical Nursing

99. (1) It is essential that the end stage renal client adhere to all aspects of the medical regimen. Only excess solutes and fluid are removed with dialysis. Blood pressure management, aspects of care concerning concomitant anemia, and phosphate/calcium/vitamin D imbalance, as well as protein restriction and fluid restriction, must be carried out at all times. The dialysis client continues to be uremic and has multisystem problems that continue despite dialysis.

Nursing Process: Evaluation
Client Needs: Health Promotion and Maintenance
Clinical Area: Medical Nursing

100. (4) Peritonitis is a grave complication with peritoneal dialysis. Hemodialysis may be necessary until infection clears. Excess fluid and protein effluent into the peritoneum also complicate care. Use of aseptic technique is essential.

Nursing Process: Evaluation
Client Needs: Physiological Integrity
Clinical Area: Medical Nursing

Surgical Nursing

1. A 45-year-old client has just been admitted to the hospital for an abdominal hysterectomy. Results of lab tests indicate that the client's white blood cell count is 9,800/cu mm. The most appropriate intervention is to

   1. Call the operating room and cancel the surgery.
   2. Notify the surgeon immediately.
   3. Take no action as this is a normal value.
   4. Call the lab and have the test repeated.

2. While the nurse is orienting a client scheduled for surgery, she states she is afraid of what will happen the next day. The most appropriate response is to

   1. Assure her that the surgery is very safe and problems are rare.
   2. Encourage her to talk about her fears as much as she wishes.
   3. Explain that her physician is one of the best and she has nothing to worry about.
   4. Explain that worrying will only prolong her hospitalization.

3. A 38-year-old female client is admitted to the emergency room after breaking her right wrist in a fall. Before administering the NSAID ketrololac tromethamine (Toradol) for pain, the nurse would assess for

   1. Any eye problems such as glaucoma.
   2. Presence of peptic ulcer disease.
   3. Currently taking birth control pills.
   4. An allergy to Tylenol.

4. When a client is being instructed in crutch walking using the swing-through gait, the most appropriate directions are

   1. "Look down at your feet before moving the crutches to ensure you won't fall as you move them."
   2. "Place one crutch forward with the opposite foot and then place the second crutch forward followed by the second foot."
   3. "Move both crutches forward then lift and swing your body past the crutches."
   4. "Use the crutch bar to balance yourself to prevent falls."

5. A cast placed on a client's leg has dried. If the drying process were completed, the nurse would observe the cast to be

   1. Dull and gray in appearance.
   2. Shiny and white in appearance.
   3. Cool to the touch and gray in appearance.
   4. Warm to the touch and white in appearance.

6. While filling out his menu for the following day, a client scheduled for a cardiac catheterization mentions to the nurse that he "always gets a rash when I eat shellfish." Following safety protocol, the most appropriate initial nursing intervention is to

1. Notify the physician.
2. Place a note on the chart regarding this reaction.
3. Ask the client if there are any other foods that cause such a reaction.
4. Notify the dietitian of the reaction and request a "no shellfish" diet.

7. The visiting home health nurse is assigned to a client who just had cataract surgery. A care plan would include instructions to

   1. Maintain bedrest for at least two days with bathroom privileges only.
   2. Keep the head up and straight and not to look down.
   3. Deep breathe and cough four times a day.
   4. Only lie on the affected side when in bed.

8. A client is on dialysis treatments three times per week. The nurse explains that the main advantage of using an internal arteriovenous fistula rather than an external arteriovenous cannula for dialysis is

   1. Accessing the internal fistula is less uncomfortable for the client.
   2. The internal fistula can be utilized immediately after insertion.
   3. There is less risk of hemorrhage from the internal fistula.
   4. It is easier to access the blood flow with the internal fistula than through the external cannula.

9. A client scheduled for colostomy surgery will have a preoperative diet ordered that will include

   1. Broiled chicken, baked potato, and wheat bread.

2. Ground hamburger, rice, and salad.
3. Broiled fish, rice, squash, and tea.
4. Steak, mashed potatoes, raw carrots, and celery.

10. The physician tells a client that he will need exploratory surgery the next day. As the nurse determines the preoperative teaching plan, which one of the following interventions is most important?

    1. Answer questions the client has about his condition or the forthcoming surgery.
    2. Explain the routine preoperative procedures: NPO, shower, medication, shave, etc.
    3. Describe the surgery and what the client will experience following surgery.
    4. Assure the client there is nothing to worry about because the physician is very experienced.

11. A 52-year-old client has had a lobectomy for cancer of the left lower lobe of the lung. He is eighteen hours postoperative. The nurse understands that the most appropriate position immediately postoperatively is

    1. Flat bedrest.
    2. Turned to the unoperative side only.
    3. Turned to the operative side only.
    4. Semi-Fowler's position, turned to either side.

12. Following a fracture of the right hip, a client has an open reduction with internal fixation using an Austin Moore prosthesis. Postoperatively the affected leg should be maintained in a position of

    1. Adduction.
    2. External rotation.

3. Internal rotation.
4. Abduction.

13. A male client has just had a cataract operation without a lens implant. In discharge teaching, the nurse will instruct the client's wife to

1. Feed him soft foods for several days to prevent facial movement.
2. Keep the eye dressing on for one week.
3. Have her husband remain in bed for three days.
4. Allow him to walk upstairs only with assistance.

14. A client has been admitted to the orthopedic unit with an intracapsular fracture of the right hip sustained after a fall on the ice. Buck's extension is applied and arrangements are being made for hip prosthesis surgery in the morning. The purpose for application of Buck's extension at this time is to

1. Reduce the fracture.
2. Relieve muscle spasm.
3. Keep the knee extended.
4. Stabilize the fractured hip.

15. Which of the following statements is true of skeletal traction?

1. Neurovascular complications are less apt to occur than with skin traction.
2. The client has less mobility than he does with skin traction.
3. Fractures can be reduced because more weight can be used than with skin traction.
4. It is preferred for children because fracture fragment alignment is so important.

16. Russell's traction is easily recognized because it incorporates a

1. Sling under the knee.
2. Cervical halter.
3. Pelvic girdle.
4. Pearson attachment.

17. When evaluating all forms of traction, the nurse knows that the direction of pull is controlled by the

1. Client's position.
2. Rope/pulley system.
3. Amount of weight.
4. Point of friction.

18. The statement that best explains the principle of hemodialysis is

1. Water passes through the membrane by osmosis.
2. Plasma proteins are eliminated from the blood by diffusion.
3. The pH of the blood is lowered by removal of nonvolatile acids.
4. Blood constituents pass from an area of higher to an area of lower concentration.

19. A client has lost about 30 percent of his total blood volume. Blood has been replaced, but his blood pressure remains low. Which of the following drugs would the nurse anticipate the physician ordering?

1. A vasopressor.
2. A vasodilator.
3. An adrenergic blocking drug.
4. A parasympatholytic drug.

20. A client scheduled for surgery is given a spinal anesthetic. Immediately following the injection, the nurse will position the client

1. On his abdomen.
2. In semi-Fowler's position.
3. In slight Trendelenburg's position.
4. On his back or side; head raised.

21. Following spinal anesthesia, a client is brought into the recovery room. The assessment data that indicates a complication of anesthesia has developed is

    1. Hiccoughs.
    2. Numbness in legs.
    3. Headache.
    4. No urge to void.

22. A client has had a partial colectomy. Surgery began at 7:30 A.M. She returned to the unit at 1:30 P.M. During a 6:00 P.M. assessment, the nurse observed all of the following. A priority concern which would require the earliest intervention is a

    1. Dressing that is moderately saturated with serosanguineous drainage.
    2. Warm and reddened area on the client's left calf.
    3. Distended bladder that is firm to palpation.
    4. Decrease in breath sounds on the right side.

23. Following surgery, the client's surgeon orders a Foley catheter to be inserted. Which one of the following interventions would the nurse carry out first?

    1. Clean the perineum from front to back.
    2. Check the catheter for patency.
    3. Explain to the client that she will feel slight, temporary discomfort.
    4. Arrange the sterile items on the sterile field.

24. After a Foley catheter was inserted for two days, it was removed by the nurse. The response considered to be normal at this time is

    1. Dribbling after the first several voidings.
    2. Urgency and frequency for several days.
    3. Frequent voidings in small amounts.
    4. Retention of urine for 10- to 12-hour periods.

25. A client is scheduled for a cystectomy and ureteroileostomy (ileal conduit). The nurse observes this client for complications in the postoperative period. Which of the following symptoms indicates an unexpected outcome and requires priority care?

    1. Edema of the stoma.
    2. Mucus in the drainage appliance.
    3. Redness of the stoma.
    4. Feces in the drainage appliance.

26. The nurse understands that it is important to obtain baseline vital signs for her client preoperatively in order to

    1. Establish a baseline postoperatively.
    2. Inform the anesthetist so he can administer appropriate preanesthesia medication.
    3. Judge the client's recovery from the effects of surgery and anesthesia when taking postoperative vital signs.
    4. Prevent operative hypotension.

27. A client requires that a bronchoscopy procedure be done. Due to his physical condition he will be awake during the procedure. As part of the pretest teaching, the nurse will instruct him that before the scope insertion his neck will be positioned so that it is

1. In a flexed position.
2. In an extended position.
3. In a neutral position.
4. Hyperextended.

28. A male, age 35, was knifed in a street fight, admitted though the emergency room, and is now in the ICU. An assessment of his condition reveals the following symptoms: respirations shallow and rapid, paradoxical pulse, CVP 15 cm H_2O, BP 90 mmHg systolic, skin cold and pale, urinary output 60–100 ml/hr for the last two hours. Analyzing these symptoms, the nurse will conclude that the client has which one of the following conditions?

    1. Hypovolemic shock.
    2. Cardiac tamponade.
    3. Wound dehiscence.
    4. Atelectasis.

29. The advantages to the client for an immediate prosthesis fitting following an amputation, are

    1. Ability to ambulate sooner.
    2. Less chance of phantom limb sensation.
    3. Dressing changes are not necessary.
    4. Better fit of the prosthesis.

30. A client has possible malignancy of the colon, and surgery is scheduled. The rationale for administering Neomycin preoperatively is to

    1. Prevent infection postoperatively.
    2. Eliminate the need for preoperative enemas.
    3. Decrease and retard the growth of normal bacteria in the intestines.
    4. Treat cancer of the colon.

31. Thrombophlebitis is a common complication following vascular surgery. Which of the following signs indicates that a possible thrombus has occurred?

    1. Kernig's sign.
    2. Hegar's sign.
    3. Homan's sign.
    4. Brudzinski's sign.

32. A nursing care plan for a client with a suprapubic cystostomy would include

    1. Placing a urinal bag around the tube insertion to collect the urine.
    2. Clamping the tube and allowing the client to void through the urinary meatus before removing the tube.
    3. Catheter irrigations every four hours to prevent formation of urinary stones.
    4. Limiting fluid intake to 1500 ml per day.

33. A 42-year-old client has been diagnosed with a right-sided acoustic neuroma. The tumor is large and has impaired the function of the seventh and eighth cranial nerves. Which of the following nursing actions will be carried out to prevent complications?

    1. Keeping a suction machine available.
    2. Use of an eyepatch or eyeshield on the right eye.
    3. Use of only cool water to wash the face.
    4. Advising the client to use only the left eye.

34. For a client who has ataxia, which of the following tests would be performed to assess the ability to ambulate?

    1. Kernig's.
    2. Romberg's.

3. Riley-Day's.
4. Hoffmann's.

35. Following a treadmill test and cardiac catheterization, the client is found to have coronary artery disease which is inoperative. He is referred to the cardiac rehabilitation unit. During his first visit to the unit he says that he doesn't understand why he needs to be there because there is nothing that can be done to make him better. The best nursing response is

1. "Cardiac rehabilitation is not a cure but can help restore you to many of your former activities."
2. "Here we teach you to gradually change your lifestyle to accommodate your heart disease."
3. "You are probably right but we can gradually increase your activities so that you can live a more active life."
4. "Do you feel that you will have to make some changes in your life now?"

36. Assessing a client who has developed atelectasis postoperatively, the nurse will be most likely to find

1. A flushed face.
2. Dyspnea.
3. Decreased temperature.
4. Severe cough.

37. A client admitted to a surgical unit for possible bleeding in the cerebrum has vital signs taken every hour to monitor her neurological status. Which of the following neurological checks will give the nurse the best information about the extent of bleeding?

1. Pupillary checks.
2. Spinal tap.
3. Deep tendon reflexes.
4. Evaluation of extrapyramidal motor system.

38. Instructions given to clients following cataract surgery include the information that

1. The eye patch will be removed in three to four days, and they will be able to use the eye without difficulty.
2. They must use only one eye at a time to prevent double vision.
3. They will be able to judge distances without difficulty.
4. Contact lenses will be fitted before discharge from the hospital.

39. Conditions known to predispose to renal calculi formation include

1. Polyuria.
2. Dehydration, immobility.
3. Glycosuria.
4. Presence of an indwelling Foley catheter.

40. Following abdominal surgery, which of the following clinical manifestations will be indicative of negative nitrogen balance?

1. Poor skin turgor from dehydration.
2. Edema or ascites of the abdomen and flank.
3. Pale color to skin.
4. Diarrhea.

41. Preoperative teaching for a client scheduled for a laryngectomy should include the fact that

1. The client will continue to be able to breathe and smell through the nose.
2. The client will be fed through a permanent gastrostomy tube.
3. The client will be able to speak again, but it will not be the same as before surgery.
4. Oral fluids will be eliminated for the first week following surgery.

42. The main complication following a nephrostomy that the nurse must assess for is

   1. Bleeding from the nephrostomy site.
   2. Cardiopulmonary involvement following the procedure.
   3. Difficulty in restoring fluid and electrolyte balance.
   4. Contamination.

43. Hemorrhage is a major complication following oral surgery and radical neck dissection. If this condition occurs, the most immediate nursing intervention would be to

   1. Notify the surgeon immediately.
   2. Treat the client for shock.
   3. Put pressure over the common carotid and jugular vessels in the neck.
   4. Immediately put the client in high-Fowler's position.

44. Following a cystoscopy, it was determined that a client with benign prostatic hypertrophy would be admitted for a transurethral resection (TUR). Preoperative nursing care will include

   1. Discussing the surgical intervention and the fact that it causes impotence.
   2. Decreasing fluid intake for at least two days to prevent bladder irritability.

3. Keeping the client NPO for at least 18 hours to prevent bowel evacuation during the surgical procedure.
4. Discussing hygienic care of the penis before surgery.

45. Assessing for immediate postoperative complications, the nurse knows that a complication likely to occur following unresolved atelectasis is

   1. Hemorrhage.
   2. Infection.
   3. Pneumonia.
   4. Pulmonary embolism.

46. One method of assessing for signs of circulatory impairment in a client with a fractured femur is to ask the client to

   1. Cough and deep breathe.
   2. Turn himself in bed.
   3. Perform bicep exercises
   4. Wiggle his toes.

47. A nursing measure to prevent the complication of deep vein thrombophlebitis following surgery would include

   1. Placing pillows under the affected limb.
   2. Wearing elastic hose at all times.
   3. Having the client sit up tid.
   4. Elevating the foot of the bed.

48. The morning of the second postoperative day following hip surgery for a fractured right hip, the nurse will ambulate the client. The first intervention is to

   1. Get the client up in a chair after dangling at the bedside.
   2. Use a walker when getting the client up.

3. Have the client put minimal weight on the affected side when getting up.
4. Practice getting the client out of bed by having her slightly flex her hips.

49. Following cholecystectomy surgery, the client has a T-tube in place. When she is returned to the unit, the nurse will ensure optimal functioning by placing her in

   1. Semi-Fowler's position.
   2. Prone position.
   3. High-Fowler's position.
   4. Sims' position.

50. A young client is in the hospital with his left leg in Buck's traction. The team leader asks the nurse to place a footplate on the affected side at the bottom of the bed. The purpose of this action is to

   1. Anchor the traction.
   2. Prevent footdrop.
   3. Keep the client from sliding down in bed.
   4. Prevent pressure areas on the foot.

Surgical Nursing
Answers with Rationale

1.   (3)   The normal WBC is 5,000 to 10,000 per cu mm. If the results were abnormally high, the surgeon would have to be notified and the surgery may be canceled. Tests with abnormal results are not routinely repeated unless the results are grossly abnormal.

    Nursing Process: Implementation
    Client Needs: Safe, Effective Care Environment
    Clinical Area: Surgical Nursing

2.   (2)   Allowing the client to express her fears results in a decrease in anxiety and a more realistic and knowledgeable reaction to the situation. Studies have shown that the less anxiety the client has about the surgery, the more positive the postoperative results.

    Nursing Process: Implementation
    Client Needs: Psychosocial Integrity
    Clinical Area: Surgical Nursing

3.   (2)   Toradol can cause GI toxicity, especially ulceration or hemorrhage in clients with a history of ulcers or bleeding. Salicylate levels can be increased in the serum and bleeding times can be prolonged with use of the drug.

    Nursing Process: Assessment
    Client Needs: Safe, Effective Care Environment
    Clinical Area: Surgical Nursing

4.   (3)   This is the procedure for using the swing-through gait. Clients are instructed to look straight ahead when walking with crutches. Looking down can lead to falls and uneven gait. Putting pressure from the arm on the crutch bar can cause nerve damage.

    Nursing Process: Implementation
    Client Needs: Health Promotion and Maintenance
    Clinical Area: Surgical Nursing

5.   (2)   The cast will be shiny and cool to the touch when dry. It will have a dull appearance when wet.

    Nursing Process: Evaluation
    Client Needs: Safe, Effective Care Environment
    Clinical Area: Surgical Nursing

6.   (1)   Because the dye used during a cardiac catheterization contains iodine, the physician must be aware of this client's reaction to iodine (shellfish). The other interventions should be carried out, but they should follow notifying the physician.

Nursing Process: Implementation
Client Needs: Safe, Effective Care Environment
Clinical Area: Surgical Nursing

7.   (2)   Keeping the head straight and avoiding looking down will prevent intraocular pressure. The nurse would practice breathing exercises with the client but will not encourage coughing, as this could cause an increase in intraocular pressure in the operative eye.

Nursing Process: Planning
Client Needs: Health Promotion and Maintenance
Clinical Area: Surgical Nursing

8.   (3)   There is an increased incidence of hemorrhaging with the external cannula. Hemorrhage results from the cannula becoming disconnected. One advantage of the external cannula is that it is painless to use. Surgery is required to establish the internal fistula and it should be allowed to heal for several weeks before being utilized.

Nursing Process: Analysis
Client Needs: Physiological Integrity
Clinical Area: Surgical Nursing

9.   (3)   The client's diet should be low residue and high calorie. Foods high in carbohydrates are usually low residue; chicken is acceptable without skin. Any salad, fresh vegetables, or grains would be considered high residue.

Nursing Process: Planning
Client Needs: Safe, Effective Care Environment
Clinical Area: Surgical Nursing

10.   (1)   It is most important to begin at the client's level of understanding, so answering questions is more essential than giving explanations until the client is ready to listen. Describing the surgery is not the nurse's responsibility, and giving false reassurance by assuring the client there is nothing to worry about is nontherapeutic.

Nursing Process: Planning
Client Needs: Psychosocial Integrity
Clinical Area: Surgical Nursing

11.   (4)   The client can be turned to both sides to increase full expansion of lung tissue postoperatively. It is best to place him in

Nursing Process: Planning
Client Needs: Safe, Effective Care Environment
Clinical Area: Surgical Nursing

semi-Fowler's position when his vital signs are stable to ensure full lung expansion.

12. (4) To prevent dislocation of the prosthesis, the legs are kept abducted with neutral rotation. Adduction, flexion and internal rotation are to be avoided.

Nursing Process: Implementation
Client Needs: Physiological Integrity
Clinical Area: Surgical Nursing

13. (4) Without a lens, the eye cannot accommodate. It is difficult to judge distance and climb stairs when the eyes cannot accommodate. Therefore, the client should walk up and down stairs only with assistance.

Nursing Process: Implementation
Client Needs: Health Promotion and Maintenance
Clinical Area: Surgical Nursing

14. (2) The purpose of Buck's extension application following hip fracture is immobilization to relieve muscle spasm at the fracture site and, thereby, relieve pain. Any movement of fracture fragments will aggravate severe muscle spasm and pain. Skin traction such as this is not used to reduce a fracture and it is not important to keep the knee extended. Bryant's or Russell's traction will stabilize a fractured femur, not the hip.

Nursing Process: Analysis
Client Needs: Physiological Integrity
Clinical Area: Surgical Nursing

15. (3) Because more weight can be applied with skeletal traction, it can be used to reduce fractures and maintain alignment. It is not used commonly in the elderly because of prolonged immobilization. It is not preferred for children because some displacement of fracture fragments is desirable to prevent growth disturbance. Frequently, clients have more mobility than they do with skin traction, because balanced suspension is often incorporated with skeletal traction.

Nursing Process: Planning
Client Needs: Physiological Integrity
Clinical Area: Surgical Nursing

16. (1) Russell's traction is a type of skin action that incorporates a sling under the knee that is connected by a rope to an overhead bar pulley. It is frequently used to

Nursing Process: Assessment
Client Needs: Safe, Effective Care Environment
Clinical Area: Surgical Nursing

treat femoral shaft fractures in the adolescent.

17. (2) The rope/pulley and weight system is arranged so that fracture fragments are in the desired approximate position for healing. The client's position should always rest in line with the traction pull. The line of pull must never be interfered with by changing the position of a pulley and extension bar.

Nursing Process: Evaluation
Client Needs: Safe, Effective Care Environment
Clinical Area: Surgical Nursing

18. (4) Blood constituents pass into the dialysate solution where these constituents are of lower concentration (diffusion). Excess fluid is removed by filtration rather than by osmosis when hemodialysis is employed. The pH of the blood is not lowered by dialysis, nor are plasma proteins removed.

Nursing Process: Analysis
Client Needs: Physiological Integrity
Clinical Area: Surgical Nursing

19. (2) Vasodilator drugs are given when volume replacement has been completed. They decrease vascular resistance, decrease the work of the heart, and improve cardiac output and tissue perfusion. Vasopressor drugs intensify shock by increasing vasoconstriction in the microcirculatory beds.

Nursing Process: Planning
Client Needs: Physiological Integrity
Clinical Area: Surgical Nursing

20. (3) Usually the client is positioned on the back following the injection. If a high level of anesthesia is desired, the head and shoulders can be lowered slightly. After 20 minutes the anesthetic is set, and the client can be positioned in any manner.

Nursing Process: Implementation
Client Needs: Safe, Effective Care Environment
Clinical Area: Surgical Nursing

21. (3) When spinal fluid is lost through a leak or the client is dehydrated, a severe headache can occur, which may last several days. Numbness and no urge to void would be expected with spinal anesthesia unless it continues for several hours postop. The complication of hiccoughs can

Nursing Process: Assessment
Client Needs: Physiological Integrity
Clinical Area: Surgical Nursing

be associated with abdominal surgery, but is not attributable to spinal anesthesia.

22.   (3)   Inability to void after surgery is a common problem resulting from anesthesia or pain medication and requires an early intervention. It is important to be aware of the client's output for several reasons: to ensure adequate intake, to detect renal problems, and to assess for blood pressure problems. Solution to this problem is catheterization with a physician's order. The dressing should be closely observed but is not presently a problem. The area on the calf may be developing thrombophlebitis and should be reported to the physician immediately. The breath sounds can be improved by turning, coughing and deep breathing.

Nursing Process: Implementation
Client Needs: Safe, Effective Care Environment
Clinical Area: Surgical Nursing

23.   (3)   It is necessary to give the client an adequate explanation for any procedure. This will result in less anxiety and more cooperation from the client.

Nursing Process: Implementation
Client Needs: Psychosocial Integrity
Clinical Area: Surgical Nursing

24.   (1)   Dribbling may be normal until the sphincter muscles regain their tone. If the catheter had been place for several weeks, (3) might have been the most appropriate response. Urgency and frequency are symptoms of a bladder infection.

Nursing Process: Evaluation
Client Needs: Physiological Integrity
Clinical Area: Surgical Nursing

25.   (4)   Edema and a red color of the stoma are expected outcomes in the immediate postoperative period, as is mucus from the stoma. The ileal conduit procedure incorporates implantation of the ureters into a portion of the ileum which has been resected from its anatomical position and now functions as a reservoir or conduit for urine. The proximal and distal ileal borders can be resumed. Feces should not be draining from the conduit.

Nursing Process: Evaluation
Client Needs: Physiological Integrity
Clinical Area: Surgical Nursing

26.	(3) It is important to have presurgery vital signs so that the client's progress can be monitored to assure that his postoperative condition is stable.

Nursing Process: Assessment
Client Needs: Safe, Effective Care Environment
Clinical Area: Surgical Nursing

27.	(4) Hyperextension brings the pharynx into alignment with the trachea and allows the scope to be inserted without trauma.

Nursing Process: Implementation
Client Needs: Health Promotion and Maintenance
Clinical Area: Surgical Nursing

28.	(2) All of the client's symptoms are found in both cardiac tamponade and hypovolemic shock except the increase in urinary output. In shock, urinary output decreases to less than 30 ml/hour; thus, this is the symptom that would distinguish hypovolemic shock from cardiac tamponade.

Nursing Process: Analysis
Client Needs: Physiological Integrity
Clinical Area: Surgical Nursing

29.	(1) When the prosthesis is in place immediately following surgery, the client can stand up several hours postoperatively and walk the next day. The operative site is closed to outside contamination and benefits from improved circulation due to ambulation.

Nursing Process: Planning
Client Needs: Safe, Effective Care Environment
Clinical Area: Surgical Nursing

30.	(3) Neomycin suppresses normal bacterial flora, thereby "sterilizing" the bowel preoperatively to decrease the possibility of postoperative infection.

Nursing Process: Planning
Client Needs: Physiological Integrity
Clinical Area: Surgical Nursing

31.	(3) On dorsiflexion of the foot, the client will experience upper posterior pain in the calf if a clot is present. This is termed Homan's sign.

Nursing Process: Assessment
Client Needs: Physiological Integrity
Clinical Area: Surgical Nursing

32.	(2) Allowing the client to void naturally will be done prior to removal of the catheter to ensure adequate emptying of the bladder. Irrigations are not recommended, as they increase the chances of the client developing a urinary tract infection. Any time a client has an indwelling

Nursing Process: Planning
Client Needs: Safe, Effective Care Environment
Clinical Area: Surgical Nursing

catheter in place, fluids should be encouraged (unless contraindicated) to prevent stone formation.

33. (2) The seventh nerve closes the eyelid. Without a patch, the cornea is subject to damage. Temperature of the water does not matter. A suction machine is not necessary.

Nursing Process: Implementation
Client Needs: Safe, Effective Care Environment
Clinical Area: Surgical Nursing

34. (2) Romberg's test is the ability to maintain an upright position without swaying when standing with feet close together and eyes closed. Kernig's sign, a reflex contraction, is pain in the hamstring muscle when attempting to extend the leg after flexing the thigh.

Nursing Process: Assessment
Client Needs: Physiological Integrity
Clinical Area: Surgical Nursing

35. (1) Such a response does not give false hope to the client but is positive and realistic. The correct answer tells the client what cardiac rehabilitation is and does not dwell upon his negativity about it.

Nursing Process: Implementation
Client Needs: Health Promotion and Maintenance
Clinical Area: Surgical Nursing

36. (2) Atelectasis is a collapse of the alveoli due to obstruction or hypoventilation. Clients become short of breath and usually experience severe pain but do not have a severe cough. The shortness of breath is a result of decreased oxygen-carbon dioxide exchange at the alveolar level.

Nursing Process: Assessment
Client Needs: Physiological Integrity
Clinical Area: Surgical Nursing

37. (1) Pupillary checks reflect function of the third cranial nerve, which stretches as it becomes displaced by blood, tumor, etc.

Nursing Process: Analysis
Client Needs: Safe, Effective Care Environment
Clinical Area: Surgical Nursing

38. (2) The function of the lens is that of accommodation, the focusing of near objects on the retina by the lens; therefore, only the remaining lens will function in this capacity, depending on whether a cataract is present.

Nursing Process: Implementation
Client Needs: Health Promotion and Maintenance
Clinical Area: Surgical Nursing

39. (2) Urinary stasis, renal infection and dehydration predispose the client to the formation of renal calculi, which may or may not require surgery.

Nursing Process: Analysis
Client Needs: Physiological Integrity
Clinical Area: Surgical Nursing

40. (2) Edema is due to insufficient nitrogen for synthesis. When this occurs, it leads to a change in the body's osmotic pressure resulting in oozing of fluids out of the vascular space. This phenomena results in the formation of edema in the abdomen and flanks.

Nursing Process: Analysis
Client Needs: Physiological Integrity
Clinical Area: Surgical Nursing

41. (3) Most of the laryngectomy clients will use esophageal speech or a mechanical device for communication. They can usually begin to take oral fluids sometime after 48 hours. They are generally fed by an intravenous or nasogastric tube prior to oral feedings. Because the larynx is removed, it will be impossible to breathe through the nose.

Nursing Process: Planning
Client Needs: Health Promotion and Maintenance
Clinical Area: Surgical Nursing

42. (1) While all the other conditions may be complications, bleeding from the site is the main concern. The procedure is done to achieve relief from infection caused by urinary stasis, which may have resulted in kidney congestion.

Nursing Process: Assessment
Client Needs: Safe, Effective Care Environment
Clinical Area: Surgical Nursing

43. (3) Putting pressure over the vessels in the neck may be life-saving because a severe blood loss can occur rapidly, leading to shock and death. The surgeon would be notified as soon as possible.

Nursing Process: Implementation
Client Needs: Safe, Effective Care Environment
Clinical Area: Surgical Nursing

44. (4) Usually, a shower with detergent soap is taken the night before and morning of surgery. Particular attention should be paid to cleansing around the glans to rid it of microorganisms. An increased fluid intake and a good diet are essential to pre-

Nursing Process: Implementation
Client Needs: Health Promotion and Maintenance
Clinical Area: Surgical Nursing

vent urinary tract infections postop.
Clients are not impotent following surgery.

45. (3) Pneumonia is a major complication of
     unresolved atelectasis and must be treated
     along with vigorous treatment for atelecta-
     sis. Hemorrhage and infection are not
     related to this condition. Pulmonary
     embolism could result from deep vein
     thrombosis.

Nursing Process: Analysis
Client Needs: Physiological Integrity
Clinical Area: Surgical Nursing

46. (4) The only activity that will indicate a
     complication that is directly related to
     impairment in circulation due to a frac-
     tured femur is the inability to wiggle his
     toes.

Nursing Process: Assessment
Client Needs: Safe, Effective Care Environment
Clinical Area: Surgical Nursing

47. (4) Elevation of the legs promotes circula-
     tion and prevents venous stasis and more
     clot formation. Nursing measures aim at
     preventing further thrombi from forming
     and the already present thrombus from
     detaching. Elastic hose are necessary when
     the client is up walking again. Placing a
     pillow under the limb could cause a bend
     at the groin with resulting decreased circu-
     lation. Elastic hose are not necessary if the
     foot of the bed is sufficiently elevated. The
     client must be kept on bedrest until the
     danger of emboli passes (4–7 days).

Nursing Process: Implementation
Client Needs: Safe, Effective Care Environment
Clinical Area: Surgical Nursing

48. (2) Postoperative hip replacement clients
     may get up the first day, but need to use a
     walker for balance. They should not bear
     any weight on the affected side, dangle or
     sit in a chair, flexing their hips. Positions
     with 60 to 90 degree flexion should be
     avoided.

Nursing Process: Implementation
Client Needs: Safe, Effective Care Environment
Clinical Area: Surgical Nursing

49. (1) Initially a low-Fowler's position, then
     a semi-Fowler's position is encouraged,
     but not high-Fowler's. The objective is to

Nursing Process: Implementation
Client Needs: Safe, Effective Care Environment
Clinical Area: Surgical Nursing

facilitate drainage, but allow a position of comfort for the client.

50.　(2)　The purpose of the footplate is to prevent footdrop while the client is immobilized in traction. This will not anchor the traction, keep the client from sliding down in bed, or prevent pressure areas.

Nursing Process: Planning
Client Needs: Safe, Effective Care Environment
Clinical Area: Surgical Nursing

Maternity & Newborn Nursing

1. Nursing care of a pregnant client who received regional anesthesia would include

   1. Walking the client to ensure medication is evenly distributed.
   2. Asking the client to turn from side to side every 15 minutes.
   3. Monitoring blood pressure every three to five minutes until stabilized.
   4. Giving the client sips of water to swallow during the procedure.

2. Assessing a client with eclampsia, the nurse knows that a cardinal symptom is

   1. Weight gain of one pound a week.
   2. Concentrated urine.
   3. Hypertension.
   4. Feeling of lassitude and fatigue.

3. The nurse would anticipate a possible complication in infants delivered by cesarean section. This condition would be

   1. Respiratory distress.
   2. Renal impairment.
   3. ABO incompatibility.
   4. Kernicterus.

4. If a client experiences a ruptured ectopic pregnancy, an expected sign or symptom would be

   1. Elevated blood glucose levels.
   2. Sudden excruciating pain in lower abdomen.
   3. Sudden hypertension.
   4. Extensive external bleeding.

5. A client, 34 weeks pregnant, has just been admitted to the labor room in the first stage of labor. Which of the following clinical manifestations would be considered abnormal and would be reported to the physician immediately?

   1. Expulsion of a blood-tinged mucous plug.
   2. Continuous contraction of two minutes duration.
   3. Feeling of pressure on perineum causing her to bear down.
   4. Expulsion of clear fluid from the vagina.

6. An eclamptic client has been receiving magnesium sulfate IM every four hours. What symptom should be assessed for in order to safely administer the next dose?

   1. Absence of deep tendon reflexes.
   2. A respiratory rate of 16 per minute.
   3. Urine output of 50 ml over the last four hours.
   4. Complaints of being thirsty.

7. An 11 lb. 6 oz. baby girl was delivered by cesarean section to a diabetic mother. The

priority assessment of the infant of a diabetic mother would be for

1. Hypoglycemia.
2. Sepsis.
3. Hyperglycemia.
4. Hypercalcemia.

8. Of the following conditions, which one is not a result of metabolic error in the fetus?

1. Phenylketonuria.
2. Maple syrup urine disease.
3. Glutamicacidemia.
4. Pyloric stenosis.

9. A client has given birth to a stillborn with congenital deformities. She knows this but says she wants to see her baby. What is the nurse's best approach?

1. "That's your right. I'll bring the baby to you."
2. "It would be better to let your husband see the baby; then he can tell you."
3. "Are you really sure you want to? You might regret it later."
4. "Let's talk about it first. Tell me what you expect."

10. Of the following conditions, the one recognized as a known teratogen is

1. Scarlet fever.
2. Rubella.
3. Coronary heart disease.
4. Dental x-rays.

11. The nurse's understanding of fetal position is that when the baby's head is at station 0 it means that the

1. Sagittal sutures can be felt in the left posterior position.

2. Biparietal diameter of the head has passed the outlet.
3. Posterior fontanels are first palpable.
4. Level of the head is felt at the ischial spines.

12. A client is gravida 3 para 2 and is in labor and delivery. After a vaginal exam, it is determined that the presenting head is at station +3. The appropriate nursing action is to

1. Continue to observe the client's contractions.
2. Check the fetal heart rate for a prolapsed cord.
3. Prepare to move the client quickly to the delivery room.
4. Check with the physician to see if an oxytocin drip is warranted.

13. Pelvic inflammatory disease (PID) is an inflammatory condition of the pelvic cavity and may involve the ovaries, tubes, vascular system, or pelvic peritoneum. The nurse explains to the client that the most common cause of PID is

1. Tuberculosis bacilli.
2. Streptococcus.
3. Staphylococcus.
4. Gonorrhea.

14. Normal menstrual cycles and ovarian function are regulated by the hormones

1. FSH and LH.
2. LH and progesterone.
3. FSH and progesterone.
4. Estrogen and progesterone.

15. As the nurse walks into the newborn nursery, she sees a baby in respiratory distress

from apparent mucus. The *first* nursing action is to

1. Carefully slap the infant's back.
2. Thump the chest and start cardiopulmonary resuscitation.
3. Pick the baby up by the feet.
4. Call the rescue squad.

16. A client, 18 weeks pregnant, is concerned because she had a fever and rash about two and one-half weeks ago. The nurse's best response is

1. "It's best to talk with the physician about that."
2. "It's unlikely the fetus would have been affected as the first trimester is the most important time."
3. "What do you think the problems are with that?"
4. "Are you thinking you may have to terminate the pregnancy?."

17. A 14 year old came to the clinic for a birth control method. She sat through the class that describes the methods available to her. After class she asked the nurse, "Which method is best for me to use?" The best response is

1. "You are so young, are you sure you are ready for the responsibilities of a sexual relationship?"
2. "Because of your age, we need your parents' consent before you can be examined and then we'll talk."
3. "Before I can help you with that question, I need to know more about your sexual activity."
4. "The physician can best help you with that after your physical examination."

18. Assessing a newborn infant, the nurse knows that postmature infants may exhibit

1. Heavy vernix, little lanugo.
2. Large size for gestational age.
3. Increased subcutaneous fat, absent creases on feet.
4. Small size for gestational age.

19. A primigravida, age 36, delivered an 8 lb. 6 oz. baby girl by cesarean section. Which one of the following nursing actions would *not* be included in the client's immediate postoperative care?

1. Taking vital signs q 15 minutes for 2 to 3 hours.
2. Checking lochia for amount and color q 15 minutes for 2 to 3 hours.
3. Assisting the client to turn, cough and deep breathe.
4. Offering oral fluids q 15 minutes for 2 to 3 hours.

20. Counseling a client who is starting to use oral contraception, the nurse explains that birth control pills work by the mechanism of

1. Inhibiting chorionic gonadotropin production.
2. Inhibiting follicle-stimulating hormone production.
3. Inhibiting progesterone and estrogen production.
4. Stimulating luteinizing hormone production.

21. Which of the following garments worn by a pregnant woman would necessitate a special nursing intervention?

1. Garter belt with nylon stockings.
2. Support panty hose.

3. Woolen athletic socks.
4. Knee-high nylon sockettes.

22. An appropriate nursing intervention to help a nursing mother care for cracked nipples would be

    1. Applying benzoin to toughen the nipples.
    2. Keeping the nipples covered with warm, moist packs.
    3. Offering to give the baby a bottle.
    4. Exposing the nipples to air as much as possible.

23. A client is very concerned because her one-day-old son, who was very alert at birth, is now sleeping most of the time. The nursing response would be

    1. "Most infants are alert at birth and then require 24–48 hours of deep sleep to recover from the birth experience."
    2. "Your son's behavior is slightly abnormal and bears careful observation."
    3. "Would you like the pediatrician to check him to ease your mind?"
    4. "Your son's behavior is definitely abnormal, and we should keep him in the nursery."

24. During a physical exam of an infant with congenital hip dysplasia, the nurse would notice which of the following characteristics?

    1. Symmetrical gluteal folds.
    2. Limited adduction of the affected leg.
    3. Femoral pulse when the hip is flexed and the leg is abducted.
    4. Limited abduction of the affected leg.

25. A neonatal nurse would be aware that small-for-gestational age infants (SGA) are

more likely to develop which of the following neonatal illnesses?

1. Hyperthermia.
2. Hyperglycemia.
3. Congenital defects.
4. Hypothermia.

26. When the mother of a new baby asks the nurse to feed her baby, the most appropriate response is to say

    1. "I'll feed him today. Maybe tomorrow you can try it."
    2. "It's not difficult at all. He is just like a normal baby, only smaller."
    3. "You can learn to feed him as well as I can; I wasn't good when I first fed a premature infant either."
    4. "It's frightening sometimes to feed an infant this small, but I'll stay with you to help."

27. A client has just delivered her first baby. Hyperbilirubinemia is anticipated because of Rh incompatibility. Hyperbilirubinemia occurs with Rh incompatibility between mother and fetus because

    1. The mother's blood does not contain the Rh factor, so she produces anti-Rh antibodies that cross the placental barrier and cause hemolysis of red blood cells in infants.
    2. The mother's blood contains the Rh factor and the infant's does not, and antibodies are formed in the fetus that destroy red blood cells.
    3. The mother has a history of previous yellow jaundice caused by a blood transfusion, which was passed to the fetus through the placenta.

4. The infant develops a congenital defect shortly after birth that causes the destruction of red blood cells.

28. If RhoGAM is given to a mother after delivering a healthy baby, the condition that must be present for the globulin to be effective is that the

   1. Mother is Rh positive.
   2. Baby is Rh negative.
   3. Mother has no titer in her blood.
   4. Mother has some titer in her blood.

29. A client in her 36th week of pregnancy is admitted to the maternity unit in an effort to control the further development of eclampsia. She is assigned to a private room. The best rationale for this room assignment is that

   1. The client is financially able to afford it.
   2. The client would be disturbed if placed in a room where another mother was in active labor.
   3. A quiet, darkened room is important to reduce external stimuli.
   4. A rigid regimen is an important aspect of eclamptic care.

30. As part of the prenatal teaching, the nurse instructs the client to immediately report any visual disturbances. The best rationale for this instruction is that the symptom is

   1. A forerunner to preeclampsia.
   2. Indicative of increased intracranial pressure.
   3. A sign of malnutrition.
   4. Indicative of renal failure.

31. Instructing the client about her nutritional needs during pregnancy, the nurse tells her that she will have an increased need for

   1. Potassium.
   2. Fat.
   3. High carbohydrate foods.
   4. Iron.

32. A client delivered a 34-week, 1550-gm female infant. The infant demonstrates nasal flaring, intercostal retraction, expiratory grunt, and slight cyanosis. The baby will be placed in a heated isolette because

   1. The infant has a small body surface for her weight.
   2. Heat increases flow of oxygen to extremities.
   3. Her temperature control mechanism is immature.
   4. Heat within the isolette facilitates drainage of mucus.

33. The nurses caring for a premature baby use careful handwashing techniques because they know premature infants are more susceptible to infection than full-term infants. Which of the following explains why premature infants are more likely to develop infection?

   1. Their liver enzymes are immature.
   2. Premature babies may receive steroid drugs and they affect the immune system.
   3. Premature infants receive few antibodies from the mother, because antibodies pass across the placenta during the last month of pregnancy.
   4. Surfactant is decreased in premature infants.

34. In the delivery room, a client has just delivered a healthy seven-pound baby boy. The physician instructs the nurse to suction the baby. The procedure the nurse would use is to

   1. Suction the nose first.
   2. Suction the mouth first.
   3. Suction neither the nose nor mouth until the physician gives further instructions.
   4. Turn the baby on his side so mucus will drain out before suctioning.

35. Signs and symptoms of infection as a complication of the postpartum period would include

   1. Dark red lochia.
   2. Bradycardia.
   3. Discomfort and tenderness of the abdomen.
   4. Generalized rash.

36. A 24-year-old client who has just learned she is pregnant tells the nurse that she smokes one pack of cigarettes a day. In counseling, the nurse encourages her to stop smoking because newborns of mothers who smoke are often

   1. Premature and have respiratory distress syndrome.
   2. Small for gestational age.
   3. Large for gestational age.
   4. Born with congenital abnormalities.

37. In evaluating a premature baby's condition, the nurse knows that the symptoms of respiratory distress syndrome (RDS) are the result of a/an

   1. Increased amount of vasodilatation in the lungs as a result of decreased oxygenation.
   2. Small surface area of the premature's lungs preventing gas exchange.
   3. Decrease in the production of surfactant in the infant's lungs leading to alveolar collapse.
   4. Increase in the amount of surfactant in the infant's lungs preventing alveolar expansion.

38. After a prolonged labor and lack of progress past a dilatation of 8 cm, the client had a cesarean delivery. She and her partner express their disappointment that they did not have a natural childbirth. The best response is to say

   1. "Most couples who have an unplanned cesarean birth feel cheated and disappointed."
   2. "You know that at least you have a healthy baby."
   3. "Maybe next time you can have a vaginal delivery."
   4. "You will be able to resume sex sooner than if you had delivered vaginally."

39. Evaluating the mother and her infant's interaction and bonding relationship in the postpartum period is an important nursing function. An indication of an unhealthy mother-infant relationship is when the mother

   1. Identifies infant characteristics that are similar to her husband's.
   2. Refuses to go to a bath demonstration.
   3. Describes only the infant's negative qualities.
   4. Asks to skip a feeding to sleep.

Maternity & Newborn Nursing
Answers with Rationale

1. (3)   Regional anesthesia, such as a caudal or epidural, may result in vasodilatation by causing blood to pool in the extremities. This may lead to maternal hypotension. Immediate treatment is to elevate both legs for a few minutes in order to return the blood to the central circulation and then turn the client on her side to reduce pressure on the veins and arteries in the pelvic area.

    Nursing Process: Implementation
    Client Needs: Safe, Effective Care Environment
    Clinical Area: Maternity Nursing

2. (3)   High blood pressure is one of the cardinal symptoms of toxemia or eclampsia along with excessive weight gain, edema and albumin in the urine.

    Nursing Process: Assessment
    Client Needs: Physiological Integrity
    Clinical Area: Maternity Nursing

3. (1)   During a normal birth, the fetus passes through the birth canal and pressure on the chest helps rid the fetus of amniotic fluid that has accumulated in the lungs. The baby delivered by cesarean section does not go through this process; thus, may develop respiratory problems.

    Nursing Process: Evaluation
    Client Needs: Physiological Integrity
    Clinical Area: Maternity Nursing

4. (2)   In a ruptured ectopic pregnancy, there may be signs of shock, excruciating pain, and little bleeding. There should be no effect on blood glucose levels.

    Nursing Process: Analysis
    Client Needs: Physiological Integrity
    Clinical Area: Maternity Nursing

5. (2)   A uterus that is contracted for more than one full minute is a sign of tetany which could lead to uterine rupture. This symptom must be reported to the physician immediately so interventions can be initiated. This other answers are all normal

    Nursing Process: Assessment
    Client Needs: Safe, Effective Care Environment
    Clinical Area: Maternity Nursing

conditions which occur with labor. The client should be cautioned against bearing down this early as it is not effective and can cause edema of the cervix.

6. (2) The respiratory rate must be maintained at a rate of at least 12 per minute as a precaution against excessive depression of impulses at the myoneural junction. When deep tendon reflexes are absent and the urine output is decreased, the medication should be held to prevent complications of depression of the CNS. If the client is complaining of being thirsty, she is experiencing a sign of magnesium toxicity.

Nursing Process: Evaluation
Client Needs: Safe, Effective Care Environment
Clinical Area: Maternity Nursing

7. (1) Infants of diabetic mothers are prone to develop hypoglycemia, respiratory distress, and hypocalcemia. The infant of a diabetic mother may develop sepsis, but usually from a cause unrelated to the diabetes itself. Hyperbilirubinemia is also fairly common in these infants.

Nursing Process: Assessment
Client Needs: Safe, Effective Care Environment
Clinical Area: Maternity Nursing

8. (4) This is an example of a congenital abnormality and does not fall into the category of a metabolic or biochemical disorder. Phenylketonuria is an inability to metabolize the amino acid, phenylalanine; maple syrup urine disease is a defective metabolism of branched chain keto acids; glutamicacidemia is an increase in total amino nitrogen.

Nursing Process: Analysis
Client Needs: Physiological Integrity
Clinical Area: Maternity Nursing

9. (4) The mother has a right to see her infant, but must have some anticipatory guidance. Finding out her expectations will help the nurse better prepare the mother to see her dead child.

Nursing Process: Implementation
Client Needs: Psychosocial Integrity
Clinical Area: Maternity Nursing

10. (2) *Teratogen* is a term denoting "monster-former," and rubella in the first trimester is known to produce monster babies. X-rays

Nursing Process: Analysis
Client Needs: Physiological Integrity
Clinical Area: Maternity Nursing

are also considered teratogens. Dental x-rays would not have high roentgens, thus they have little chance of being dangerous.

11.   (4)   The head is at station 0 when it is felt at the level of the ischial spines. Levels above the ischial spines are referred to as minus: –1, –2, –3. Levels below the ischial spines are referred to as plus: +1, +2, +3.

Nursing Process: Analysis
Client Needs: Health Promotion and Maintenance
Clinical Area: Maternity Nursing

12.   (3)   If the head is +3, it is just about crowning, and because the client is a multi-para, it would be reasonable to assume delivery is imminent. Answers (1) and (4) are not appropriate nursing actions and answer (2) is wrong because there is no data suggesting a prolapsed cord.

Nursing Process: Implementation
Client Needs: Safe, Effective Care Environment
Clinical Area: Maternity Nursing

13.   (4)   Gonorrhea accounts for 65 to 75 percent of all cases of PID. Streptococcus, staphylococcus, and Tb bacilli are less frequent causes.

Nursing Process: Implementation
Client Needs: Health Promotion and Maintenance
Clinical Area: Maternity Nursing

14.   (1)   Normal menstrual cycles and ovarian function are regulated by FSH and LH, which are produced in the hypothalamus.

Nursing Process: Analysis
Client Needs: Physiological Integrity
Clinical Area: Maternity Nursing

15.   (3)   The airway must be cleared before anything else can help. Of the choices, (3) is the best for clearing the airway by creating a gravity or postural drainage situation.

Nursing Process: Implementation
Client Needs: Safe, Effective Care Environment
Clinical Area: Maternity Nursing

16.   (3)   Although the first trimester is the danger period with German measles, the nurse should first ascertain the client's concerns before she gives any direction. Answer (4) is putting words in the client's mouth.

Nursing Process: Implementation
Client Needs: Psychosocial Integrity
Clinical Area: Maternity Nursing

17.   (3)   Consultation with a client on the best form of birth control for her is dependent on the frequency of intercourse, number of partners, and her own motivation and reli-

Nursing Process: Implementation
Client Needs: Health Promotion and Maintenance
Clinical Area: Maternity Nursing

ability. The other responses cut off the client and do not form a therapeutic relationship.

18. (4) Babies that are postmature often look as though they have lost weight. They exhibit long nails, little subcutaneous fat, and the skin is very dry. Often, meconium is stained green or yellow.

Nursing Process: Assessment
Client Needs: Physiological Integrity
Clinical Area: Maternity Nursing

19. (4) Oral fluids are usually withheld after surgery until normal conscious levels are reached and bowel sounds are heard. Giving oral fluids before normal consciousness returns can lead to vomiting and aspiration. A C-section is also considered a surgical procedure, and normal postop as well as postpartum care should be given.

Nursing Process: Planning
Client Needs: Safe, Effective Care Environment
Clinical Area: Maternity Nursing

20. (2) Birth control pills are small doses of estrogen and progesterone that maintain sufficient levels in the body to inhibit the pituitary from producing the follicle-stimulating hormone.

Nursing Process: Implementation
Client Needs: Health Promotion and Maintenance
Clinical Area: Maternity Nursing

21. (4) These stockings are held up by elastic bands around the leg and may cause constriction of blood vessels. Frequently, women are more susceptible to varicose veins, and this would aggravate the problem. Any tightly constrictive clothing on the legs should be avoided by everyone, and especially by pregnant women.

Nursing Process: Implementation
Client Needs: Health Promotion and Maintenance
Clinical Area: Maternity Nursing

22. (4) Keeping the nipples dry is the best treatment. Massé cream or pure lanolin may be applied sparingly but never harsh agents such as benzoin or alcohol. Teach the mother to use general hygiene practices—wash the breasts once daily; do not use soap as it removes natural oils. To prevent further problems with engorgement, bottles should not be offered.

Nursing Process: Implementation
Client Needs: Safe, Effective Care Environment
Clinical Area: Maternity Nursing

23.   (1)   Normally most newborns are alert at birth and then require deep sleep to recover from the birth experience. This should be explained first, and then if the client is still concerned, the nurse could offer to have the pediatrician talk to her.

Nursing Process: Implementation
Client Needs: Health Promotion and Maintenance
Clinical Area: Maternity Nursing

24.   (4)   Abduction is limited in the affected leg. The nurse would also find asymmetrical gluteal folds and an absent femoral pulse when the affected leg is abducted.

Nursing Process: Assessment
Client Needs: Physiological Integrity
Clinical Area: Maternity Nursing

25.   (4)   A large proportion of body surface to body weight increases susceptibility to hypothermia. These infants are also more prone to hypoglycemia. Congenital defects are not neonatal illnesses.

Nursing Process: Analysis
Client Needs: Physiological Integrity
Clinical Area: Maternity Nursing

26.   (4)   The nurse, while recognizing and accepting this mother's apprehension, assures her that she will have assistance and gives her confidence to feed the baby while remaining with her. This is good client teaching.

Nursing Process: Implementation
Client Needs: Health Promotion and Maintenance
Clinical Area: Maternity Nursing

27.   (1)   Rh antigens from the fetus enter the bloodstream of the mother, including the production of anti-Rh antibodies in the mother. These anti-Rh antibodies cross the placenta, enter the fetal circulation, and cause hemolysis. The red blood cells are destroyed and broken down faster than the products of hemolysis, including bilirubin, can be excreted. Serum bilirubin rises quickly.

Nursing Process: Analysis
Client Needs: Physiological Integrity
Clinical Area: Maternity Nursing

28.   (3)   RhoGAM will not work if there is any titer in the blood; thus it is important to administer it within 72 hours after delivery or abortion if the mother shows no evidence of antibody production. The mother would be Rh negative and the baby Rh positive for RhoGAM to be needed.

Nursing Process: Analysis
Client Needs: Physiological Integrity
Clinical Area: Maternity Nursing

29.   (3)   An important aspect of the treatment of preeclampsia is absolute quiet, and only a private room could accomplish this objective.

Nursing Process: Planning
Client Needs: Safe, Effective Care Environment
Clinical Area: Maternity Nursing

30.   (1)   Visual disturbance is a symptom of pre-eclampsia, and the client must immediately be put under a physician's care to prevent further development of eclampsia.

Nursing Process: Planning
Client Needs: Health Promotion and Maintenance
Clinical Area: Maternity Nursing

31.   (4)   During pregnancy there is an increased need for calories, protein, iron, calcium, and other minerals and vitamins. A high fat, high carbohydrate diet is not recommended because it may cause excessive weight gain and fat deposits, which are difficult to lose after pregnancy.

Nursing Process: Implementation
Client Needs: Health Promotion and Maintenance
Clinical Area· Maternity Nursing

32.   (3)   The premature infant has poor body control of temperature and needs immediate attention to keep from losing heat. Reasons for heat loss include little subcutaneous fat and poor insulation, large body surface for weight, immaturity of temperature control, and lack of activity.

Nursing Process: Analysis
Client Needs: Physiological Integrity
Clinical Area: Maternity Nursing

33.   (3)   Lacking antibodies can lead to infection in the premature. Immaturity of the liver is responsible for hyperbilirubinemia. White cell count would be related to potential infection. Lack of surfactant occurs in prematures who have respiratory distress syndrome.

Nursing Process: Analysis
Client Needs: Physiological Integrity
Clinical Area: Maternity Nursing

34.   (2)   It is important to suction the mouth first. If the nose were to be suctioned first, stimulation of the delicate receptors in the nose could cause the infant to aspirate mucus from the mouth.

Nursing Process: Planning
Client Needs: Safe, Effective Care Environment
Clinical Area: Maternity Nursing

35.   (3)   The major symptoms of infection would be rapid pulse, foul-smelling lochia or discharge, and discomfort and tender-

Nursing Process: Assessment
Client Needs: Physiological Integrity
Clinical Area: Maternity Nursing

ness of the abdomen. A generalized rash would not be a sign of postpartum infection but would indicate a virus infection, such as measles, or an allergic reaction to a medication or food. A rash should never be ignored; rather it should be charted and its cause investigated.

36.   (2)   Women who smoke have almost twice the chance of delivering a low-birth weight infant (less than 2500 grams) than non-smokers.

Nursing Process: Implementation
Client Needs: Psychosocial Integrity
Clinical Area: Maternity Nursing

37.   (3)   An adequate amount of surfactant is necessary to keep the alveoli expanded. A decrease in the amount of surfactant results in alveolar collapse, atelectasis, and RDS.

Nursing Process: Evaluation
Client Needs: Physiological Integrity
Clinical Area: Maternity Nursing

38.   (1)   It is important to recognize their grief and let them know it's normal. They need to work through their grief before they can cope with other information.

Nursing Process: Implementation
Client Needs: Psychosocial Integrity
Clinical Area: Maternity Nursing

39.   (3)   An unhealthy relationship may be developing if the mother cannot find any good qualities to describe. Identification of family characteristics is usually a sign of healthy attachment. The mother's need to "take in" in the early postpartum period is seen in her refusal to attend classes and her need for sleep and is normal.

Nursing Process: Analysis
Client Needs: Psychosocial Integrity
Clinical Area: Maternity Nursing

40.   (1)   The first action is to turn the Pitocin off. If the fetal heart rate has dropped in response to the prolonged contraction, turning the mother and administering oxygen may be necessary.

Nursing Process: Implementation
Client Needs: Safe, Effective Care Environment
Clinical Area: Maternity Nursing

41.   (4)   The premature infant's poorly developed ability to control respirations is a frequent problem. Additional respiratory support with oxygen will decrease poten-

Nursing Process: Analysis
Client Needs: Physiological Integrity
Clinical Area: Maternity Nursing

tial hypoxemia. The oxygen will also help oxygenate the systemic circulation if the infant has a tendency for hypoventilation.

42. (4)   Insulin does not cross into the milk. The mother's calorie intake needs to be adjusted with increased protein intake. Insulin must be adjusted and care must be exercised during weaning. Breast feeding may actually have an antidiabetogenic effect and this requires less insulin.

Nursing Process: Analysis
Client Needs: Health Promotion and Maintenance
Clinical Area: Maternity Nursing

43. (1)   Jaundice (icterus neonatorum) is a normal newborn condition that appears 48–72 hours after birth and begins to subside on the sixth to seventh day. If the levels go above 13 mgm per 100 ml, it is considered to be beyond the "safe" physiologic limit. The condition is caused by the breakdown of excess fetal red blood cells after birth.

Nursing Process: Analysis
Client Needs: Health Promotion and Maintenance
Clinical Area: Maternity Nursing

44. (3)   The optimum weight gain for both mother's and baby's health is about 25 pounds. Dieting is contraindicated. There is a lower incidence of prematurity, stillbirths, and low birth-weight infants with a weight gain of at least 25 pounds.

Nursing Process: Implementation
Client Needs: Health Promotion and Maintenance
Clinical Area: Maternity Nursing

45. (1)   Primiparas normally go through effacement before dilatation of the cervix. Multiparas tend to dilate and efface simultaneously.

Nursing Process: Analysis
Client Needs: Physiological Integrity
Clinical Area: Maternity Nursing

46. (2)   From the assessment findings of the lochia and fundus, the new mother is progressing normally during the postpartum period. The breast signs indicate normal engorgement which occurs about three days after birth. With stable vital signs, infection is not likely to be a problem. Applying warm packs and wearing a nursing bra will reduce discomfort.

Nursing Process: Analysis
Client Needs: Health Promotion and Maintenance
Clinical Area: Maternity Nursing

47.   (4)   An infant's normal breathing pattern is irregular. Staying with the client helps give her support, and the nurse can reassure her that the infant is all right.

Nursing Process: Implementation
Client Needs: Psychosocial Integrity
Clinical Area: Maternity Nursing

48.   (3)   Amniocentesis cannot be done until adequate amniotic fluid is available, which is at about 14 weeks gestation. It usually is done for genetic counseling purposes before 18 weeks, as the test result requires 2–4 weeks, and elective abortion after 22 weeks is contraindicated. Chorionic Villus Sampling (CVS) may replace this test as diagnostic information is available from 8–12 weeks.

Nursing Process: Analysis
Client Needs: Health Promotion and Maintenance
Clinical Area: Maternity Nursing

49.   (2)   The venereal disease syphilis is again becoming increasingly prevalent. It may cause abortion early in pregnancy and may be passed to the fetus after the fourth month of pregnancy, causing congenital syphilis in the infant. Gonorrhea and herpes virus II may be passed to the infant during delivery, but syphilis is usually passed to the infant in utero.

Nursing Process: Implementation
Client Needs: Health Promotion and Maintenance
Clinical Area: Maternity Nursing

50.   (2)   It is important that the mother pant, not push, to avoid rapid delivery of the head. Closing her eyes and counting will not be sufficient distraction to avoid pushing. Breathing naturally at this point is also not appropriate.

Nursing Process: Implementation
Client Needs: Safe, Effective Care Environment
Clinical Area: Maternity Nursing

Pediatric Nursing

1. A 7-month-old infant is tentatively diagnosed with mental retardation. The parents have come into the hospital for further assessment and counseling. During the nursing assessment, the observation that will assist in diagnosing mental retardation is that the infant

   1. Is unable to sit unsupported for brief periods.
   2. Is able to approach a toy and grasp it.
   3. Frequently rolls from back to stomach.
   4. Can grasp a spoon and bring it to his mouth.

2. Following a child's treatment for poisoning in the emergency room, the nurse asks the mother how the child got all of the bruises. She replied that he is always falling down and hurting himself. The next action the nurse should take is to

   1. Report the suspected child abuse to the authorities.
   2. Continue evaluating the circumstances.
   3. Ask the psychiatrist to talk with the mother.
   4. Ask the mother to bring her boyfriend in for a conference.

3. A mother calls to the pediatric hot line and tells the nurse that her three year old has a virus and a fever. She asks how much aspirin she should give child. The best response is

1. "You'll have to call your physician."
2. "Give her no more than three baby aspirin every four hours."
3. "Give her Tylenol, not aspirin."
4. "Follow directions on the aspirin bottle for her age and weight."

4. An infant was born with spina bifida and has remained on the pediatric unit for observation. The most important assessment would be to

   1. Measure head circumference daily.
   2. Monitor for contractures.
   3. Observe for signs of infection.
   4. Observe intake and output.

5. A five year old with suspected epiglottitis has just been admitted to the pediatric unit. His temperature is 102° F, he has difficulty swallowing, and has inspiratory stridor. The most important immediate intervention is to

   1. Check the mouth for a gag reflex.
   2. Sit the child in an upright position.
   3. Monitor vital signs.
   4. Give the child sips of ice water.

6. Which one of the following characteristics of acute glomerulonephritis is it essential for the nurse to know in order to deliver comprehensive care to a 5-year-old child?

1. Polyuria (increased urine output) is a clinical manifestation of this disorder.
2. Acute glomerulonephritis is usually preceded by a streptococcal infection of the upper respiratory tract or skin.
3. It is necessary to monitor for hypotension and tachycardia.
4. Fluid overload is a common clinical manifestation.

7. The best place to check the pulse of an infant is at the

   1. Carotid artery.
   2. Apex of the heart.
   3. Brachial artery.
   4. Temporal artery.

8. Proper depth of compressions for infant CPR would be

   1. ½ to 1 inch.
   2. ¼ to ¾ inch.
   3. 1 to 1 ½ inches.
   4. 1½ to 2 inches.

9. A systolic blood pressure of 60 mmHg or less would indicate shock in which of the following client age groups?

   1. 5 years old or younger.
   2. 5 to 12 years old.
   3. 12 to 16 years old.
   4. 16 to 20 years old.

10. Which of the following statements would the nurse make to a mother of a new baby about infant nutrition?

    1. Eggs are a good source of iron and can be introduced at six months.
    2. Solid foods can be introduced in the sixth week of life.
    3. Rice cereal is the least allergenic of the cereals for infants.
    4. Only one new food should be introduced per day.

11. When providing diversional activities for a child in isolation, the nurse will remember that

    1. Any articles brought into the unit should be washable.
    2. These children are always on bedrest.
    3. The room is usually darkened to protect the child's eyes.
    4. Most children are satisfied with books.

12. In children, the period of negativism begins when the child

    1. Can manipulate his or her parents.
    2. Copies negative behavior of siblings.
    3. Is struggling between dependence and independence.
    4. Is learning manual skills.

13. Which of the following procedures is contraindicated in infantile eczema?

    1. Have the child vaccinated to prevent childhood diseases.
    2. Cover the child's hands and feet with cotton materials.
    3. Apply open wet dressings or corn starch.
    4. Adhere strictly to elimination diet.

14. Which one of the following therapeutic approaches would be appropriate in the nursing/medical management of a 12 year old with juvenile rheumatoid arthritis?

1. Encourage prolonged periods of complete joint immobilization.
2. Apply warm compresses to the affected joint and night splints.
3. Discourage the child's active participation in his care in the initial phases of the disease.
4. Allow as much salicylates as necessary for control of pain.

15. Considering a 17-month-old child's developmental level, the most effective technique to reestablish nutritional status after the immediate postoperative period would be

   1. Semisoft foods qid.
   2. Finger foods at frequent intervals.
   3. Regular diet put into a blender and given in liquid state.
   4. A high-roughage diet.

16. An two-year-old toddler was diagnosed with iron-deficiency anemia. Which one of the following statements best describes the anemias of childhood?

   1. The clinical manifestations of anemia are directly related to the decrease in oxygen-carrying capacity of the blood.
   2. Significant deficiencies of all vitamins will result in reduced production of red blood cells.
   3. A 2-year-old child with a hemoglobin of 5 gm/100 ml will not manifest signs and symptoms of the disorder.
   4. All anemias in childhood are potentially terminal.

17. The nurse has just completed the nursing assessment of a 4-year-old child. Which one of the following findings is most characteristic of thrombocytopenia?

   1. Petechiae, hematuria, purpura.
   2. Urticaria, epistaxis, hypertension.
   3. Purpura, tachycardia, hypotension.
   4. Vertigo, petechiae, bradycardia.

18. When determining if a child has Down's syndrome characteristics, which of the following would *not* be present?

   1. Abnormal palmar creases.
   2. Protruding tongue.
   3. Low-set ears.
   4. Loose joints and flaccid muscles.

19. A special, controlled diet instituted relatively early after birth may prevent or limit mental retardation in children with the condition of

   1. Cretinism.
   2. Down's syndrome.
   3. Phenylketonuria (PKU).
   4. Tay-Sachs disease.

20. A mother with a 4-month-old infant comes to the clinic for a well-baby examination. The nurse advises the mother to change the formula she is feeding the baby to one that contains iron. The nurse explains the reason for this is

   1. Iron is required by the infant's eyes as they begin to focus and develop.
   2. The infant requires extra iron to grow.
   3. The infant's iron source from the mother is depleted.
   4. The infant requires more iron for the breakdown of bilirubin.

21. A 1-month-old child manifests all of the following signs and symptoms. Which of these is most suggestive of a complication of a central nervous system infection?

   1. Separation of cranial sutures.
   2. Depressed anterior fontanel.
   3. Oliguria.
   4. Photophobia.

22. During a routine physical examination, the following reflexes are noted in a 9-month-old child. Which of the following is an abnormal finding?

   1. Parachute reflex.
   2. Neck righting reflex.
   3. Rooting and sucking reflex.
   4. Moro reflex.

23. A three month old is admitted to the hospital with a diagnosis of chalasia. He has had severe weight loss because of frequent vomiting. To minimize vomiting, the nurse would place the infant

   1. In a prone position after feeding.
   2. On his abdomen with his head to one side.
   3. On his left side with his head elevated.
   4. On his right side with his head elevated.

24. A first-grader was sent to the school nurse by her teacher because the teacher feared the child had lice in her hair. The most effective way of recognizing lice instead of dandruff is to know that

   1. Prepubescent children rarely have dandruff.
   2. There will be an area of alopecia on the nape of her neck.
   3. The child is scratching her head almost incessantly.
   4. Lice would not fall off the hair shaft when the hair is moved.

25. What anatomical condition must be present in order for an infant with complete transposition of the great vessels to survive at birth?

   1. Coarctation of the aorta.
   2. Large septal defect.
   3. Pulmonic stenosis.
   4. Mitral stenosis.

26. In addition to assessing for hemorrhage, the most important objective in client care following a tonsillectomy is prevention of

   1. Coughing.
   2. Swallowing blood.
   3. Aspiration of mucus.
   4. Airway constriction.

27. The statement that most accurately describes childhood brain tumors is

   1. The majority of tumors are diagnosed during infancy and can be successfully treated with surgery, radiation and chemotherapy.
   2. The majority of brain tumors are located in the posterior fossa; hence, signs of intracranial pressure are not evident.
   3. Most childhood brain tumors are highly malignant.
   4. Most childhood brain tumors initially manifest themselves in five to seven years; the symptoms are directly related to the area of the brain involved.

28. The diet regimen the nurse will follow for a child with acute glomerulonephritis is

    1. Low sodium, low calorie.
    2. Low potassium, low protein.
    3. Fluid intake of 1000 ml/24 hours.
    4. Low calcium, low potassium.

29. Assessing a child with a possible cardiac condition, the nurse knows that a child with a large patent ductus arteriosus would exhibit which of the following symptoms?

    1. Squats a great deal.
    2. Becomes cyanotic or exertion.
    3. Is acyanotic but has difficulty breathing after physical activity.
    4. Has breathing difficulty and is cyanotic with slight activity.

30. A four week old was admitted to the Infant Surgical Unit for correction of pyloric stenosis. In assessing the infant, which one of the following clinical manifestations is not consistent with the diagnosis of pyloric stenosis?

    1. Palpable olive-size mass in the upper right quadrant.
    2. Visible peristaltic waves passing left to right during and after feeding.
    3. Severe projectile vomiting after each feeding.
    4. Fluid overload, demonstrated by bulging fontanels, widely separated cranial sutures, and urine specific gravity of 1.002.

31. Which of the following clinical profiles present in a 2-week-old neonate would alert the nurse to a possible renal disorder?

    1. Low-set ears, periorbital edema, hypertension, palpable abdominal mass.
    2. Tachycardia, urine specific gravity of 1.005, polyuria.
    3. Hypotension, dyspnea, dependent edema.
    4. Lethargy, depressed fontanels, mongolian spots.

32. The nurse is caring for a toddler in the hospital who was toilet trained at home. He wets his pants. The best response to this situation is to say

    1. "It's okay; try not to wet your pants next time."
    2. "That's okay; now let's get you cleaned up."
    3. "I know you understand how to use the toilet; what happened?"
    4. "Your mom told me you don't wet anymore; what's wrong?"

33. A client gave birth to a baby who weighed only 5 pounds and is considered premature. One of the most important principles in providing nutrition is to

    1. Use a regular nipple with a large hole.
    2. Feed every 4–6 hours.
    3. Use a premie nipple for bottle feeding.
    4. Use milk high in fat for the formula.

34. A 6-week-old infant with a diagnosis of a fever of unknown origin is admitted to the unit. The nurse enters the room and finds him sleeping. A priority assessment on admission is to obtain his vital signs. The nurse would begin this assessment by

    1. Taking his axillary temperature.
    2. Taking his apical pulse.

3. Taking his rectal temperature.
4. Counting his respirations.

35. To obtain an apical pulse on an infant, the diaphragm of the stethoscope is placed at the apex of the heart. When placing the diaphragm on the infant's chest, it should be located

   1. At the left nipple, where the heart's point of maximum impulse is located.
   2. To the left of the midclavicular line, at the third to fourth intercostal space.
   3. At the left edge of the sternum and fifth intercostal space.
   4. At the left midclavicular line and fifth intercostal space.

36. When obtaining an infant's respiratory rate, the nurse should count his respirations for one full minute because

   1. Young infants are abdominal breathers.
   2. Infants do not expand their lungs fully with each respiration.
   3. Activity will increase the respiratory rate.
   4. The rhythm of respiratory rates is irregular in infants.

37. An eight year old with an acute asthma attack is admitted to the hospital. Epinephrine is administered. The nursing assessment of the child will probably reveal

   1. Noisy, hoarse inspirations.
   2. Wheezing on expiration.
   3. Labored abdominal breathing.
   4. Flail chest with inspiratory wheeze.

38. A 10-year-old child in respiratory difficulty is admitted to the emergency room and given epinephrine with oxygen ordered prn. The nurse observes that he is short of breath with circumoral cyanosis and sweating. The nursing action will be to

   1. Notify the physician immediately.
   2. Encourage the child to lie down and administer oxygen.
   3. Reassure the child that the medication will begin working soon.
   4. Encourage the child to sit upright and administer oxygen.

39. A definitive diagnosis to determine if a child has bacterial meningitis is based on the

   1. Clinical manifestations and history of exposure.
   2. Blood culture.
   3. Lumbar puncture.
   4. Serum white blood cell count.

40. Once a child has had one poison ingestion, statistically he is nine times more likely to have another poisoning episode within the year. To prevent further poisoning incidents, the most important information the nurse should give to the child's mother is to

   1. Keep purses out of the child's reach.
   2. Never give medications to others in front of the child.
   3. Keep all cabinets locked at all times.
   4. Keep medicine only in high cupboards.

41. A nine year old is hospitalized to undergo evaluation. Her history indicates that she has frequent severe respiratory infections. The tentative diagnosis is cystic fibrosis. The nurse anticipates that the child will have a test used in the diagnosis of cystic fibrosis called

1. Sweat chloride test.
2. Blood glucose analysis.
3. Sputum culture.
4. Stool analysis for fat content.

42. An infant warmer is used in the newborn nursery to ensure maintenance of adequate body temperature. The major safety factor involved with the use of the warmer is for the nurse to

    1. Ensure the warmer is on manual control.
    2. Tape the thermometer skin probe in place.
    3. Inspect the skin under the temperature probe at routine intervals.
    4. Adjust temperature of the warmer each day to ensure it is set at 102° F.

43. Working with children who have acyanotic heart defects, the nurse is aware that

    1. Occurrence of cardiac failure is rare after the age of six months.
    2. Bacterial endocarditis is not a complication of acyanotic congenital heart disease.
    3. An infant or young child with acyanotic heart disease requires alteration in their activity level by their parents.
    4. Children with congenital heart disease are usually asymptomatic.

44. The nurse explains to the mother of a one year old that the child is more likely to have otitis media than her 13-year-old brother because

    1. Her hands are often contaminated when she crawls on the floor.
    2. She is still "cutting" new teeth.

3. The angle of the child's eustachian tube is straighter than her brother's.
4. She is not old enough to have learned how to "clear" her nasal passages.

45. At the age of one and one-half, a child returns to the hospital for a cleft palate repair. A very important factor in preparing the child for this experience is

    1. Always allowing her a choice.
    2. Never leaving her with strangers.
    3. Giving her affection and a feeling of security.
    4. Reminding her of her previous hospital experience.

46. With a diagnosis of hemophilia B, part of the teaching plan for a child's parents will include treatment measures to control minor bleeding episodes. These will include

    1. Topical coagulants, cold packs, and constant pressure to affected areas.
    2. Elevation of the affected area, oral anticoagulants, and warm compresses.
    3. Gentian violet, ice packs, and pressure dressings.
    4. Bedrest, topical coagulants, and cold compresses.

47. A mother of a 3-month-old infant asks the nurse if her baby can eat solid food now so she can sleep through the night. The appropriate response is to say

    1. "Infants obtain all the nutrients they need from the formula and they really can't digest foods well at that early age."
    2. "Infants at age three months do not usually sleep through the night, so solid food probably will not help this problem."

3. "It would be best to give the baby her bath at night to relax her and then she might sleep through the night."

4. "It sounds like she's not getting enough food to satisfy her, so it is probably a good idea to start introducing solid food."

48. Evaluating a 1-month-old infant's social developmental skills, the nurse should observe that the infant

1. Actively follows movements of familiar persons with her eyes.
2. Responds to "No, No."
3. Turns her head to a familiar noise.
4. Discriminates between family and strangers.

49. As the nurse enters the room of a 7-year-old autistic child, she sees him banging his head against the wall. The first action is to

1. Call the attendant to hold the child so that he cannot hurt himself.
2. Go to him and immediately get between the child and the wall.
3. Move slowly toward him talking softly but making sure to get his attention.
4. Immediately call an attendant to put a helmet on the child.

50. While a one year old is hospitalized with bronchitis, she is receiving care for the respiratory condition. An appropriate toy for her would be a

1. Book with pop-up pages.
2. Set of blocks.
3. Mobile hanging from the crib.
4. Terry cloth teddy bear.

Pediatric Nursing
Answers with Rationale

1. (1) At six months a child should be sitting with minimal support. Often with retarded children, their flaccid muscles and loose joints prevent the attainment of simple developmental milestones. The ability to sit is one of the most important milestones in development.

    Nursing Process: Assessment
    Client Needs: Physiological Integrity
    Clinical Area: Pediatric Nursing

2. (2) The nurse does not have enough data or information to report this as child abuse, so she should continue the assessment. When she has sufficient data to suspect child abuse, then the nurse will notify the designated authorities so that they may investigate the case fully. The nurse is legally responsible to report any suspected case of child abuse.

    Nursing Process: Implementation
    Client Needs: Psychosocial Integrity
    Clinical Area: Pediatric Nursing

3. (3) Children from two months to adolescence are advised not to take aspirin with a virus infection due to the connection to Reye's Syndrome, an acute encephalopathy condition. Tylenol is the treatment of choice for any virus infection.

    Nursing Process: Implementation
    Client Needs: Safe, Effective Care Environment
    Clinical Area: Pediatric Nursing

4. (1) While all of the assessments would be done, the most important is to measure head circumference daily. An increase in size would indicate a neurological condition developing (hydrocephalus is a frequent complication). Infection might occur in the urinary tract; I & O is also related to the possible urological complications. Contractures could be prevented through proper positioning.

    Nursing Process: Assessment
    Client Needs: Safe, Effective Care Environment
    Clinical Area: Pediatric Nursing

5.   (2)   The most important intervention is to keep the child upright; supine position could occlude the airway and cause respiratory arrest. The nurse would never check the gag reflex because it could cause further spasms of the epiglottis. The child should be NPO and the hydration status frequently monitored. Vital signs are important, but positioning to facilitate breathing takes precedence.

Nursing Process: Implementation
Client Needs: Safe, Effective Care Environment
Clinical Area: Pediatric Nursing

6.   (2)   This is important to understand because antibiotics are one of the primary aspects of care if the disorder was preceded by an infection of group-A beta-hemolytic streptococci. (1) and (4) are wrong because there is decreased urine output with edema formation. Answer (3) is a complication.

Nursing Process: Analysis
Client Needs: Physiological Integrity
Clinical Area: Pediatric Nursing

7.   (3)   The brachial artery should be used in checking the pulse of an infant. Apical pulse observation may give incomplete data because there is not adequate blood circulation The carotid arteries are difficult to locate in an infant.

Nursing Process: Implementation
Client Needs: Safe, Effective Care Environment
Clinical Area: Pediatric Nursing

8.   (1)   The proper depth of compression for infant CPR is ½ to 1 inch. This is done mid-sternum, using only two fingers or the thumbs, if the chest is encircled by the rescuers hands.

Nursing Process: Planning
Client Needs: Safe, Effective Care Environment
Clinical Area: Pediatric Nursing

9.   (2)   A systolic blood pressure of 60 mmHg or less found in children 5 to 12 years old would indicate shock.

Nursing Process: Analysis
Client Needs: Physiological Integrity
Clinical Area: Pediatric Nursing

10.   (3)   Rice cereal is the least allergic food. The latest research indicates that solid food should not be given until six months. This may prevent allergies later in life, and the infant's digestive system has had time to mature. Egg yolks, not whole eggs, could

Nursing Process: Implementation
Client Needs: Health Promotion and Maintenance
Clinical Area: Pediatric Nursing

be introduced because the whites of the egg may cause an allergy. Each new food should be given once a week, not one per day.

11.   (1)   Things that go into the room will have to be disinfected before they are removed, so they should be washable. The children are not always on bedrest, nor does the room necessarily have to be dark.

Nursing Process: Planning
Client Needs: Safe, Effective Care Environment
Clinical Area: Pediatric Nursing

12.   (3)   Negativism begins as the child learns to do some things independently and then becomes frustrated by things he or she cannot do. This period begins at about two years and is normal for this stage of development.

Nursing Process: Planning
Client Needs: Psychosocial Integrity
Clinical Area: Pediatric Nursing

13.   (1)   The vaccine can cause vaccinia, which can superimpose the pustular eruptions of the viral infection on the eczema. Eliminating foods that exacerbate the problem is helpful, but not using a specific diet. Soaks with Burrow's solution or normal saline is the treatment of choice.

Nursing Process: Planning
Client Needs: Health Promotion and Maintenance
Clinical Area: Pediatric Nursing

14.   (2)   Warm compresses will help to relieve the pain and night splints are important. During an exacerbation of this childhood disorder, hospitalization is usually required; however, affected joints should *not* be immobilized for extended periods of time as residual effects (joint atrophy) will ensue. Active participation in care should be encouraged in all stages of the disease. Unlimited salicylates could be dangerous to the child.

Nursing Process: Implementation
Client Needs: Safe, Effective Care Environment
Clinical Area: Pediatric Nursing

15.   (2)   The developmental period is the autonomy stage. The child wants to do things for himself and will respond well to finger foods offered frequently. If the child will eat a variety of nutritious finger foods,

Nursing Process: Implementation
Client Needs: Physiological Integrity
Clinical Area: Pediatric Nursing

the nutritional status will be reestablished more effectively.

16.   (1)   Clinical manifestations of fatigability, anorexia, weakness, and tachycardia are a result of vitamin B_{12} and folic acid deficiency. These result in reduced production of red blood cells, and a 2-year-old child will manifest symptoms of this disorder.

Nursing Process: Analysis
Client Needs: Physiological Integrity
Clinical Area: Pediatric Nursing

17.   (1)   Thrombocytopenia (a platelet count 50,000 or below) is characterized by petechiae, purpura and, on occasion, spontaneous hematuria. The lower the platelet count, the greater the risk of spontaneous bleeding.

Nursing Process: Assessment
Client Needs: Safe, Effective Care Environment
Clinical Area: Pediatric Nursing

18.   (3)   Although low-set ears are a sign of congenital defects, they are usually associated with some kidney problem. The other characteristics will be present with Down's syndrome.

Nursing Process: Assessment
Client Needs: Physiological Integrity
Clinical Area: Pediatric Nursing

19.   (3)   A strictly controlled diet, eliminating protein because the infant cannot metabolize the amino acid, phenylalanine, will prevent or limit mental retardation. A special formula is used for the infant and a special diet must be followed until adulthood.

Nursing Process: Planning
Client Needs: Health Promotion and Maintenance
Clinical Area: Pediatric Nursing

20.   (3)   Between three and five months, the infant has used up the iron provided by the mother and requires further supplementation if bottle feeding.

Nursing Process: Implementation
Client Needs: Health Promotion and Maintenance
Clinical Area: Pediatric Nursing

21.   (1)   Meningitis is a common central nervous system infection of infancy and early childhood. Increased intracranial pressure, which can accompany meningitis, accounts for separation of the cranial sutures, bulging fontanels, and/or projectile vomiting. Oliguria and photophobia are not symptoms common to CNS infection.

Nursing Process: Assessment
Client Needs: Physiological Integrity
Clinical Area: Pediatric Nursing

22.   (4)   The Moro reflex begins to fade at the third or fourth month. Thus, if found in a nine month old, it would be abnormal. The remaining reflexes would be normal development.

Nursing Process: Assessment
Client Needs: Safe, Effective Care Environment
Clinical Area: Pediatric Nursing

23.   (4)   The greater curvature of the stomach is toward the left side so this position affords less pressure. Elevation of the head would lessen the tendency to vomit.

Nursing Process: Implementation
Client Needs: Safe, Effective Care Environment
Clinical Area: Pediatric Nursing

24.   (4)   Lice secrete a cementlike substance which allows them to hold tenaciously onto the hair shaft. Dandruff will easily brush off. Alopecia, loss of hair, will not occur.

Nursing Process: Assessment
Client Needs: Health Promotion and Maintenance
Clinical Area: Pediatric Nursing

25.   (2)   Because complete transposition results in two closed blood systems, the child can survive only if a large septal defect is present.

Nursing Process: Analysis
Client Needs: Physiological Integrity
Clinical Area: Pediatric Nursing

26.   (4)   Trauma to the airway may cause a severe inflammatory response resulting in blockage. Therefore, the goal is to prevent airway constriction. Application of an ice collar, keeping the client in semi-Fowler's position, and encouraging fluids would be the treatment of choice.

Nursing Process: Planning
Client Needs: Safe, Effective Care Environment
Clinical Area: Pediatric Nursing

27.   (4)   Although childhood tumors, most of which occur between five to seven years of age, are often treated with radiation, chemotherapy and/or surgery, the overall prognosis is not favorable. Surgery is not always indicated because of the location and extensiveness of these tumors.

Nursing Process: Analysis
Client Needs: Physiological Integrity
Clinical Area: Pediatric Nursing

28.   (2)   A diet restricted from potassium and protein is necessary for all children who demonstrate some degree of renal failure. For severe renal failure, protein is totally restricted.

Nursing Process: Implementation
Client Needs: Health Promotion and Maintenance
Clinical Area: Pediatric Nursing

29. (3) PDA is acyanotic. If the ductus is large and much blood is shunted into the pulmonary circulation, there may be growth retardation and limitation of physical activity. Squatting occurs with cyanotic disorders.

Nursing Process: Assessment
Client Needs: Physiological Integrity
Clinical Area: Pediatric Nursing

30. (4) Pyloric stenosis presents in early infancy with projectile vomiting after feeding. Dehydration and electrolyte imbalances are possible complications if therapy is not performed; therefore, fluid overload is not a symptom.

Nursing Process: Assessment
Client Needs: Safe, Effective Care Environment
Clinical Area: Pediatric Nursing

31. (1) Embryologically, the ears and kidneys are formed at the same time; therefore, if a child presents with low-set ears or any defect in the ears, renal disease is also suspected. In addition, there are certain syndromes characterized by both renal and ear malformations. Periorbital edema is seen in neonates with renal and/or cardiac disease. A palpable abdominal mass in a neonate could indicate Wilms' tumor, a malignant tumor of embryonic origin.

Nursing Process: Assessment
Client Needs: Physiological Integrity
Clinical Area: Pediatric Nursing

32. (2) The nurse knows that children tend to regress when under the stress of hospitalization, so it is important not to make a judgment or imply that the child should know better. The best approach is to be matter-of-fact with no blame.

Nursing Process: Implementation
Client Needs: Psychosocial Integrity
Clinical Area: Pediatric Nursing

33. (3) A regular nipple is too hard and will make it difficult for the infant to suck, causing unnecessary fatigue. A premie soft nipple should be used.

Nursing Process: Planning
Client Needs: Safe, Effective Care Environment
Clinical Area: Pediatric Nursing

34. (4) Counting respirations before disturbing the child will give the most accurate number. As soon as a child is touched (or even approached, if awake) his respiratory and apical rate will increase. The nurse

Nursing Process: Implementation
Client Needs: Safe, Effective Care Environment
Clinical Area: Pediatric Nursing

should take respirations first, apical pulse
next, and rectal temperature last.

35.   (2)   This is the appropriate location on an
infant's chest for an apical pulse. Over 7,
the apical pulse is located at answer (4).

Nursing Process: Planning
Client Needs: Safe, Effective Care Environment
Clinical Area: Pediatric Nursing

36.   (4)   Infants breathe in an irregular pattern
with varying depth and rate so that a one
minute count is appropriate. (1), (2) and (3)
are true statements, but not the correct
answer.

Nursing Process: Analysis
Client Needs: Safe, Effective Care Environment
Clinical Area: Pediatric Nursing

37.   (2)   The hallmark of asthma is wheezing.
Wheezing is an expiratory sound. There is
no vocal cord involvement so "hoarse" is
unlikely. Abdominal breathing does not
occur with asthma.

Nursing Process: Assessment
Client Needs: Physiological Integrity
Clinical Area: Pediatric Nursing

38.   (4)   The child's immediate situation needs
to be addressed before calling the physician. Epinephrine is usually effective
immediately. Breathing is more effective in
an upright position, and oxygen is indicated from the symptoms.

Nursing Process: Implementation
Client Needs: Safe, Effective Care Environment
Clinical Area: Pediatric Nursing

39.   (3)   Examination of the cerebrospinal fluid
is the only definitive way to verify bacterial meningitis.

Nursing Process: Analysis
Client Needs: Physiological Integrity
Clinical Area: Pediatric Nursing

40.   (3)   The other answers are also necessary
information but keeping cabinets locked is
critical. It is not enough to keep only medicine in high cupboards because other products, such as cleaning materials, can be poison. The child's mother should also be
given the telephone number of a poison
control center.

Nursing Process: Implementation
Client Needs: Health Promotion and Maintenance
Clinical Area: Pediatric Nursing

41.   (1)   Cystic fibrosis children produce
abnormally high levels of sodium chloride
in their sweat. Though answers (3) and (4)
might be used during the diagnostic

Nursing Process: Planning
Client Needs: Physiological Integrity
Clinical Area: Pediatric Nursing

workup, they do not definitively diagnose the disease.

42. (3) The probe can cause irritation. If this occurs, the probe is placed in a different location. An infant's skin is very delicate and becomes irritated easily.

Nursing Process: Implementation
Client Needs: Safe, Effective Care Environment
Clinical Area: Pediatric Nursing

43. (1) Cardiac failure rarely occurs after the age of six months. If the child has gone six months without failure, then either the cardiac problem is not severe or the child is compensating successfully. Bacterial endocarditis is a possible complication (2) and usually a child sets his own pace of activity (3).

Nursing Process: Analysis
Client Needs: Physiological Integrity
Clinical Area: Pediatric Nursing

44. (3) It is easier for infectious agents to travel from the nasopharyngeal area to the middle ear in younger than in older children because the eustachian tube is straighter when they are younger.

Nursing Process: Implementation
Client Needs: Physiological Integrity
Clinical Area: Pediatric Nursing

45. (3) A child needs extra assurance at this age. Children suffer separation anxiety and need to feel that someone is close to protect them.

Nursing Process: Planning
Client Needs: Health Promotion and Maintenance
Clinical Area: Pediatric Nursing

46. (1) Local measures which sometimes help control minor bleeding episodes are topical coagulants, constant pressure, and cold packs (which cause vasoconstriction) to the bleeding areas.

Nursing Process: Planning
Client Needs: Physiological Integrity
Clinical Area: Pediatric Nursing

47. (1) Studies have indicated that breast milk or formula will provide sufficient nutrition to infants up to six months and even one year. Many pediatricians begin introducing solid food about six months of age, as infants cannot easily digest food before this time. Sleeping patterns for infants vary on an individual basis and the

Nursing Process: Implementation
Client Needs: Safe, Effective Care Environment
Clinical Area: Pediatric Nursing

introduction of solid food does not ensure
a full night's sleep.

48.   (1)   Actively following movements would
occur at one month. Responding to "No"
and turning the head in response to a noise
begins at four months, and discrimination
between family and strangers appears at
five months of age.

Nursing Process: Analysis
Client Needs: Psychosocial Integrity
Clinical Area: Pediatric Nursing

49.   (3)   It is crucial to establish a relationship
with the child so talking is important. It is
also necessary to get the attention of an
autistic child, for without their attention,
they continue the maladaptive behavior.
The other three responses are nontherapeutic and may be perceived as threatening by the child, so it is better to move in
slowly as a first action.

Nursing Process: Implementation
Client Needs: Safe, Effective Care Environment
Clinical Area: Pediatric Nursing

50.   (4)   Because the child is in a mist tent, she
will need a toy that can get wet, then dry
out. A book (1) might not last in this misty
environment. The blocks (2) would be difficult to play with and the mobile (3) is for
a younger child.

Nursing Process: Planning
Client Need: Psychosocial Integrity
Clinical Area: Pediatric Nursing

Psychiatric Nursing

1. A depressed client refuses to get out of bed, go to activities, or participate in any of the unit's programs. The most appropriate nursing action is to

   1. Tell her the rules of the unit are that no client can remain in bed.
   2. Suggest she may be hungry later so she had better get out of bed.
   3. Tell her that the nurse will assist her out of bed and help her to dress.
   4. Allow her to remain in bed until she feels ready to join the other clients.

2. A client with depression was placed on the tricyclic medication, Elavil, one week before she was admitted to the hospital. Her depression has not lifted. The nurse concludes, from her understanding of this medication, that Elavil

   1. Has not yet become effective and it may be as long as two or three more weeks before the depression lifts.
   2. Will not work for this client's depression so another antidepressant should be ordered.
   3. Must be discontinued at least one week before another medication is ordered.
   4. May be having a reverse effect on this client and will cause a greater level of depression.

3. When encouraged to join an activity, a depressed client on the psychiatric unit refuses and says, "What's the use?" The approach by the nurse that would be most effective is to

   1. Sit down beside her and ask her how she is feeling.
   2. Tell her it is time for the activity, help her out of the chair, and go with her to the activity.
   3. Convince her how helpful it will be to engage in the activity.
   4. Tell her that this is a self-defeating attitude and it will only make her feel worse.

4. When a depressed client becomes more active and there is evidence that her mood has lifted, an appropriate goal to add to the nursing care plan is to

   1. Encourage her to go home for the weekend.
   2. Move her to a room with three other clients.
   3. Monitor her whereabouts at all times.
   4. Begin to explore the reasons she became depressed.

5. Which of the following behaviors would indicate improvement in coping for a client?

   1. Going to the dining room to eat.
   2. Initiating interaction with another client.
   3. Sleeping frequently during the day.
   4. Turning off the TV to listen to voices.

6. When a client's hallucinations become more insistent and demanding, and difficult to ignore, the nurse assesses his mental status as

   1. Improving.
   ✓ 2. Deteriorating.
   3. Remaining the same.
   4. Showing more evidence of paranoia.

7. During the last 15 years, suicide has increased dramatically in the age group of

   1. Menopausal women.
   ✓ 2. Adolescents.
   3. Elderly men.
   4. Children under age 12.

8. Group therapy has been an accepted method of treatment for psychiatric clients for several years. The best rationale for this form of treatment is

   1. It is the most economical—one staff member can treat many clients.
   2. The format of the therapy is realistic and does not deal with unconscious material.
   3. It enables clients to become aware that others have problems and that they are not alone in their suffering.
   ✓ 4. It provides a social milieu similar to society in general, where the client can relate to others and validate perceptions in a realistic setting.

9. A 60-year-old male client has been admitted to the psychiatric unit, with symptoms ranging from fatigue, an inability to concentrate, and an inability to complete everyday tasks, to refusal to care for himself and preferring to sleep all day. One of the first interventions should be aimed at

   1. Developing a good nursing care plan.

   2. Talking to his wife for cues to help him.
   3. Encouraging him to join activities on the unit.
   ✓ 4. Developing a structured routine for him to follow.

10. A client becomes very dejected and states that life isn't worth living and no one really cares what happens to him. The best response from the nurse would be

   1. "Of course, people care. Your wife comes to visit every day."
   2. "Let's not talk about sad things. Why don't we play Ping-pong?"
   ✓ 3. "I care about you, and I am concerned that you feel so down."
   4. "Tell me, who doesn't care about you?"

11. A client makes a suicide attempt on the evening shift. The staff intervenes in time to prevent harm. In assessing the situation, the most important rationale for the staff to discuss the incident is that

   1. They need to re-enact the attempt so that they understand exactly what happened.
   2. The staff needs to file an incident report so that the hospital administration is kept informed.
   ✓ 3. The staff needs to discuss the client's behavior prior to the attempt to determine what cues in his behavior might have warned them that he was contemplating suicide.
   4. Because the client made one suicide attempt, there is high probability he will make a second attempt in the immediate future.

12. A nurse observes a client sitting alone in her room crying. As the nurse approaches her, the client states, "I'm feeling sad. I don't

want to talk now." The nurse's best response would be

1. "It will help you feel better if you talk about it."
2. "I'll come back when you feel like talking."
3. "I'll stay with you a few minutes."
4. "Sometimes it helps to talk."

13. A client with the diagnosis of manic episode is racing around the psychiatric unit trying to organize games with the clients. An appropriate nursing intervention is to

1. Have the client play Ping-Pong.
2. Suggest video exercises with the other clients.
3. Take the client outside for a walk.
4. Do nothing, as organizing a game is considered therapeutic.

14. When assessing a client for possible suicide, an important clue would be if the client

1. Is hostile and sarcastic to the staff.
2. Identifies with problems expressed by other clients.
3. Seems satisfied and detached.
4. Begins to talk about leaving the hospital.

15. A male client on the psychiatric unit becomes upset when a visitor does not show up and breaks a chair. The first nursing intervention should be to

1. Stay with the client during the stressful time.
2. Ask direct questions about the client's behavior.
3. Set limits and restrict the client's behavior.
4. Plan with the client for how he can better handle frustration.

16. A client with a diagnosis of obsessive-compulsive disorder constantly does repetitive cleaning. The nurse knows that this behavior is probably most basically an attempt to

1. Decrease the anxiety to a tolerable level.
2. Focus attention on nonthreatening tasks.
3. Control others.
4. Decrease the time available for interaction with people.

17. A client has been admitted with a diagnosis of delirium tremens (DTs). The nurse knows that the primary reason the client is so fearful and apprehensive is because

1. He has a serious mental illness.
2. He may die, as 15 percent of the people with DTs do die.
3. His illusions and hallucinations are very real to him.
4. He has to give up alcohol until the symptoms recede.

18. A client is experiencing a high degree of anxiety. It is important to recognize if additional help is required because

1. If the client is out of control, another person will help to decrease his anxiety level.
2. Being alone with an anxious client is dangerous.
3. It will take another person to direct the client into activities to relieve anxiety.
4. Hospital protocol for handling anxious clients requires at least two people.

19. A 56-year-old client is tentatively diagnosed as having Korsakoff's syndrome. In developing a strategy to care for this client, the nurse knows that this condition is a/an

1. Neurological condition common with alcohol poisoning.
2. Neurological degeneration caused by vitamin deficiency.
3. Organic brain lesion brought on by repeated hepatitis attacks.
4. State resulting from severe, long-term psychosis.

20. Three days after admission for depression, a 54-year-old female client approaches the nurse and says, "I know I have cancer of the uterus. Can't you let me stay in bed and have some peace before I die?" In responding, the nurse must keep in mind that

    1. The client must be postmenopausal.
    2. Thoughts of disease are common in depressed clients.
    3. Clients suffering from depression can be demanding, making many requests of the nurse.
    4. Antidepressant medications frequently cause vaginal spotting.

21. As a depressed client begins to participate in her treatment program, an indication that she is ready for discharge will be when she has

    1. Formulated a plan to return home and continue therapy.
    2. Talked to her boss about returning to work.
    3. Identified her weak areas and is working on them.
    4. Asked the staff for advice about her future.

22. As the nurse is talking with a male client on a psychiatric unit, he begins to make sexual advances. He puts his arm around her and

tells her that he bets she is a great lover. The most therapeutic response is

1. "Whether I am or am not a good lover is not relevant."
2. "This subject is inappropriate, and if you continue, I will end our discussion."
3. "If you continue this discussion, I will notify the physician."
4. "Let's talk about something else. We are here to discuss your problems."

23. The nurse observes a client's daughter, who is visiting her mother, sitting alone and crying. When approached, the daughter states, "I'm really concerned about Mom." The nurse's best response would be

    1. "Are you concerned about her hospitalization?"
    2. "Tell me what's concerning you."
    3. "Would you like to talk with the social worker?"
    4. "Would you like to talk to her physician?"

24. Of the following approaches to a client with organic brain syndrome, the most therapeutic would be to

    1. Use short, concrete, specific interactions.
    2. Give complete explanations to the client about his problems.
    3. Provide a flexible therapy schedule.
    4. Confront the client whenever he loses contact with reality.

25. In assisting in the treatment of a person on a "bad trip" from LSD ingestion, the nurse would

    1. Stay with the client.
    2. Ask him what help he would like to have.

3. Encourage verbalization of feelings and perceptions.
4. Provide ongoing orientation.

26. A schizophrenic client is admitted to the psychiatric unit. As the nurse approaches the client with medication, he refuses it, accusing the nurse of trying to kill him. The nurse's best strategy would be to tell him that

1. "It is not poison and you must take the medication."
2. "I will give you an injection if necessary."
3. "You may decide if you want to take the medication by mouth or injection, but you must take it."
4. "It's all right if you don't take the medication right now."

27. A client with the diagnosis of schizophrenia has improved and is now able to attend group therapy meetings. One day she jumps up and runs out after the group has been laughing at a story one of the clients told. She states, "You are all making fun of me." This client is displaying

1. Symbolic rejection.
2. Hallucinations.
3. Depersonalization.
4. Ideas of reference.

28. A client with the diagnosis of organic brain syndrome, dementia type, confabulates when talking with the nurse. The nurse's best response and the rationale for it is to

1. Tell him she knows he is distorting the situation and not telling the truth because she knows alcoholics need to have moral values reinforced.

2. Sit him down and repeatedly give him the correct version of his activity until he remembers it, because one way of learning is to have something repeatedly stressed.
3. Constantly reiterate the correct story each time he confabulates because a realistic goal with this client is to correct memory distortion.
4. Accept his stories without challenge as he is unable, because of organic damage, to recall accurately.

29. A 50-year-old client has just been admitted to the psychiatric unit with a diagnosis of depression. The nurse can best approach her by saying

1. "You have just been admitted, and I'd like to show you the unit."
2. "Would you like to come with me to occupational therapy and see if you can find a project you would enjoy?"
3. "My name is Mary. I will introduce you to all of the other clients."
4. "My name is Mary. I am a nurse on this floor and I will be spending some time with you."

30. The nurse is assigned to work with a client during his drug crisis. While all of the following areas need to be assessed, which one is most important?

1. Contextual—events leading to the crisis.
2. Behavioral—level of awareness and thought processes.
3. Psychological—level of emotional stability and maturational development.
4. Physical—level of degeneration and effect on the body.

31. An antisocial client refuses to participate in unit activities, staying in his room reading until late at night. When he is on the unit, he makes fun of the other clients, calling them "nuts" or "stupid." Considering his diagnosis and behavior, the nursing plan that would be most effective for the staff to follow is to

  1. Let the client know the rules on the unit.
  2. Allow the client to isolate himself so that he does not upset the other clients.
 ✓ 3. Confer with the client, the staff, and his psychiatrist about his lack of participation on the unit.
  4. Require the client's participation in activities.

32. A client on the psychiatric unit agrees to sign a contract specifying his level of therapy involvement, according to a behavior modification plan. This plan will help implement

 ✓ 1. Reinforcement parameters.
 ✓ 2. Limit setting.
  3. Milieu therapy.
  4. Interpersonal psychotherapy.

33. A client with a diagnosis of schizophrenia who threatened a neighbor with a knife was placed on a 72-hour hold by the courts and the psychiatrist. The hold is up, and the psychiatrist and court must determine if the client is

  1. Gravely disabled and unable to take care of himself.
 ✓ 2. A danger to himself and others.
  3. Able to pay for his hospitalization and treatment.
  4. Willing to remain in treatment if he is discharged.

34. If a depressed client refuses medication on the fourth day of her admission to the hospital, the best approach is to

  1. Tell her it is all right not to take the medication.
  2. Tell her the medication is really like vitamins.
 ✓ 3. Allow her to express her fears about taking the medication.
  4. Tell her she will lose her unit privileges if she refuses the medication.

35. A client tells the nurse that she is having a great deal of difficulty talking to her husband. She says, "He treats me like a child. Nothing I say seems to matter to him." The best response is

  1. "Tell me more about how you and your husband communicate."
 ✓ 2. "How do you feel about his reactions to you?"
  3. "He sounds very childish himself."
  4. "Why do you think he treats you like a child?"

36. When an agitated schizophrenic client quiets down, she exhibits catatonic behavior or waxy flexibility (i.e., her limbs may be placed in any position, and she will maintain that stance). A nursing care plan should emphasize

  1. Increased sensory stimulation (for example, talking loudly) to break through her stupor.
 ✓ 2. Much nonverbal, nurturing care, such as bathing and feeding.
  3. Increased privacy in response to her nonverbal message, "Leave me alone."
  4. A protective, custodially oriented regimen of care.

37. A client in a long-term care facility has the diagnosis of Alzheimer's disease. His care plan should include the goal of assisting him to participate in activities that provide him a chance to

    1. Interact with other clients.
    2. Compete with others.
    3. Succeed at something.
    4. Get a sense of continuity.

38. A client, age 70, is admitted with the diagnosis of organic brain syndrome, dementia type. Assessing his condition, the nurse would expect that his prognosis is

    1. Good, because the condition tends to be reversible.
    2. Unpredictable because the condition may reverse.
    3. Poor because symptoms are reduced intellectual capacity, emotional stability, memory, and judgment.
    4. Poor because the condition will rapidly progress.

39. As a male nurse is coming on duty, one of the clients meets him in the elevator and says, "You look like a wreck today." The best response would be

    1. "You don't look so good yourself."
    2. "If you can't say anything nice, perhaps you shouldn't say anything at all."
    3. "I don't understand what you mean by that."
    4. "I was a little rushed this morning."

40. The nurse is in the day room with a group of clients when a client, who has been quietly watching TV, suddenly jumps up screaming and runs out of the room. The nurse's priority intervention would be to

    1. Turn off the TV, and ask the group what they think about the client's behavior.
    2. Follow after the client to see what has happened.
    3. Ignore the incident because these outbursts are frequent.
    4. Send another client out of the room to check on the agitated client.

41. A client believes that there is a little black box in his abdomen and that there is a little man in it who controls his bowel movements. This symptom is an example of

    1. Somatic displacement.
    2. Ideas of reference.
    3. Somatic delusion.
    4. Illusions of grandeur.

42. A nurse approaches a schizophrenic client with her medication and hands it to her. She reaches for it, then draws her hands back, then reaches for it again. She repeats this behavior several times. The most appropriate intervention would be

    1. Put the pill in the client's mouth for her.
    2. Gently put the medication in her hand and direct her hand to her mouth while reassuring that it's all right to take the medication.
    3. Give medications to the other clients and come back to her.
    4. Tell the client that she is acting peculiarly, and that she needs to take the medication.

43. A 50-year-old male client has a history of many hospitalizations for schizophrenic dis-

order. He has been on long-term pheno-thiazines (Thorazine), 400 mg/day. The nurse assessing this client observes that he demonstrates a shuffling gait, drooling, and exhibits general dystonic symptoms. From these symptoms and his history, the nurse concludes that the client has developed

✓1. Tardive dyskinesia.
2. Parkinsonism.
3. Dystonia.
4. Akathisia.

44. A client's deafness has been diagnosed as conversion disorder. Nursing interventions should be guided by which one of the following?

1. The client will probably express much anxiety about her deafness and require much reassurance.
✓2. The client will have little or no awareness of the psychogenic cause of her deafness.
3. The client's need for the symptom should be respected; thus, secondary gains should be allowed.
4. The defense mechanisms of suppression and rationalization are involved in creating the symptom.

45. A student failed her psychology final exam and spent the entire evening berating the teacher and the course. This behavior would be an example of

1. Reaction-formation.
2. Compensation.
✓3. Projection.
4. Acting out.

46. A client is constantly trying to manipulate the staff as a way of getting his needs met.

Which response to the client would indicate that the nurse understands the psychodynamic principle behind the manipulation?

1. "I won't allow you to manipulate me."
✓2. "I won't be able to do as you ask, but I will stay with you and talk."
3. "If this behavior doesn't stop, I shall have to tell your physician."
4. "Let's focus on your anxiety so we can deal with all this manipulation."

47. In planning nursing care for the individual with a somatoform or psychosomatic illness, the nurse needs to consider which of the following general concepts?

1. The nurse must incorporate concepts of adaptation, stress, body image, and anxiety.
2. The area of symptom formation may be symbolic to the client.
3. Psychosomatic illnesses may be life threatening.
✓4. All of the above concepts are important.

48. The most effective nursing intervention for a severely anxious client who is pacing vigorously would be to

1. Instruct her to sit down and quit pacing.
2. Place her in bed to reduce stimuli and allow rest.
3. Allow her to walk until she becomes physically tired.
✓4. Give her prn medication and walk with her at a gradually slowing pace.

49. A client has been in the hospital for four weeks. He is dying of terminal cancer. During this time he has never mentioned his condition or the fact that he is dying. The

nurse's knowledge of the dying process leads to the conclusion that the client is

1. In the grieving process and does not wish to talk.
2. Still in the denial phase.
3. Depending on his family for support and talks to them.
4. Afraid that by talking about dying it will become reality.

50. A new staff nurse is on an orientation tour with the head nurse. A client approaches her and says, "I don't belong here. Please try to get me out." The staff nurse's best response would be

1. "What would you do if you were out of the hospital?"
2. "I am a new staff member, and I'm on a tour. I'll come back and talk with you later."
3. "I think you should talk with the head nurse about that."
4. "I can't do anything about that."

Psychiatric Nursing
Answers with Rationale

1.   (3) Be positive, definite and specific about expectations. Do not give depressed clients a choice or try to convince them to get out of bed. Physically assist the client to get up and dressed to mobilize her.

Nursing Process: Implementation
Client Need: Psychosocial Integrity
Clinical Area: Psychiatric Nursing

2.   (1) Tricyclics may take one to four weeks to be effective and, because it has only been a week, at least two more weeks must be allowed for evaluation of the medication. If after several weeks it has not helped the depression, it must be discontinued for several weeks (dependent on the half-life of the drug) before another antidepressant is given.

Nursing Process: Analysis
Client Need: Psychosocial Integrity
Clinical Area: Psychiatric Nursing

3.   (2) The nursing intervention is directed toward mobilizing the client without asking her to make a decision or trying to convince her to go. The nurse must be direct, specific and not take no for an answer.

Nursing Process: Implementation
Client Need: Safe, Effective Care Environment
Clinical Area: Psychiatric Nursing

4.   (3) The goal is to implement suicide precautions because the danger of suicide is when the depression lifts and the client has the energy to formulate a plan. The nurse would not encourage her to go home where she could not be observed constantly. She could be moved into a room with other clients, but this is not the priority concern.

Nursing Process: Planning
Client Need: Psychosocial Integrity
Clinical Area: Psychiatric Nursing

5.   (2) If a client can initiate interaction with another client, it indicates he is not totally absorbed in himself, too depressed to initiate, or too absorbed in delusions or halluci-

Nursing Process: Evaluation
Client Need: Psychosocial Integrity
Clinical Area: Psychiatric Nursing

nations to interact. All of the other choices do not indicate improvement in coping.

6. (2)   The more demanding and absorbing hallucinations (hearing voices) become, the more the client's condition may be deteriorating. Secondarily, this may indicate increased paranoia. Paranoid schizophrenia is only one form of this condition, and hallucinations occur in all types of schizophrenia.

Nursing Process: Assessment
Client Need: Psychosocial Integrity
Clinical Area: Psychiatric Nursing

7. (2)   The number of suicides has increased dramatically in the adolescent age group in the last 15 years. As more elderly are living longer, the number of suicides has also increased, but it is proportional.

Nursing Process: Analysis
Client Need: Psychosocial Integrity
Clinical Area: Psychiatric Nursing

8. (4)   Because many people's problems occur in an interpersonal framework, the group setting is a way to correct faulty perceptions, as well as to work on more effective ways of relating to others.

Nursing Process: Analysis
Client Needs: Psychosocial Integrity
Clinical Area: Psychiatric Nursing

9. (4)   While a good nursing care plan is important, the priority would be to get the client mobilized. Even without a specific diagnosis, the nurse will realize that part of what is happening with the client is a depressed mood. Providing a structured plan of activities for the client to follow will help his mood to lift and provide a focus so that he will not be centered on internal suffering.

Nursing Process: Implementation
Client Needs: Safe, Effective Care Environment
Clinical Area: Psychiatric Nursing

10. (3)   A depressed person needs to experience that someone is concerned for his welfare and that there is a person he can relate to during his hospitalization. Answers (1) and (2) negate the client's feelings and answer (4) may focus on uncomfortable thoughts that will deepen the depression.

Nursing Process: Implementation
Client Needs: Psychosocial Integrity
Clinical Area: Psychiatric Nursing

11. (3) Even though all of the reasons are important and should not be ignored, the most important task for the staff is to assess the client's behavior and to identify cues that might indicate an impending suicide attempt.

Nursing Process: Assessment
Client Needs: Psychosocial Integrity
Clinical Area: Psychiatric Nursing

12. (3) Simply offering comfort by staying with the client and being open for communication is the most therapeutic. The other responses place an additional burden on the client if she does not wish to talk.

Nursing Process: Implementation
Client Needs: Psychosocial Integrity
Clinical Area: Psychiatric Nursing

13. (3) Engaging the client in a large muscle activity, like walking with the nurse, will direct the client's energy, but not be too stimulating as would a competitive game such as Ping-Pong.

Nursing Process: Implementation
Client Needs: Safe, Effective Care Environment
Clinical Area: Psychiatric Nursing

14. (3) Most suggestible of suicide is the sudden sense of satisfaction or relief (perhaps from finally making the decision to commit suicide) and detachment. Hostility, identifying with others, or thinking of the future do not as clearly suggest suicidal thinking.

Nursing Process: Evaluation
Client Needs: Safe, Effective Care Environment
Clinical Area: Psychiatric Nursing

15. (3) The first intervention is to set firm, clear limits on his behavior. The nurse would also remain with the client until he calms down and then encourage him to discuss his feelings rather than act out.

Nursing Process: Implementation
Client Needs: Psychosocial Integrity
Clinical Area: Psychiatric Nursing

16. (1) The primary reason for the compulsive activity is to decrease the anxiety caused by obsessive thoughts. The client is not trying to focus her attention on tasks, control others or lessen interaction with others.

Nursing Process: Analysis
Client Needs: Psychosocial Integrity
Clinical Area: Psychiatric Nursing

17. (3) A client experiencing DTs may have illusions and/or hallucinations and these are very frightening to him because they seem real and the client does not recognize that they are part of his illness.

Nursing Process: Planning
Client Needs: Psychosocial Integrity
Clinical Area: Psychiatric Nursing

18. (1)   If the client and/or the situation gets out of control, anxiety will only increase. Additional help may prevent this from occurring.

Nursing Process: Analysis
Client Needs: Psychosocial Integrity
Clinical Area: Psychiatric Nursing

19. (2)   Korsakoff's syndrome (also called polyneuritic psychosis) is a form of organic brain syndrome that is associated with long term alcohol abuse and a deficiency of vitamin B complex, especially thiamine. (2) is more specific than answer (1). This condition is not caused from a lesion, hepatitis (3), or psychosis (4).

Nursing Process: Analysis
Client Needs: Physiological Integrity
Clinical Area: Psychiatric Nursing

20. (2)   Concern with having a life-threatening disease is a common issue with depressed clients, related to the extreme feeling of guilt. While demanding behavior may be a symptom, it is not the issue here.

Nursing Process: Analysis
Client Needs: Psychosocial Integrity
Clinical Area: Psychiatric Nursing

21. (1)   A plan to return home and continue therapy shows that the client has begun to realistically and responsibly deal with her problems. Talking to her boss is positive but not as comprehensive as (1). Identifying and working on weak areas usually are intermediate steps toward discharge. In asking the staff for advice, the client is not ready or willing to accept responsibility for herself.

Nursing Process: Evaluation
Client Needs: Health Promotion and Maintenance
Clinical Area: Psychiatric Nursing

22. (2)   It is important to give the client feedback that his discussion is inappropriate and to set firm, clear limits. He needs to understand that he cannot manipulate the nurse and that the nurse will not accept inappropriate behavior.

Nursing Process: Implementation
Client Needs: Psychosocial Integrity
Clinical Area: Psychiatric Nursing

23. (2)   The nurse should offer on-the-spot support to visiting family members. They are important components of the therapeutic process and need assistance in dealing

Nursing Process: Implementation
Client Needs: Psychosocial Integrity
Clinical Area: Psychiatric Nursing

with their thoughts and feelings about the client.

24.   (1)   Organic brain syndrome clients need specific, concrete instructions and a safe, consistent environment with reality orientation. Confrontation and environmental instability further confuse the client by increasing his anxiety level. Giving too much information is confusing.

Nursing Process: Planning
Client Needs: Safe, Effective Care Environment
Clinical Area: Psychiatric Nursing

25.   (1)   The client needs to have external stimuli decreased but does not need to be isolated. It is much less traumatic if the nurse remains with the client. Encouraging verbalization or answering questions during this period would not be therapeutic.

Nursing Process: Implementation
Client Needs: Psychosocial Integrity
Clinical Area: Psychiatric Nursing

26.   (3)   Giving the client a choice of how he would like to take his medication, while being firm that he must take it, gives the client a sense of control and helps to reduce the power struggle. Telling the client that the medication is not poison will do little to persuade him to comply. Answer (2) would represent a punishment. The client must take his medication; therefore, distractor (4) is not appropriate.

Nursing Process: Implementation
Client Needs: Safe, Effective Care Environment
Clinical Area: Psychiatric Nursing

27.   (4)   Ideas of reference or misinterpretation occurs when the client believes that an incident has a personal reference to one's self when, in fact, it is not at all related.

Nursing Process: Analysis
Client Needs: Psychosocial Integrity
Clinical Area: Psychiatric Nursing

28.   (4)   Confabulation is filling in memory gaps caused by organic deterioration of brain cells. Attempts to correct stories, re-educate or refute may increase anxiety, thus being unproductive and/or detrimental. It would also lower the client's self-esteem.

Nursing Process: Planning
Client Needs: Psychosocial Integrity
Clinical Area: Psychiatric Nursing

29.   (4)   Acknowledge the client by introduc-
       ing yourself and start a one-to-one rela-
       tionship by spending time with her. Let the
       client know that the nurse cares about her
       by staying with her.

Nursing Process: Implementation
Client Needs: Psychosocial Integrity
Clinical Area: Psychiatric Nursing

30.   (4)   The most important safety considera-
       tion is the physical condition of the client.
       If this client is hydrated and in a reason-
       ably good physical state, the other parame-
       ters can be explored.

Nursing Process: Assessment
Client Needs: Physiological Integrity
Clinical Area: Psychiatric Nursing

31.   (3)   In dealing with manipulative behavior,
       it is important that all members of the team
       and the client are clear about expectations.
       (1) is nontherapeutic as it pits the nurse
       against the client. (2) is not a reasonable
       choice because the client is not involved in
       treatment. (4) is nontherapeutic.

Nursing Process: Planning
Client Needs: Safe, Effective Care Environment
Clinical Area: Psychiatric Nursing

32.   (2)   This plan is more directly an example
       of limit setting, which specifies behaviors,
       actions, and their consequences. In milieu
       therapy, the group would formulate the
       contract, and in psychotherapy the thera-
       pist would take responsibility for setting
       limits with the client.

Nursing Process: Planning
Client Needs: Safe, Effective Care Environment
Clinical Area: Psychiatric Nursing

33.   (2)   The staff and court must determine if
       the client is a danger to self and others.
       Answer (1) may be a correct answer, but
       the client was admitted to the hospital for
       threatening a neighbor. Answers (3) and
       (4) are not pertinent to the decision.

Nursing Process: Implementation
Client Needs: Psychosocial Integrity
Clinical Area: Psychiatric Nursing

34.   (3)   It is important that the client's con-
       cerns and fears be acknowledged before
       planning a subsequent intervention.
       Adequate information about the medica-
       tion may dispel her fears so that a second
       intervention may not be necessary.

Nursing Process: Implementation
Client Needs: Safe, Effective Care Environment
Clinical Area: Psychiatric Nursing

35. (2) The client needs to recognize her feelings, and this response will assist her to do so. Answer (1) keeps the conversation on the cognitive level and does not deal with her feelings. (3) is making a judgment. (4) is asking for an intellectual analysis which may or may not help the client and which may cause her to feel she must justify herself.

Nursing Process: Implementation
Client Needs: Psychosocial Integrity
Clinical Area: Psychiatric Nursing

36. (2) The nurturing care is an attempt to provide for some of the client's unmet needs during this phase of isolation. It is also a way of beginning to establish a relationship. Sensory overstimulation would probably only increase the client's isolation, and privacy would add to her withdrawal. Custodial care would not adequately meet the client's needs.

Nursing Process: Planning
Client Needs: Psychosocial Integrity
Clinical Area: Psychiatric Nursing

37. (3) It is essential that the client participate in activities that provide him with immediate success and increase his self-esteem. Interaction with others is important but is secondary to improving his self-esteem.

Nursing Process: Planning
Client Need: Psychosocial Integrity
Clinical Area: Psychiatric Nursing

38. (3) Dementia has a poor prognosis, is usually progressive and irreversible, and the symptoms are closely related to the patient's basic personality. All of the characteristics in (3) fit the picture of organic brain syndrome. The condition may or may not progress rapidly, but will generally deteriorate.

Nursing Process: Assessment
Client Need: Physiological Integrity
Clinical Area: Psychiatric Nursing

39. (3) Asking for clarification of such a statement might reveal more feelings than implied by the casual comment. This type of statement may be indicative of anger or projected feelings. Answer (1) is sarcastic, and (2) and (4) cut off further exploration of what the client may really be saying. It

Nursing Process: Implementation
Client Needs: Psychosocial Integrity
Clinical Area: Psychiatric Nursing

would not be appropriate to continue with a personal explanation of why the nurse looks bad.

40.   (2)   The immediate priority is to find the client and assess what further intervention may be needed. Whether or not the behavior has happened frequently in the past is irrelevant, because the behavior exhibited now is significant and should be followed up. Sending another client is inappropriate as an immediate intervention may be necessary.

Nursing Process: Implementation
Client Needs: Safe, Effective Care Environment
Clinical Area: Psychiatric Nursing

41.   (3)   Clients who complain of bodily dysfunction, such as their brains decaying, electricity being run through their feet, or someone controlling their bodily functions, are displaying somatic delusions. It is usually associated with schizophrenia.

Nursing Process: Analysis
Client Needs: Psychosocial Integrity
Clinical Area: Psychiatric Nursing

42.   (2)   This type of behavior is indicative of ambivalence (common with the diagnosis of schizophrenia) on the client's part. When a client is experiencing indecision and fear, it is often helpful to be gently directive and reassuring so the pressure of decision-making is relieved. Answer (1) is taking total control, which the client's behavior does not dictate.

Nursing Process: Implementation
Client Needs: Safe, Effective Care Environment
Clinical Area: Psychiatric Nursing

43.   (1)   Tardive dyskinesia usually develops late in treatment and may occur in up to 50 percent of chronic schizophrenics with the long-term use of phenothiazine drugs. Antiparkinson drugs such as Artane and Cogentin are of no help in decreasing the symptoms of shuffling gait, drooling and general dystonia. Parkinsonism, dystonia and akathisia are also extrapyramidal effects of phenothiazine use, but these conditions are reversible with drugs.

Nursing Process: Analysis
Client Needs: Physiological Integrity
Clinical Area: Psychiatric Nursing

44. (2) This disorder has an unconscious mechanism in place; thus, there is a relative lack of distress or anxiety regarding the symptom. The client is likely to demonstrate "la belle indifference," an unconcerned, indifferent attitude toward the loss of function with no awareness of the psychogenic cause. Answer (3) is incorrect as secondary gains should be minimized. Answer (4) is incorrect as repression and displacement are the operating mechanisms.

Nursing Process: Analysis
Client Needs: Psychosocial Integrity
Clinical Area: Psychiatric Nursing

45. (3) The client is placing blame on others and not taking responsibility for her own behavior. Reaction-formation is preventing "dangerous" feelings from being expressed by exaggerating the opposite attitude. Compensation is covering up a weakness by emphasizing a desirable trait. Acting out is not a defense mechanism.

Nursing Process: Analysis
Client Needs: Psychosocial Integrity
Clinical Area: Psychiatric Nursing

46. (2) It is important to set limits but not to reinforce low self-esteem, so staying with the client would be therapeutic. It is the responsibility of the nurse to directly handle this situation, so answer (3) is inappropriate. The other options are nontherapeutic.

Nursing Process: Evaluation
Client Needs: Psychosocial Integrity
Clinical Area: Psychiatric Nursing

47. (4) Psychosomatic illnesses involve the "holism" of the individual; thus, all three of the concepts are important. If the nurse considers all of these concepts in planning nursing care, interventions will be therapeutic.

Nursing Process: Planning
Client Needs: Psychosocial Integrity
Clinical Area: Psychiatric Nursing

48. (4) This client is in severe anxiety heading for a panic level. She requires immediate medication, constant attention, and a gradual lessening of activity according to her expressed level of energy. With moderate anxiety, directed activity helps to reduce the level.

Nursing Process: Implementation
Client Needs: Safe, Effective Care Environment
Clinical Area: Psychiatric Nursing

49.　(2)　The fact that he has not talked about dying in a month, or even about his illness, leads the nurse to suspect denial. In this situation, the nurse would not confront him with reality but wait until he is ready to talk.

Nursing Process: Analysis
Client Needs: Safe, Effective Care Environment
Clinical Area: Psychiatric Nursing

50.　(2)　As a new staff member, the nurse should clarify who she is and why she is there. She also should acknowledge the client's attempt to initiate interaction by offering to talk at a more appropriate time. Answer (1) might be used in a later interaction, but is not appropriate at this time.

Nursing Process: Implementation
Client Needs: Safe, Effective Care Environment
Clinical Area: Psychiatric Nursing

Adjunct Topics

Pharmacology

1. Following surgery, a client has an order for Nubain (Nalbuphine HCl) for moderate to severe pain. The assessment for possible adverse reactions should include observing for

   1. Blurred vision, palpitations and urinary retention.
   2. Increased pulse rate, drowsiness, and nausea.
   3. Increased confusion, tachycardia and anorexia.
   4. Irregular pulse, hypotension and oliguria.

2. The nurse is assigned to a client who is receiving mydriatic eye drops. Which of the following symptoms indicates a systemic anticholinergic effect?

   1. Complaints of light headedness and headache.
   2. Respirations becoming more shallow.
   3. Sweating and blurred vision.
   4. Decreased pulse and blood pressure.

3. A female client with a history of multiple sclerosis has orders for dantrolene sodium (Dantrium). The nurse will know the client understands the action of the drug when she says

   1. "I need to use a sunscreen when I go outside."
   2. "I can't take any other medications when I'm on this drug."
   3. "I take this drug only when my spasms are bad."
   4. "I should see a marked change in my muscle strength within two to three days."

4. Bethanechol chloride (Urecholine) is ordered prn for a client following a transurethral resection (TUR). Which of the following conditions would be present for the nurse to administer this drug?

   1. Complaints of bladder spasms.
   2. Complaints of severe pain.
   3. Inability to void.
   4. Frequent episodes of painful urination.

5. Which one of the statements is most accurate about the drug cimetidine (Tagamet) and should be discussed with clients who take the medication?

   1. Tagamet should be taken with an antacid to decrease GI distress, a common occurrence with the drug.
   2. Tagamet should be used cautiously with clients on Coumadin because it could inhibit the absorption of the drug.

3. Tagamet should be taken on an empty stomach for better absorption.

4. Tagamet is usually prescribed for long-term prevention of gastric ulcers.

6. A 60-year-old male client with chronic osteoarthritis is severely debilitated. Betamethasone (Celestone) therapy has been ordered for him. The nurse will advise the client to take a single, daily dose of the drug

1. At bedtime with a glass of milk.
2. With orange juice at bedtime.
3. With milk in the morning.
4. On an empty stomach in the morning.

7. A client is receiving lithium carbonate for manic behavior. Administration of this medication should be guided by

1. Maintaining a therapeutic dose of 900 mgm tid.
2. Encouraging regular blood studies (serum lithium levels) until the maintenance dose is stabilized.
3. Telling the client that a lag of seven to ten days can be expected between the initiation of lithium therapy and the control of manic symptoms.
4. Telling the client that muscle weakness indicates severe toxicity and the physician should be notified.

8. Some clients with severely active lupus erythematosus are managed with steroids. A positive response to steroid therapy would be evidenced by

1. An increase in platelet count.
2. A normal gamma globulin count.
3. A decrease in anti-DNA titer.
4. Negative syphilis serology.

9. A client in liver failure from cirrhosis with ascites is receiving spironolactone. The expected outcome when this drug is given, is

1. Increased urine sodium.
2. Increased urinary output.
3. Decreased potassium excretion.
4. Prevention of metabolic alkalosis.

10. A client with a fractured right hip has Buck's traction applied and orders for prophylactic anticoagulant therapy. The nurse anticipates that the physician will order

1. Aspirin.
2. Dextran.
3. Heparin.
4. Coumadin.

11. A client with a urinary tract infection is given an aminoglycoside (gentamicin) antimicrobial therapy. The nurse understands that this drug is more active when the urine is

1. Concentrated.
2. Dilute.
3. Alkaline.
4. Acid.

12. A client with the diagnosis of systemic lupus erythematosus is placed on Plaquenil, an antimalarial drug, to reduce skin inflammation. A toxic reaction to this drug that the nurse will teach the client to report is

1. Muscle cramps.
2. Decreased visual acuity.
3. Cardiac arrhythmias.
4. Joint pain.

13. A client with thrombophlebitis has orders for continuous heparin infusion. The nurse will have the antidote available, which is

    1. Vitamin K.
    2. Protamine sulfate.
    3. Mephyton.
    4. Calcium gluconate.

14. The physician orders dexamethasone (Decadron) to be administered to a client with a head injury. Based on nursing knowledge of this medication, the nurse would question the physician if he did not order which of the following additional medications?

    1. Morphine sulfate.
    2. Sodium bicarbonate.
    3. Cimetidine.
    4. Levophed.

15. A male client is currently taking Digitalis 0.25 mg daily, Lasix 100 mg daily, Acyclovir 10 mg qid, and Tagamet 300 mg qid. Which one of the following drugs has potential side effects that are the most life-threatening?

    1. Digitalis.
    2. Lasix.
    3. Acyclovir.
    4. Tagamet.

16. When a client is taking the drug baclofen, the most accurate information the nurse should tell him about the drug is that he should

    1. Not drive a car until he knows if any CNS effects occur with the use of the drug.
    2. Take the medication on an empty stomach for better absorption.

3. Notify the physician if diarrhea occurs.
4. Notify the physician if any side effects occur.

17. Which of the following actions would *not* be carried out when administering a medication using the Z-track method?

    1. Placing 0.3 to 0.5 ml of air into the syringe.
    2. Using a 3-inch needle.
    3. Inserting the needle and injecting medication without aspirating.
    4. Pulling skin laterally away from the injection site before inserting the needle.

18. A 68-year-old client has an IV infusing at 50 ml per hour. The IV administration set delivers 15 gtts/ml. When adjusting the flow rate, the nurse would regulate the rate at

    1. 4 drops per minute.
    2. 8 drops per minute.
    3. 12 drops per minute.
    4. 25 drops per minute.

19. After a client begins taking a prescribed antianxiety agent, the nurse would observe her for side effects of

    1. Sedation and slurred speech.
    2. Photosensitivity and muscular rigidity.
    3. Tremors and hypertension.
    4. A paradoxical reaction and hypoactivity.

20. When administering Valium (a benzodiazepine drug) to a client, the nurse needs to consider that

    1. Valium has sedative properties.
    2. There are no important side effects to consider because it is a one-time dose.

3. Valium should never be mixed with foods containing tyramine.
4. Valium directly affects the blood pressure as a vasoconstrictor.

21. The drug that will most likely be used in the treatment of malignancy of the prostate is

    1. Chorionic gonadotropin.
    2. Cytoxan.
    3. Diethylstilbestrol (DES).
    4. Nitrogen mustard.

22. A 65 year old with the diagnosis of organic brain syndrome has orders for Seconal at bedtime. The nurse's understanding of this drug is that it has the effect on the body of

    1. Tranquilization.
    2. Sedation.
    3. Mood elevation.
    4. Stimulation.

23. A client has developed agranulocytosis as a result of medications he is taking. In counseling the client, the nurse knows that one of the most serious consequences of this condition is

1. The potential danger of excessive bleeding even with minor trauma.
2. Generalized ecchymosis on exposed areas of the body.
3. High susceptibility to infection.
4. Extreme prostration.

24. The instructions to a client whose physician recently ordered nitroglycerin are that this medication should be taken

    1. Every two to three hours during the day.
    2. Before every meal and at bedtime.
    3. At the first indication of chest pain.
    4. Only when chest pain is not relieved by rest.

25. The nurse is counseling a client taking corticosteroids who has developed an infectious process. How would the infection affect the medication dosage?

    1. Corticosteroid dose would be increased.
    2. Corticosteroid dose would be discontinued.
    3. Corticosteroid dose would be decreased.
    4. There would be no change in dosage.

Nutrition

1. Evaluating the teaching plan for a client recently placed on a low sodium diet by her physician, the nurse will know the client understands the plan when she states

    1. "I will call the dietician if I can't remember."
    2. "I will look at the list of foods I can have."

    3. "I will read the label on the food product."
    4. "I will cook without adding salt to the food."

2. The nurse asks a client to list the snacks he likes that are allowed on his low fat, low sodium, low cholesterol diet. The nurse real-

izes that further dietary teaching is necessary when one of his choices is

1. Buttermilk.
2. Jam sandwich.
3. Apple.
4. Applesauce.

3. Clients with hepatitis may have a regular diet ordered, unless they become increasingly symptomatic. The diet will then be modified to decrease the amount of

1. Carbohydrates.
2. Fats.
3. Fluids.
4. Protein.

4. The nurse will know that her teaching has been effective when the client responds that a low fiber diet allows the inclusion of

1. Whole grain breads, seeds and legumes.
2. Fresh fruits and vegetables.
3. Bran and whole grain cereals.
4. Cooked vegetables, fruits and refined breads.

5. The nurse questions the dietary department about the lunch delivered for a client with the diagnosis of cirrhosis when she finds on his tray

1. A tuna sandwich.
2. French fries.
3. A ham sandwich.
4. A milkshake.

6. Clients with a history of pancreatitis have dietary restrictions. While evaluating diet history with these clients, the nurse will

determine that they understand food restrictions when they know they should avoid

1. Noodles.
2. Vegetable soup.
3. Baked fish fillet.
4. Cheddar cheese sandwiches.

7. A 28-year-old client has just learned that her pregnancy test is positive. The nurse will reinforce nutritional counseling by telling the client that her diet should

1. Maintain iron intake and increase calorie intake by 500 calories.
2. Increase iron and increase calorie intake by 300 calories.
3. Increase iron and multivitamins but maintain calorie intake.
4. Decrease iron but increase calorie intake by 200–300 calories.

8. A client with cirrhosis and ascites is placed on a sodium restricted diet to help control the ascites. In order for this plan to be effective, it is important that the client also

1. Restrict his fluid intake.
2. Increase his potassium intake.
3. Increase his fluid intake.
4. Decrease his potassium intake.

9. A client with acute pancreatitis required nasogastric tube intubation due to persistent vomiting and paralytic ileus. Following NG tube removal, oral feeding should include foods which are

1. High in fat.
2. High in protein.
3. High in carbohydrate.
4. Clear liquid.

10. The most appropriate sugar substitute for the Insulin-Dependent Diabetes Mellitus, type I (IDDM) client is

   1. Corn sugar.
   2. Honey.
   3. Aspartame.
   4. Fructose.

11. The diabetic client understands his diet when he says that he should obtain the greatest percentage of calories from

   1. Fats.
   2. Complex carbohydrates.
   3. Simple carbohydrates.
   4. Protein.

12. When a client is in early prehepatic coma, the dietary regimen will be changed to include how much protein per day?

   1. 20–40 gm.
   2. 50–70 gm.
   3. 75–95 gm.
   4. 100–120 gm.

13. The nurse will know the client understands his low-purine diet when he states

   1. "I will need to limit the number of fruit servings each day."
   2. "Organ meats will need to be eliminated from my diet."
   3. "I can only drink white wine because red wine is high in purine."
   4. "Beef, chicken and pork are high in purine; therefore, I can only have them once in a while."

14. Which of the following statements would be correct counseling a client about the postoperative diet he would receive?

   1. A client undergoing major surgery may have a soft diet the day of surgery.
   2. Approximately 2800 calories are required daily for tissue repair, so this will be his caloric intake.
   3. Daily fluid intake should be 1500 ml for an uncomplicated surgical procedure.
   4. A mechanical, soft diet should be given the first postoperative day.

15. The nurse's diet instructions for a client with a colostomy will be

   1. According to his own individual needs and similar to his preoperative diet.
   2. Low in fiber with a large amount of fluids.
   3. High in fiber with large amounts of fluids and supplemental vitamin K.
   4. Elimination of milk products.

16. Discharge planning for a client with a partial colectomy will include which one of the following dietary principles?

   1. High residue, force fluids.
   2. Low residue, no dairy products.
   3. High fiber, no spices.
   4. Regular, no dairy products.

17. The nurse will know that the client understands presurgical instructions for hemorrhoid surgery if his diet is

   1. Low-roughage.
   2. High-fiber.
   3. High-carbohydrate.
   4. Low-fiber.

18. A client with chronic lymphocytic leukemia is started on chemotherapy. Monitoring the administration of these drugs, the nurse would

1. Offer a liquid diet before the treatments.
2. Offer fluids and foods high in bulk and fiber.
3. Instruct the client to use a medium firm toothbrush for oral hygiene.
4. Instruct the client to use dental floss daily.

19. The nurse's discharge teaching for a client with acute pancreatitis will include advising him to take

   1. Vitamin K.
   2. Fat soluble vitamins.
   3. Vitamin C.
   4. Vitamin B_{12}.

20. A client, age 54, has been diagnosed as having lung cancer. The tumor is inoperable and he will undergo radiation therapy. Because of the GI complications associated with radiation, the client will be placed on a diet of

   1. High protein, high carbohydrate, low residue.
   2. High protein, high residue.
   3. High protein, high residue, low sodium.
   4. Low protein, low residue, high calcium.

21. A 53-year-old client with Crohn's disease is placed on total parenteral nutrition (TPN). The fluid in the present TPN bottle should be infused by 8 A.M. At 7 A.M. the nurse observes that it is empty and another TPN bottle has not yet arrived on the unit. The nursing action is to attach a bottle of

   1. D_{25} and water.
   2. D_5 and water.
   3. D_{10} and water.
   4. D_{45} and water.

22. A client has injured her eyes with a chemical and must have eye patches in place for several weeks. When her food tray arrives, the most helpful nursing intervention would be to

   1. Feed the client or assign an aid to feed her.
   2. Explain that her tray is here and put her hands on it.
   3. Tell her to think of a clock and describe which food is where and put the fork in her hand.
   4. Ask her if she would prefer a liquid diet.

23. A client will have a central vein infusion to maintain nutritional status while his gastrointestinal tract is being bypassed. The nurse would expect that the site of catheter insertion for a protein and glucose concentration of 15% would be in the

   1. Jugular vein.
   2. Right subclavian vein.
   3. Right subclavian artery.
   4. Left arm artery access.

24. A client's physician has ordered intralipid therapy for his client. In carrying out this order, the nurse understands that monitoring for side effects is important. Which of the following side effects would necessitate that the nurse immediately notify the physician?

   1. Dyspnea and chills.
   2. Hyperlipemia.
   3. Eczema-like rash and dry, scaly skin.
   4. Erythema and edema at the insertion site.

25. A client has had abdominal surgery and the physician has ordered a bland diet three days postsurgery. Which of the following

diet trays would have portions removed because it does not adhere to the dietary regimen?

1. Scrambled eggs, cereal and white toast.
2. Baked potato, cottage cheese and coffee.
3. Cream soup, jello and white toast.
4. Cooked cereal, boiled egg and milk

Legal Issues

1. The civil rights of a client would not be jeopardized in which one of the following situations?

    1. Trying to forcibly detain a client who may suffer great harm by leaving the hospital.
    2. Giving emergency medical care to a client without his or her consent or the consent of the family.
    3. Giving a psychiatric client's letters addressed to the President of the United Sates to his physician.
    4. Giving the client's insurance broker access to his chart.

2. The primary purpose and criteria of licensure is to

    1. Limit practice.
    2. Define the scope of practice.
    3. Protect the public.
    4. Outline legislative action.

3. One of the elements of negligence is breach of the standard of care. "Standard of care" may be defined as

    1. Nursing competence as defined by the State Nurse Practice Act.
    2. Degree of judgment and skill in nursing care given by a reasonable and prudent professional nurse under similar circumstances.
    3. Health services as prescribed by community ordinances.
    4. Giving care to clients in good faith to the best of one's ability.

4. The decision as to whether or not a nurse can lawfully restrain a client is made by the

    1. Nurse.
    2. Family.
    3. Hospital administrator.
    4. Physician.

5. The physician wrote a medication order for a client. The nurse thought the dosage was incorrect. She questioned the physician who said it was all right. Still questioning, she asked another nurse, who said it was all right. The nurse gave the medicine, and the client died from an overdose. Who is liable?

    1. The physician and the two nurses.
    2. The physician.
    3. The nurse who gave the medication.
    4. Both the physician and the nurse who gave the medication.

6. Which of the following best describes the function and purpose of the unusual occurrence (incident) report?

1. A legal part of the chart used to furnish data about the incident.
2. A hospital record used to record the details of the incident for possible legal reference.
3. A legal hospital business record which is subject to subpoena and can be used against the hospital personnel.
4. A hospital record that is entered into the client's chart if he or she dies.

7. If the nurse is involved in a situation in which he or she must countersign the charting of a paraprofessional, which of the following will most aid in decreasing legal liability?

   1. Read the document before it is signed.
   2. Have personal knowledge of the information contained in the document.
   3. Make sure the information is accurate.
   4. Check with a second nurse to see if information is accurate.

8. The nurse transcribing the physician's order finds it difficult to read. Which of the following people should the nurse consult for clarification of the order?

   1. The head nurse who is familiar with the physician's writing.
   2. Another nurse working with the nurse.
   3. The physician who wrote the order.
   4. The nursing supervisor.

9. Which of the following would not constitute negligent conduct?

   1. A medication error.
   2. Failure to follow a physician's order.
   3. Failure to challenge a physician's order.
   4. Disagreeing with a physician.

10. The nurse is asked to do a TV commercial for hand lotion. In this commercial she will wear her nurse's uniform and advocate the use of this lotion by nurses in their work setting. In doing this the nurse is violating

    1. Consumer fraud laws.
    2. The nurse practice act.
    3. The code of ethics for nurses.
    4. None of the above.

11. Nurse practice acts include

    1. A definition of nursing practice.
    2. Qualifications for licensure.
    3. Grounds for revocation of a license.
    4. All of the above.

12. Client's rights are

    1. Specifically written into many laws.
    2. A position paper that was developed by the American Hospital Association.
    3. A declaration of the World Health Organization.
    4. Not supported by statutory law.

13. Which of the following statements concerning nursing liability is true?

    1. A physician may assume personal liability for the negligent acts of the nurse.
    2. The nurse is responsible for her own negligent acts.
    3. The doctrine of respondeat superior always protects the nurse.
    4. Malpractice insurance will always cover the damages assessed against the nurse.

14. Which of the following might negate liability on the part of the nurse in a negligent action?

1. The client consented to the act.
2. The harm was not reasonably foreseeable.
3. The nurse had not been taught to do the procedure in nursing school.
4. Other foreseeable acts occurred which added to the client's injury.

15. The nurse's liability in terms of the client's consent to receive health services is to

1. Be certain that the physician has prepared the client.
2. Ensure that the client is fully informed before being asked to sign a consent form.
3. Check that the client understands the details of the surgery.
4. The nurse would not be liable—the physician would be.

Adjunct Topics
Answers with Rationale

Pharmacology

1. (1)   These are symptoms associated with adverse reactions to Nubain. Drowsiness, nausea, confusion, bradycardia, and anorexia are also adverse reactions. Tachycardia, irregular pulse and hypotension are not symptoms associated with adverse effects of Nubain.

    Nursing Process: Assessment
    Client Needs: Safe, Effective Care Environment
    Clinical Area: Surgical Nursing

2. (3)   Sweating and blurred vision are signs of a systemic anticholinergic effect. In addition to these symptoms the client may experience loss of sight, difficulty breathing, flushing, or eye pain. If these symptoms occur, the medication must be discontinued and the physician notified.

    Nursing Process: Evaluation
    Client Needs: Physiological Integrity
    Clinical Area: Medical Nursing

3. (1)   This drug has the potential for photosensitivity; therefore, the client should protect her skin by wearing a hat and using sunscreen.

    Nursing Process: Evaluation
    Client Needs: Health Promotion and Maintenance
    Clinical Area: Medical Nursing

4. (3)   Urecholine stimulates the parasympathetic nervous system. It increases the tone and motility of the smooth muscles of the urinary tract. It is used frequently following a TUR when the client has a lack of muscle tone and is unable to void. Bladder spasms can be relieved with Belladonna or opium suppositories.

    Nursing Process: Assessment
    Client Needs: Physiological Integrity
    Clinical Area: Surgical Nursing

5. (2)   Tagamet can interfere with the absorption of Coumadin and several other drugs such as Dilantin, Lidocaine or

    Nursing Process: Analysis
    Client Needs: Health Promotion and Maintenance
    Clinical Area: Medical Nursing

Inderal; therefore, the serum levels of the drugs should be monitored closely. Tagamet should not be taken within one hour of an antacid, because this will interfere with the absorption. It is best to take the drug with food. Tagamet is usually ordered for short-term treatment of duodenal and active gastric ulcers.

6. (3) A single dose in the morning promotes better results and less toxicity. It is given with milk to reduce gastrointestinal irritation.

Nursing Process: Implementation
Client Needs: Safe, Effective Care Environment
Clinical Area: Medical Nursing

7. (3) There will be 7 to 10 days before the client will experience a decrease in the manic symptoms. A therapeutic dose is 300 mg tid; regular blood studies must be continued throughout drug therapy; muscle weakness is an expected side effect and does not indicate toxicity.

Nursing Process: Planning
Client Needs: Safe, Effective Care Environment
Clinical Area: Psychiatric Nursing

8. (3) Anti-DNA antibody levels correlate most specifically with lupus disease activity. A positive response to steroids would show a decrease in these levels. Twenty percent of clients with lupus develop a positive syphilis serology, and many have hypergammaglobulinemia and a decreased platelet count.

Nursing Process: Evaluation
Client Needs: Physiological Integrity
Clinical Area: Medical Nursing

9. (1) The primary action of spironolactone is to increase urine sodium and thereby cause diuresis. It is also potassium sparing and helps counteract metabolic alkalosis by this mechanism.

Nursing Process: Evaluation
Client Needs: Physiological Integrity
Clinical Area: Medical Nursing

10. (3) Anticoagulant prophylaxis would be initiated with intermittent heparin therapy which is effective immediately. Dextran is frequently given postoperatively and aspirin is used in the recovery period

Nursing Process: Planning
Client Needs: Physiological Integrity
Clinical Area: Surgical Nursing

during hospitalization to prevent venous thrombosis.

11.   (3)   Aminoglycoside antibiotics are more active when the urine is alkaline and the client may receive soda bicarbonate to accomplish creating this environment.

Nursing Process: Analysis
Client Needs: Physiological Integrity
Clinical Area: Medical Nursing

12.   (2)   Retinal damage can occur with the use of Plaquenil; the client should be assessed regularly for visual acuity.

Nursing Process: Evaluation
Client Needs: Health Promotion and Maintenance
Clinical Area: Medical Nursing

13.   (2)   The heparin antidote is protamine sulfate. Answers (1) and (3) are antidotes to coumarin derivatives.

Nursing Process: Implementation
Client Needs: Safe, Effective Care Environment
Clinical Area: Medical Nursing

14.   (3)   Dexamethasone (Decadron) is an anti-inflammatory corticosteroid used in the treatment and prevention of cerebral edema. It is a very potent drug, often prescribed preoperatively and continued postoperatively for the neurosurgery client. Because the drug is irritating to the gastrointestinal tract, it should be administered with antacids such as Maalox or Mylanta, or with drugs used to reduce gastric secretions such as cimetidine (Tagamet) or rantidine (Zantac). The nurse must be alert for signs of toxic side effects associated with steroid administration. In particular, the nurse must know that the drug must never be abruptly withdrawn and a gradual tapering of the dose is necessary.

Nursing Process: Evaluation
Client Needs: Safe, Effective Care Environment
Clinical Area: Medical Nursing

15.   (2)   Although each of these drugs has significant side effects, Lasix has the potential for life-threatening cardiac arrhythmias. Potassium is lost as a result of the drug use. 100 mg is a large dose and, thus, a low serum potassium level could easily occur leading to ventricular arrhythmias.

Nursing Process: Evaluation
Client Needs: Safe, Effective Care Environment
Clinical Area: Medical Nursing

16. (1) Several CNS related side effects are common. These include drowsiness, dizziness, headache, and confusion. Therefore, until the client knows if he will experience these side effects, he should not drive a car. Constipation is a common side effect and, thus, a mild laxative should also be ordered. The drug causes nausea and GI distress, so it should be taken with milk or meals.

Nursing Process: Implementation
Client Needs: Health Promotion and Maintenance
Clinical Area: Medical Nursing

17. (3) Pulling back on the plunger, or aspirating, would ensure that the needle had not entered a blood vessel. Therefore, this action would be included in the Z-track method.

Nursing Process: Implementation
Client Needs: Safe, Effective Care Environment
Clinical Area: Medical Nursing

18. (3) To calculate the drip factor, multiply the hourly rate times the drop factor (50 ml times 15). Divide the answer by 60 minutes (750 / 60 = 12.5 gtts/min). Round off answer to 12.

Nursing Process: Implementation
Client Needs: Safe, Effective Care Environment
Clinical Area: Medical Nursing

19. (1) Sedation and slurred speech are the primary side effects. Photosensitivity, an increased susceptibility to sunlight and sunburn, is a common side effect of antipsychotic medications. Muscular rigidity is not a side effect of these medications; in fact, the antianxiety agents often act as muscle relaxants.

Nursing Process: Assessment
Client Needs: Physiological Integrity
Clinical Area: Medical Nursing

20. (1) Valium has sedative properties, and the client needs to be warned about possible side effects. For example, driving while taking Valium is dangerous. Also important, is to inform the client about the life-threatening danger of mixing this drug with alcohol.

Nursing Process: Analysis
Client Needs: Safe, Effective Care Environment
Clinical Area: Psychiatric Nursing

21. (3) DES is used to treat cancer of the prostate. It antagonizes the androgens required by the androgen-dependent

Nursing Process: Planning
Client Needs: Physiological Integrity
Clinical Area: Medical Nursing

neoplasm. Cytoxan and nitrogen mustard are used in Hodgkin's disease. HCG is used for treatment of undescended testicles in young boys.

22. (2) Seconal is a common barbiturate used for sleeplessness. It has a sedative effect on the CNS. Its use should be monitored because of potential addiction or overdose.

Nursing Process: Evaluation
Client Need: Physiological Integrity
Clinical Area: Medical Nursing

23. (3) Agranulocytosis is characterized by neutropenia (decreased number of lymphocytes) which lowers the body defenses against infection. Granulocytes are the first barrier to infection in the body.

Nursing Process: Analysis
Client Needs: Physiological Integrity
Clinical Area: Medical Nursing

24. (3) Nitroglycerin should be taken whenever the client feels a full, pressure feeling or tightness in his chest, not waiting until chest pain is severe. It can also be taken prophylactically before engaging in an activity known to cause angina in order to prevent an anginal attack.

Nursing Process: Implementation
Client Needs: Health Promotion and Maintenance
Clinical Area: Medical Nursing

25. (1) Infectious processes increase the body's need for steroids. During times of stress (infection) the dose needs to be increased to prevent adrenal insufficiency in previously steroid-dependent clients.

Nursing Process: Analysis
Client Needs: Safe, Effective Care Environment
Clinical Area: Medical Nursing

Nutrition

1. (3) The most appropriate response is answer (3). Clients should be instructed to read labels before purchasing canned, frozen or processed foods because they are usually very high in sodium. A list of foods will provide guidance, but she should know the sodium content of food. Not adding salt to cooking is also important, but not as critical as (3).

Nursing Process: Evaluation
Client Needs: Health Promotion and Maintenance
Clinical Area: Medical Nursing

2. (1) Buttermilk contains large amounts of fat and must be avoided. Fruits and whole grains are encouraged.

Nursing Process: Evaluation
Client Needs: Health Promotion and Maintenance
Clinical Area: Medical Nursing

3. (4) With liver cell damage, the liver cannot break down and eliminate the protein. Protein needs to be decreased until symptoms dissipate.

Nursing Process: Planning
Client Needs: Physiological Integrity
Clinical Area: Medical Nursing

4. (4) Bran, fresh fruits and whole grains and seeds are included in a high-fiber diet. Cooked vegetables and fruits as well as refined breads are included in a low-fiber diet.

Nursing Process: Evaluation
Client Needs: Health Promotion and Maintenance
Clinical Area: Medical Nursing

5. (3) Ham is high in sodium and can increase fluid retention leading to edema. Cirrhosis clients are prone to edema as the osmotic pressures change due to a decrease in plasma albumin.

Nursing Process: Implementation
Client Needs: Safe, Effective Care Environment
Clinical Area: Medical Nursing

6. (4) Clients with this condition must not consume foods high in fat content because there are inadequate pancreatic enzymes to digest the fat. High fat content also causes pain two to four hours after ingestion. Suggested diet is high in calories and protein.

Nursing Process: Evaluation
Client Needs: Physiological Integrity
Clinical Area: Medical Nursing

7. (2) During pregnancy iron supplements must be added to the diet because studies have found that pregnant women cannot assimilate enough iron from their regular diet. Calories are increased by 300 to be certain that the mother-to-be and fetus have enough nutritional intake.

Nursing Process: Implementation
Client Needs: Health Promotion and Maintenance
Clinical Area: Maternity Nursing

8. (1) It is important that fluids be restricted as well, because unrestricted fluid intake leads to a progressive decrease in serum sodium from dilution. Electrolyte imbalance with potential neurologic complications could result.

Nursing Process: Planning
Client Needs: Physiological Integrity
Clinical Area: Medical Nursing

9.   (3)   Foods which are high in carbohydrate are given, because those with high protein or fat content stimulate the pancreas. Alcohol is forbidden.

Nursing Process: Planning
Client Needs: Health Promotion and Maintenance
Clinical Area: Medical Nursing

10.   (3)   Aspartame is the only calorie-free sweetener listed; the others are nutritive, their average caloric value being 20 kcal per teaspoon. When an equal volume of honey and sugar are compared, honey provides about one and one-third times as many kcal as does table sugar.

Nursing Process: Planning
Client Needs: Health Promotion and Maintenance
Clinical Area: Medical Nursing

11.   (2)   The diabetic's diet should be between 50 and 65 percent carbohydrate calories with only 5 percent of these being sucrose. Fat recommendation is less than 30 percent of calories and protein should be 0.8 mg/kg per day.

Nursing Process: Evaluation
Client Needs: Health Promotion and Maintenance
Clinical Area: Medical Nursing

12.   (1)   In the early stages, protein intake will be reduced to 20–40 gm because high protein intake elevates blood ammonia. Protein will need to be reduced further if the coma state progresses.

Nursing Process: Planning
Client Needs: Health Promotion and Maintenance
Clinical Area: Medical Nursing

13.   (2)   Organ meats, wine, yeast, scallops, and mussels are all high in purine and must be eliminated from the diet of the client who has gout.

Nursing Process: Evaluation
Client Needs: Health Promotion and Maintenance
Clinical Area: Medical Nursing

14.   (2)   A daily intake of 2800 calories is required for usual/general tissue repair, whereas 6000 calories may be required for extensive tissue repair. Fluid intake is 2000–3000 ml/day for uncomplicated surgery. Diet progresses from nothing by mouth the day of surgery to a general diet within a few days.

Nursing Process: Implementation
Client Needs: Health Promotion and Maintenance
Clinical Area: Surgical Nursing

15.   (1)   Diets are individualized and clients are generally able to eat the same foods they enjoyed preoperatively. Fresh fruits

Nursing Process: Implementation
Client Needs: Safe, Effective Care Environment
Clinical Area: Surgical Nursing

may cause diarrhea in some, but not all, individuals.

16. (2) The low residue diet will put less strain on the colon and eliminating dairy products initially is important because these products cause mucus.

Nursing Process: Planning
Client Needs: Health Promotion and Maintenance
Clinical Area: Surgical Nursing

17. (2) A high-fiber diet produces a soft stool without mechanically irritating the hemorrhoidal area. Foods include bran and complex carbohydrates.

Nursing Process: Evaluation
Client Needs: Health Promotion and Maintenance
Clinical Area: Surgical Nursing

18. (2) Food and fluids would not be given 4–6 hours before treatments. Because of possible problems with constipation, the foods need to be high in bulk and fiber. Oral hygiene will be accomplished using the most nonirritating means.

Nursing Process: Implementation
Client Needs: Safe, Effective Care Environment
Clinical Area: Medical Nursing

19. (2) Because the client will be on a low fat diet to decrease pancreatic activity, he will need supplements of the fat soluble vitamins. A well balanced diet should meet the other nutritional needs.

Nursing Process: Planning
Client Needs: Health Promotion and Maintenance
Clinical Area: Medical Nursing

20. (1) Clients undergoing external radiation therapy may develop gastrointestinal irritation and can bleed. They need calories and protein but not rough, high residue foods which further irritate the GI tract.

Nursing Process: Planning
Client Needs: Physiological Integrity
Clinical Area: Surgical Nursing

21. (3) In order that the client not experience a sudden drop in blood sugar, the solution nearest most TPN solution concentrations is D_{10}/W. D_{25}/W and D_{45} could cause osmotic diuresis or fluid overload.

Nursing Process: Implementation
Client Needs: Physiological Integrity
Clinical Area: Medical Nursing

22. (3) The most helpful intervention is to assist the client to help herself, allowing her to be as independent as possible. Feeding her or changing the diet to liquid would not be as therapeutic.

Nursing Process: Implementation
Client Needs: Health Promotion and Maintenance
Clinical Area: Medical Nursing

23. (2) The most common placement site is the right subclavian vein. The jugular vein might be used as an alternative for high concentration IV infusions, but it is more difficult to access. The arm is used for insertion of an arterial line for arterial blood gas samples and monitoring.

Nursing Process: Planning
Client Needs: Physiological Integrity
Clinical Area: Medical Nursing

24. (1) Dyspnea, chills, fever, and cyanosis are all side effects which necessitate stopping the infusion and notifying the physician. It may be an allergic reaction or the client's inability to tolerate the lipid infusion. Answer (2) is a liver function test and the physician should be notified if results are abnormal, but this would occur after the infusion. Eczema and dry skin are signs of fatty acid deficit. Erythema and edema need to be monitored and perhaps the IV insertion site changed.

Nursing Process: Evaluation
Client Needs: Safe, Effective Care Environment
Clinical Area: Medical Nursing

25. (2) Coffee is one food eliminated from a bland diet because it is chemically irritating to the stomach. All of the other foods are allowed on a bland diet. Other foods eliminated are raw, spicy, gas-forming, very hot or very cold foods, alcohol, and carbonated drinks.

Nursing Process: Analysis
Client Needs: Safe, Effective Care Environment
Clinical Area: Medical Nursing

Legal Issues

1. (2) Key elements of a client's rights are consent, confidentiality and involuntary commitment.

2. (3) The primary purpose of licensing nurses, both RN and LVN, is to safeguard the public by determining that the nurse is a safe and competent practitioner.

3. (2) Nursing actions are evaluated against a set of standards referred to as standards of performance.

4. (4) To administer any form of restraint, there must be physician's order.

5. (4) The professional nurse, as well as the physician who wrote the order, are held responsible (liable) for harm resulting from their negligent acts.

6. (2) The most accurate answer is (2). The other purposes are to help document the quality of care and to identify areas where more inservice education is needed.

7. (2) To sign a document without having personal knowledge of what occurred would open the possibility of liability.

8. (3) Because the nurse will be responsible (and liable) if she transcribes the order incorrectly, the physician who wrote the order should be consulted.

9. (4) Because the nurse is a licensed professional with an education based on a defined body of knowledge, he or she has the right, indeed the responsibility, to dis

agree with the physician. This is especially so when the health and welfare of the client is involved.

10. (3) The code of ethics is a set of formal guidelines for governing professional action. This situation is not illegal—it is unethical.

11. (4) The nurse practice act is a series of statutes enacted by a state to regulate the practice of nursing in that state. It includes all of these plus education.

12. (1) All but ten states have some provision for the rights of clients written into a law; and, these rights can be enforced by the law.

13. (2) The nurse is responsible for her or his own negligent acts; however, legal doctrine holds that an employer is also liable for negligent acts of employees.

14. (2) If basic rules of human conduct are not violated, the elements of liability may not exist. There must be certain elements of liability present; for example, there must exist a causal relationship between harm to the client and the act by the nurse. There must be some damage or harm sustained by the client and there must be a legal basis—such as statutory law—for finding liability.

15. (2) The client must be fully informed of potentially harmful effects of the treatment. If this is not done, it could result in the nurse's being personally liable.